CONTENTS

Chapter One

WEIGHT LOSS AND OPTIMAL HEALTH

he DASH diet (Dietary Approaches to Stop Hypertension) is an eating regimen prescribed by numerous specialists to normally bring down one's circulatory strain. A few people lean toward not to take drugs and rather start on the DASH diet to recover their circulatory strain levels down to typical.

Be that as it may, beginning an exacting diet doesn't mean you need to surrender each food you've at any point delighted in. As a matter of fact, the DASH diet despite everything leaves space for a portion of your top choices, regardless of whether it implies a marginally more advantageous interpretation of them. Here are some delectable foods and drinks you can at present appreciate while on the DASH diet.

Chips

While you shouldn't enjoy oily, singed potato chips, you can, in any case, appreciate the heated chips. It's essential to eat everything with some restraint, yet prepared chips accompany far less fat, calories, and sodium than their seared partners. It's anything but difficult to discover heated chips in the market; however, stay with the first flavor. The additional powder on the prepared chips regularly implies included salt.

Burgers

Rather than an 80% lean meat burger, go with 98% lean hamburger burger or a turkey burger. Swap out a standard bun for an entire wheat bun; you'll despite everything get the succulent kind of a burger yet on a lot more advantageous scale. Red meats are fine with some restraint; however, in case you're a burger sweetheart, you should devour, for the most part, turkey burgers. Veggie burgers can be sound; however, be cautious - they're frequently stacked with sodium.

Solidified Yogurt

Dessert contains a great deal of included sugar; however, solidified yogurt is a more beneficial, still-sweet other option. In addition, "froyo" places are famous these days, so you can whirl your own solidified yogurt, at that point load it up with foods grown from the ground fixings. It's the ideal method to fulfill a sweet tooth, and it's something the DASH diet won't expect you to surrender.

Chocolate Milk

For whatever length of time that your chocolate milk isn't made with entire milk, you can, in any case, enjoy every so often. The DASH diet needs you to constrain sugars, so this one should just be a sweet treat for once in a while. Be that as it may, you don't have to totally surrender it, since there are sound chocolate milk blends, (for example, Ovaltine), you'll despite everything get the low-fat or nonfat dairy benefits the DASH diet needs.

Hummus

Bean-based plunges, for example, hummus, are empowered by the diet. Furthermore, who doesn't cherish getting some sound saltines and enjoying hummus? Different plunges, for example, salsa and guacamole, can be sound however frequently contain a ton of sodium. In the event that you need one of these, make it yourself. Thusly you're in charge of how a lot of salt it contains.

Sushi

There are three things to recall when requesting sushi: Order dark colored rice, keep away from tempura, and breaking point the soy sauce. An avocado roll or fish move with darker rice is an exceptionally sound lunch. Be that as it may, on the off chance that you request anything singed (tempura) and burden it with soy sauce, you're destroying the sushi's sustenance. Soy sauce is stacked with sodium. Also, white rice contains the basic sugars you're attempting to stay away from.

Red wine

A glass of red wine every night can really advance heart wellbeing, so there is no compelling reason to surrender it on the DASH diet. Red wine contains resveratrol, which can be useful for your heart, yet just with some restraint. Stick with only one glass for each night.

Coffee

Uplifting News: Coffee is as yet your companion on the DASH diet, be that as it may, don't stack it up with entire milk and sugar, add some skim milk to your espresso and maintain a strategic distance from the sugar to keep it DASH-accommodating, it will give you the caffeine help you need without veering you off your good dieting course.

Food to Eat

The DASH diet stresses vegetables, products of the soil fat dairy foods and moderate measures of entire grains, fish, poultry, and nuts.

Notwithstanding the standard DASH diet, there is additionally a lower sodium adaptation of the diet. You can pick the rendition of the diet that meets your wellbeing needs:

- Standard DASH diet. You can devour up to 2,300 milligrams (mg) of sodium daily.
- Lower sodium DASH diet. You can expend up to 1,500 mg of sodium daily.

The two variants of the DASH diet expect to lessen the measure of sodium in your diet contrasted and what you may get in a Dash of the mill American eating regimen, which can add up to an astounding 3,400 mg of sodium daily or more.

The standard DASH diet meets the proposal from the Dietary Guidelines for Americans to keep day by day sodium admission to fewer than 2,300 mg daily.

The American Heart Association prescribes 1,500 mg daily of sodium as a maximum point of confinement for all grown-ups. On the off chance that you aren't sure what sodium level is directly for you, converse with your primary care physician.

The two variants of the DASH diet incorporate loads of entire grains, organic products, vegetables, and low-fat dairy items. The DASH diet likewise incorporates some fish, poultry, and vegetables, and energizes a modest quantity of nuts and seeds a couple of times each week.

You can eat red meat, desserts, and fats in limited quantities. The DASH diet is low in immersed fat, Tran's fat, and absolute fat.

Here's a gander at the prescribed servings from every nutrition class for the 2,000-caloric-a-day DASH dict.

Grains: 6 to 8 servings every day

Grains incorporate bread, oat, rice, and pasta. Instances of one serving of grains incorporate 1 cut entire wheat bread, 1-ounce dry oat, or 1/2 cup cooked oat, rice or pasta.

- Focus on entire grains since they have more fiber and supplements than do refined grains. For example, utilize dark colored rice rather than white rice, entire wheat pasta rather than customary pasta, and entire grain bread rather than white bread. Search for items marked "100% entire grain" or "100% entire wheat."
- Grains are normally low in fat. Keep them along these lines by maintaining a strategic distance from spread, cream, and cheddar sauces.

Vegetables: 4 to 5 servings per day

Tomatoes, carrots, broccoli, sweet potatoes, greens, and different vegetables are loaded with fiber, nutrients, and such minerals as potassium and magnesium. Instances of one serving incorporate 1 cup crude verdant green vegetables or 1/2 cup cut-up crude or cooked vegetables.

- Don't consider vegetables just as side dishes - a healthy mix of vegetables served over darker rice or entire wheat noodles can fill in as the fundamental dish for a supper.
- Fresh and solidified vegetables are both acceptable decisions. When purchasing solidified and canned vegetables, pick those named as low sodium or without included salt.
- To increment the quantity of servings you fit in day by day, be inventive. In a pan-fried food, for example, cut the measure of meat down the middle and get serious about the vegetables.

Organic products: 4 to 5 servings every day

Numerous organic products need little readiness to turn into a sound piece of a feast or bite. Like vegetables, they're stuffed with fiber, potassium, and magnesium and are ordinarily low in fat - coconuts are a special case.

Instances of one serving incorporate one medium organic product, 1/2 cup crisp, solidified or canned natural product, or 4 ounces of juice.

- Have a bit of organic product with suppers and one as a tidbit; at that point balance, your day with a pastry of new natural products beat with a spot of low-fat yogurt.
- Leave on consumable strips at whatever point conceivable. The strips of apples, pears, and most natural products add fascinating surface to plans and contain sound supplements and fiber.
- Remember that citrus foods grown from the ground, for example, grapefruit can associate with specific drugs, so check with your primary care physician or drug specialist to check whether they're OK for you.
- If you pick canned natural products or juice, ensure no sugar is included.

Dairy: 2 to 3 servings per day

Milk, yogurt, cheddar, and other dairy items are significant wellsprings of calcium, nutrient D, and protein. However, the key is to ensure that you pick dairy items that are low-fat or sans fat on the grounds that else they can be a significant wellspring of fat, and a large portion of it is immersed.

Instances of one serving incorporate 1 cup skim or 1 percent milk, 1 cup low-fat yogurt, or 1/2 ounces part-skim cheddar.

- Low-fat or sans fat solidified yogurt can assist you with boosting the measure of dairy items you eat while offering a sweet treat. Include natural products for a sound bend.

- If you experience difficulty processing dairy items, pick without lactose items, or consider taking an over-the-counter item that contains the catalyst lactase, which can diminish or forestall the side effects of lactose bigotry.
- Go simple on normal and even without fat cheeses since they are regularly high in sodium.

Lean meat, poultry, and fish: 6 one-ounce servings or less a day

Meat can be a rich wellspring of protein, B nutrients, iron, and zinc. Pick lean assortments and focus on close to 6 one-ounce servings daily. Reducing your meat part will permit space for more vegetables.

Instances of one serving incorporate 1 egg or 1 ounce of cooked meat, poultry, or fish.

- Trim away skin and fat from poultry and meat and afterward heat, cook, flame broil, or meal as opposed to searing in fat.
- Eat heart-solid fish, for example, salmon, herring, and fish. These kinds of fish are high in omega-3 unsaturated fats, which are sound for your heart.

Nuts, seeds, and vegetables: 4 to 5 servings every week

Almonds, sunflower seeds, kidney beans, peas, lentils, & different foods right now great wellsprings of magnesium, potassium, and protein. They're additionally brimming with fiber and phytochemicals, which are plant intensifies that may ensure against certain malignant growths and cardiovascular ailment.

Serving sizes are little and are planned to be expended just a couple of times each week on the grounds that these foods are higher in calories.

Instances of one serving incorporate 1/3 cup nuts, 2 tablespoons seeds or nut spread, or 1/2 cup cooked beans or peas.

- Nuts in some cases get negative criticism in view of their fat substance; however, they contain sound sorts of fat - monounsaturated fat and omega-3 unsaturated fats. Nuts are high in calories, in any case, so eat them with some restraint. Have a go at adding them to sautés, plates of mixed greens, or oats.
- Soybean-based items, for example, tofu and tempeh, can be a decent option in contrast to meat since they contain the entirety of the amino acids your body needs to make a total protein, much the same as meat.

Fats and oils: 2 to 3 servings per day

Fat enables your body to ingest fundamental nutrients and helps your body's invulnerable framework. Be that as it may, an excessive amount of fat builds your danger of coronary illness, diabetes, and stoutness.

The DASH diet takes a stab at a sound parity by constraining absolute fat to fewer than 30 percent of everyday calories from fat, with attention on the more beneficial monounsaturated fats.

Instances of one serving incorporate 1 teaspoon delicate margarine, 1 tablespoon mayonnaise or 2 tablespoons plate of mixed greens dressing.

- Saturated fat and Tran's fat are the primary dietary offenders in expanding your danger of coronary corridor ailment. The Dash helps keep your day by day immersed fat to under 6 percent of your all-out calories by constraining utilization of meat, margarine, cheddar, entire milk, cream and eggs in your diet, alongside foods produced using grease, strong shortenings, and palm and coconut oils.
- Avoid trans-fat, normally found in such prepared foods as saltines, heated merchandise, and seared things.
- Read nourishment marks on margarine and serving of mixed greens dressing with the goal that you can pick foods that are most minimal in immersed fat and free of Tran's fat.

Desserts: 5 servings or fewer seven days

You don't need to expel desserts altogether while following the DASH diet - simply chill out on them. Instances of one serving incorporate 1 tablespoon sugar, jam or jam, 1/2 cup sorbet, or 1 cup lemonade.

- When you eat desserts, pick those that are sans fat or low-fat, for example, sorbets, natural product frosts, jam beans, hard sweet, graham wafers, or low-fat treats.
- Artificial sugars, for example, aspartame (NutraSweet, Equal) and sucralose (Splenda) may help fulfill your sweet tooth while saving the sugar. However, recollect that you, despite everything, must utilize them reasonably. It's OK to swap an eating regimen cola for a normal cola, however not instead of an increasingly nutritious drink, for example, low-fat milk or even plain water.
- Cut back on included sugar, which has no dietary benefit, however, and it can pack on calories.

Dash diet: Alcohol and Caffeine

Drinking an excess of liquor can expand circulatory strain. The Dietary Guidelines for Americans prescribe that men limit liquor to close to two beverages every day and ladies to one or less.

The DASH diet doesn't address caffeine utilization. The impact of caffeine on circulatory strain stays misty. Be that as it may, caffeine can cause your circulatory strain to ascend in any event briefly.

In the event that you as of now have hypertension or on the off chance that you think caffeine is influencing your pulse, converse with your primary care physician about your caffeine utilization.

Dash Diet and Weight Reduction

While the DASH diet isn't a get-healthy plan, you may, without a doubt, lose undesirable pounds since it can help manage you toward more advantageous nourishment decisions.

The DASH diet, for the most part, incorporates around 2,000 calories every day. In case you're attempting to get in shape, you may need to eat fewer calories. You may likewise need to modify your serving objectives dependent on your individual conditions - something your human services group can enable you to choose.

Tips to Curtail Sodium

The foods at the center of the DASH diet are normally low in sodium. So just by following the DASH diet, you're probably going to diminish your sodium admission. You additionally diminish sodium further by:

- Using sans sodium flavors or flavorings with your nourishment rather than salt
- Not including salt when cooking rice, pasta or hot grain
- Rinsing canned foods to expel a portion of the sodium
- Buying foods named "no salt included," "sans sodium," "low sodium" or "low sodium"

One teaspoon of table salt has 2,325 mg of sodium. At the point when you read nourishment marks, you might be astounded at exactly how much sodium some handled foods contain.

Indeed, even low-fat soups, canned vegetables, prepared to-eat grains, and cut turkey from the neighborhood store - foods you may have thought about sound - frequently have loads of sodium.

You may see a distinction in taste when you pick low-sodium nourishment and refreshments. On the off chance that things appear to be excessively dull, progressively present low-sodium foods and cut back on table salt until you arrive at your sodium objective. That will give your sense of taste time to alter.

Utilizing sans salt flavoring mixes or herbs and flavors may likewise facilitate the progress. It can take a little while for your taste buds to become accustomed to less salty foods.

Putting the bits of the DASH diet together

Attempt these procedures to begin on the DASH diet:

- Change bit by bit. On the off chance that you currently eat just a couple of servings of organic products or vegetables daily, attempt to include a serving at lunch and one at supper. As opposed to changing to every single entire grain, start by making a couple of your grain servings entire grains. Expanding organic products, vegetables, and entire grains bit by bit can likewise help forestall swelling or the Dashs that may happen in the event that you aren't accustomed to eating an eating regimen with loads of fiber. You can likewise attempt over-the-counter items to help decrease gas from beans and vegetables.

- Reward victories and pardon slip-ups. Prize yourself with a nonfood treat for your achievements - lease a film, buy a book, or get together with a companion. Everybody slips, particularly when discovering some new information. Recall that changing your way of life is a long haul process. Discover what set off your mishap, and afterward, simply get back on track with the DASH diet.
- Add physical action. To support your pulse, bringing down endeavors considerably more, consider expanding your physical action notwithstanding following the DASH diet. Consolidating both the DASH diet and physical activity makes it more probable that you'll diminish your circulatory strain.
- Get support in the event that you need it. In case you're experiencing difficulty adhering to your diet, converse with your PCP or dietitian about it. You may get a few hints that will assist you with adhering to the DASH diet.

Keep in mind, good dieting isn't a win or bust recommendation. What's most significant is that, by and large, you eat more beneficial foods with a lot of assortment - both to keep your eating regimen nutritious and to maintain a strategic distance from fatigue or boundaries. What's more, with the DASH diet, you can have both.

Food to Avoid

Foods to stay away from when following the DASH diet incorporate high sugar, high-fat tidbits, and foods high in salt, for example,

- Candy
- Cookies
- Chips
- Salted nuts
- Sodas
- Sugary refreshments
- Pastries
- Snacks
- Meat dishes
- Prepackaged pasta and rice dishes (barring macaroni and cheddar since it is a different classification)

- Pizza
- Soups
- Salad dressings
- Cheese
- Cold cuts and relieving meats
- Bread and rolls
- Sandwiches
- Sauces and flavors
- Soups

Utilizing a salt substitute made with potassium not just fills in as a substitute in cooking and on the table; however, the extra potassium can assist lower with blooding pressure. Individuals who are on circulatory strain prescriptions that expansion potassium ought to request that their primary care physicians assist them with observing the blood level of potassium (K) while they are making changes.

Shouldn't Something Be Said About Red Meat And Coronary Illness?

While not explicitly suggested, grass-encouraged hamburger and bison would fit within these parameters. Grass-nourished meat has a totally different synthesis than a regular grain-sustained hamburger. Grass-encouraged meat is high in omega-3s and is increasingly like fish, healthfully. Grain-encouraged red meat is high in omega 6s and soaked fat, the two of which are elevated aggravation and add to coronary illness, hypertension, and corpulence. Red meat that isn't grass-sustained isn't permitted.

Chapter Two

WHAT IS THE DASH DIET?

*D*ash represents a Dietary Approach to Stop Hypertension. Dash diet has been clinically demonstrated to diminish pulse inside about fourteen days in people following the diet. It isn't just known to help deal with the circulatory strain but on the other hand, is intended for health improvement plans, assists with forestalling heart illnesses, stroke, diabetes, and a few types of malignant growth.

This diet, created by the US National Heart, Lung, and Blood Institute, is intended to lessen hypertension. It is the medicinal network's most acknowledged meaning of a heart-solid diet since it involves supplements like potassium, calcium, protein, and fiber that help lessen hypertension.

The DASH diet advocates:

- Fresh foods are grown from the ground;
- Whole grains;
- Lean protein; and is
- Low in fat and sodium.

High fat, sugar and salt foods are untouchable, as is liquor, however, it is in any case considered simple to follow, and, so is useful for long haul supporters, for example, those of us who wish to decrease our hypertension normally. Or on the other hand, at any rate, we need to make our professionally prescribed medicine increasingly powerful with the goal that we can take less of it to accomplish a similar outcome.

Who Ought to Follow A DASH Eating Plan?

Truth be told, a DASH eating plan can be a piece of any smart dieting plan. Not just will it assist lower with blooding pressure, yet it will offer extra heart medical advantages, including bringing down LDL cholesterol and irritation.

How Does the DASH Eating Plan Work?

The diet comprises of foods that are low in sodium and comprises of an assortment of food sources that are wealthy in supplements like potassium, calcium, and magnesium are known to assist lower with blooding pressure. The eating regimen is wealthy in fiber that again assists with bringing down circulatory strain and knock off the additional pounds, which will thus help with bringing down pulse.

Would It Be A Good Idea For You To Follow A DASH Eating Plan?

- Grains like entire wheat, darker rice, grain, oats, quinoa are stuffed with supplements like proteins, B nutrients and follow minerals, fiber, and cell reinforcements, which has been appeared to decrease the danger of a few sicknesses. Notwithstanding, prepared grains need most supplements and ought to be dodged.
- Include without fat or low-fat milk, yogurt, Greek yogurt, paneer in your eating regimen rather than full-fat choices. For the individuals who are lactose bigoted, without lactose, milk and milk items are an alternative.
- Nuts like almonds, pecans, pistachios, and so forth., beans, dals, and seeds like the sunflower seeds, melon seeds, and so on are a piece of a good dieting DASH diet. They are wealthy in dietary fiber protein, omega 3 unsaturated fats, nutrients and minerals like zinc and magnesium, and so on. Albeit nuts contain the sound fats, it is astute to eat them in limited sums as they are high in calories. Likewise, keep away from salted or nectar cooked nuts for their high sodium and sugar content.
- Lean meat, egg, poultry, and fish with some restraint instead of meats with high immersed fat substance. Handled meats, for example, bacon, ham, frankfurters, salami, and so forth contain a lot of sodium, subsequently limit the admission. Incidental admission of red meat is allowed.
- Fruits and vegetables are normally wealthy in potassium, which assumes a significant job in bringing down circulatory strain. On the off chance that you are one who isn't partial to products of the soil roll out the improvement slowly. Include an additional natural product or vegetable in the day notwithstanding what you are as of now having a beginning. Favor an entirely organic product to juices. Unsweetened dried organic products like raisins, cranberries, dried figs, and so forth are acceptable travel decisions. Ensure there is a vegetable at every dinner.
- The diet ought to be low in immersed fats and absolute fats. A diet high in soaked fats builds the danger of coronary illness and

hypertension. Fats are significant for the ingestion of fat-dissolvable nutrients and help in building the body's resistant framework. Utilization of oils like olive oil, rice-wheat oil, and mustard oil ought to be advanced in every feast and trans fats which are normally found in handled and seared nourishment ought to have stayed away from.

Tips to Make Dash Work Faster
To make this eating regimen work far superior here are some extra tips:

- Reducing liquor admission may help diminish circulatory strain. Thus, hold the liquor admission under check.
- Aerobic practice alongside the DASH diet works quicker in bringing down circulatory strain.
- Read nourishment names to pick items that are lower in sodium.
- Stress can raise pulse regardless of whether the eating regimen is sound. Consequently, stress the executives' procedures like contemplation, yoga, and so on will help keep the pulse under check.
- Poor rest builds pulse. Along these lines, 7-8 hours of sound rest will help in keeping the pulse in charge.
- If you are somebody who smokes, at that point stopping it would assist lower with blooding pressure.
- Take your prescription as endorsed.
- Limit the salt admission to 1 teaspoon daily.

Putting forth a way of life change is an attempt. It is a long haul responsibility which one needs to make for good wellbeing. Rolling out little improvements will get quicker outcomes than rolling out sensational improvements at the same time and losing the dedication en route. Before jumping on to the DASH diet counsels a nutritionist who can help you in chalking out an individual program for yourself.

If you are at present experiencing hypertension, at that point, you ought to consider going on the DASH diet. Dash represents Dietary Approaches to Stop Hypertension. The objective of this diet is, obviously, to help bring down your circulatory strain by eating foods that are high in calcium, magnesium, and potassium. Studies have indicated that these supplements help to decrease an individual's circulatory strain.

Before you choose in the event that you need to begin a DASH diet, you should talk about your primary care physician to ensure that it is directly for you. Additionally, your PCP can likewise help you in settling on the correct decisions with the goal that your DASH diet will be a triumph.

As expressed before, for the eating regimen to be viable, you need to eat foods that are high in calcium, magnesium, and potassium. Instances of foods that are high in these three supplements are organic products, vegetables, nuts, and low-fat dairy items. In any case, taking enhancements as opposed to eating these foods won't be powerful in helping you lessen your hypertension. You have to devour these supplements from normal foods.

Other than eating loads of products of the soil, you will likely need to build your admission of entire grain foods and lessen the measure of sodium in your eating regimen. You could likewise remember fish and poultry for your eating regimen too. It's ideal to counsel with your primary care physician to figure out what might be the perfect sum for you.

Like beginning any diet, it very well may be somewhat of a test. Yet, you can be effective in the event that you make infant strides as opposed to making one major emotional change. A ton of times, in the event that you do it at the same time, you begin to miss the foods that you cherished previously; however, you can never again have. Accordingly, you wind up surrendering. By doing it gradually, you will have the option to cause your eating regimen to turn out to be a piece of your day by day schedule.

The best approach to do small steps is to present pieces of your diet in your standard supper and set objectives for yourself. For instance, in the event that you appreciate pizza, you can purchase instant outside layer and include low-fat cheddar and include loads of vegetables that are high in supplements like broccoli, tomatoes, or spinach. Or on the other hand, you could have crude vegetables with low-fat yogurt plunge as opposed to having sleek potato chips. Concerning defining objectives, you could disclose to yourself that you intend to nibble on in any event one organic product every day as opposed to having treats or sweet.

On the off chance that you are experiencing hypertension, at that point the DASH diet is presumably something beneficial. Make certain to visit your PCP to check whether this is something that you can do and follow the rules that your PCP gives. Eating well and following a strong exercise plan will assist you in lowering your hypertension.

Plan

There are two DASHES diet intends to look over - DASH diet and Low sodium DASH diet. The main contrast between both the eating regimens is that the individuals who follow the Low sodium DASH diet should be wary about their sodium admission.

Dash Diet Plan:

The DASH diet plan doesn't include the prohibitive requests of different eating regimens. To follow the arrangement, you have to expand the day by day admission of organic products, vegetables, and dairy items. You ought to likewise expend entire grains, fish, poultry, and nuts. Attempt to expend less than 2300 milligrams of sodium daily. The DASH diet plan constrains the admission of fats, sugar-based beverages, and red meat.

- **Grains**

In a perfect world, one ought to expend six to eight servings of grains day by day. Attempt to concentrate on entire grains as they have more fiber and supplements than refined grains. Search for items that are marked 100% entire grain or entire wheat.

• Organic products

You ought to eat in any event 4 to 5 servings of natural products to raise the degrees of vitality and fiber in the body. Eat organic products like pears, apples, and grapefruit with strip as these contain high groupings of cancer prevention agents and fiber. Four servings can incorporate a medium-sized natural product, ¼ cup of dried organic product, 4 ounces of juice, and ½ cup of slashed organic products. While picking canned juice, ensure no sugar is added to it.

• Vegetables

Individuals following the DASH diet ought to devour 4 to 5 servings of vegetables every day. Vegetables like sweet potatoes, broccoli, carrots, tomatoes, and green verdant vegetables are high in fiber, nutrients, potassium, and magnesium. While buying canned vegetables, pick one with low sodium content.

• Dairy

Milk and its items are a fantastic wellspring of calcium; protein, and Vitamin D. Pick low-fat dairy items over entire milk. Attempt to eat in any event 2 to 3 servings of non-fat dairy items day by day. On the off chance that you experience difficulty with processing milk items, choose sans lactose items.

• Meat

Meat is a rich wellspring of protein, iron, zinc and B complex nutrients. The DASH diet proposes control of meat utilization. Try not to fuse multiple servings of meat day by day. Ensure that the meat is lean and skinless. Eat angles like salmon, fish, and herring for a sound heart.

• Nuts and seeds

The DASH diet prescribes eating four to five servings of beans, nuts, and seeds week after week. Nuts have awful notoriety of inferable from their high-fat substance. They contain monounsaturated fats and omega 3 unsaturated fats, which are profoundly useful for wellbeing. Almonds, cashews, pistachio, sunflower seeds, peas, lentils, and beans are acceptable wellsprings of potassium, fiber, and magnesium.

- **Fundamental oil**

Fat causes the body to assimilate basic nutrients that guide the safe framework. However, an excessive amount of fat can expand the danger of heart sicknesses, weight, and diabetes. The DASH diet restricts one's everyday fat utilization to 27% or less. It prescribes curtailing to a few servings per day. One serving of delicate margarine or vegetable oil, alongside 1 tablespoon of mayonnaise or 2 tablespoons of a plate of mixed greens dressing are sufficient for the afternoon. The DASH diet keeps the day by day farthest point of soaked fats to fewer than 7% by limiting the utilization of meat, spread, cheddar, eggs, and entire milk.

- **Desserts**

You don't have to oust desserts totally from your eating regimen. Those heavenly desserts ought to be restricted to five servings or even less seven days. Pick low-fat servings like natural product frosts, jam beans, low-fat treats and granola bars. Fake sugars ought to be utilized sparingly.

Low Sodium DASH Diet Plan:

The Low sodium DASH diet plan prescribes diminishing the measure of sodium admission. While following the Low sodium DASH diet plan, you have to constrain the sodium admission to 1500 milligrams every day. Lessening the sodium admission will bring down the circulatory strain significantly further. The Low sodium DASH diet plan is suggested for individuals experiencing wellbeing conditions like constant kidney ailments, diabetes, and cardiovascular illnesses and for those matured 50 years or more.

- You can decrease the sodium admission by utilizing without sodium flavors and flavorings rather than salt.
- Avoid including salt while cooking pasta, rice, and hot grain.
- Purchase items named as 'without sodium' and 'no salt included'. You can likewise flush canned foods to evacuate a portion of the sodium.
- While starting with the Low sodium DASH diet, start gradually and roll out continuous improvements. Embrace the customary DASH diet plan that permits 2400 milligrams of salt every day, for example around 1 teaspoon daily. At that point step by step bring down the salt admission to 1500 milligrams for every day.

At first low, sodium foods appear to be too insipid to even consider eating. You can maintain a strategic distance from the dullness by including heart-accommodating herbs and flavors. Present the low sodium foods progressively and cut back on table salt until you arrive at your objective. It will take a little while for your taste buds to become accustomed to less salty nourishment.

Dietary Benefit

The DASH diet is plentiful in a few minerals like calcium, zinc, iron, manganese, and potassium. These supplements help to direct the pulse.

- **Fat**

The DASH diet is low in soaked fat and cholesterol. Soaked fats, including trans-fats, are connected with the expanded danger of heart sicknesses. This eating regimen gives 20 to 35% of the everyday calories from fat. Soaked fats ought to be constrained to only 7% of the day by day calorie consumption according to the DASH diet.

- **Protein**

The DASH diet gives a lot of protein. Lentils, vegetables, and meat can assist you with meeting your day by day protein prerequisite. Adequate degrees of protein in the diet can likewise assist with bringing down pulse.

- **Sugars**

The DASH diet can assist you with meeting you are every day prescribed estimation of starches. The eating regimen suggests 4 servings of grains that can assist you with meeting the everyday esteem.

- **Fiber**

You have to get in any event 25 to 35 grams of fiber to complete the everyday capacities. Fiber will keep you full for a more extended time, forestalling corpulence. The DASH diet gives more than the suggested measure of fiber. Fiber is likewise basic to keep the circulatory strain and glucose levels stable.

- **Potassium**

The DASH is one of only a handful of scarcely any weight control plans that can assist you with meeting the day by day suggested measure of potassium. Potassium, which is extremely fundamental right now, the capacity of salt to raise circulatory strain, it likewise checks bone misfortune, forestalling osteoporosis.

- **Calcium**

The prescribed dietary measure of calcium is 1000 milligrams to 1300 milligrams. You will likely face no trouble in meeting your everyday calcium necessity with the DASH diet. Calcium causes you to construct and keep up solid bones.

- **Nutrient B12**

The DASH diet gives an adequate measure of Vitamin B 12. Nutrient B12 is required for appropriate cell digestion.

Dash Diet Benefits

The DASH diet gives a sound method for eating and offers a few medical advantages other than bringing down the circulatory strain.

- **Heart wellbeing**

A thorough DASH diet is demonstrated to expand the great cholesterol and decline the terrible cholesterol. This eating regimen works best for individuals experiencing modestly hypertension and pre-hypertension. It doesn't show any sensational outcomes for individuals experiencing serious hypertension.

- **Diabetes**

A few examinations have demonstrated that following the DASH eating example can assist with controlling diabetes.

- **Weight reduction**

Other than helping the heart, the DASH diet can likewise assist with getting more fit. A calorie-deficiency diet will, in the end, lead one to lose abundant fat from the body. This eating regimen additionally urges one to fuse expanded physical movement that further encourages the individual to get more fit. The blend of solid foods and exercise adds to the general wellbeing of an individual. This eating regimen can assist you with losing 500 calories for each day.

- **Keeps you full**

The DASH diet puts a great deal of significance on satiety. It suggests lean protein and fiber-rich foods grown from the ground, which keep you full for a more drawn out time. It additionally decreases calorie admission, supporting a sound weight reduction.

- **Different advantages**

Different advantages of the DASH diet incorporate diminished danger of malignant growth, osteoporosis, maturing, and mental maladies.

There is no wellbeing hazard related to the DASH diet. Truth be told, the eating regimen is reasonable and prescribed for an amazing remainder. Do counsel your primary care physician in the event that you experience the ill effects of any wellbeing condition.

Chapter Three

21 DAY ACTION PLAN

*D*o you need your husband to shed pounds? Or on the other hand, do you need the family to embrace a superior, more advantageous way of life? You need to start by making some sound supper plans. It is ideal to make around 4-5 dinner plans and afterward to pivot them with the goal that you can get a ton of assortment in your suppers. Here are a few hints for dinner designs that are sound for your family:

At the point when you make sound dinner arrangements, ensure a certain something: breakfast. It's the most significant supper of the day, and it is additionally the most overlooked one. Take care that your family has a solid breakfast. You can incorporate sound grains, grows, new products of the soil in the morning meal. It is ideal to have three dinners every day and two snacks between them. Eating more may sound unfortunate, yet eating littler parts all the more regularly is really more beneficial. It builds digestion and consumes fatter. Also, it decreases the propensity to eat out at night.

Ensure you remember a few starches for sound feast plans. Despite the fact that a great many people believe that carbs are awful, yet your body needs some of them to work appropriately. You need some vitality to work, and sugars are the wellspring of that vitality. You can choose entire wheat alternatives like bagel, waffles, or toasts. Additionally, on the off chance that you have developing children, ensure you remember calcium for your morning meal. It is useful for ladies too. Have a little glass of skimmed milk or some yogurt. Remember eggs for breakfast as they are a magnificent wellspring of protein.

For the primary bite, pick something light and little. However, it ought to be fulfilled with the goal that it keeps your family full till lunch. You can have nuts for energy; however, attempt to abstain from swelling ones (like cashews). You can pick almonds and pecans. Additionally, low sugar enhanced water would be a decent option. At that point for lunch, incorporate protein-rich eating regimen, similar to tofu burger, vegetables, and organic products. You can likewise have destroyed cheddar alongside child spinach leaves and a tomato cut.

For the second nibble of the day, incorporate several natural products. You can likewise give them some cheddar cuts. What's more, in the event that they ache for salt, pack a few little pretzels. Plan the supper to be light since they are resting after it. You can have a few organic products, serving of mixed greens, and a light protein dish. There ought to be in any event a one-hour hole among eating and dozing. Along these lines, your body will process the nourishment effectively, and you can have better rest.

21 DAY ACTION PLAN: DAY 1

Protein breakfast salmon and eggs on toast formula

- Breakfast: Protein Salmon and Eggs on Toast
- Lunch: Chicken Pesto Pita
- Supper: Southwestern Spaghetti Squash with a green plate of mixed greens

DAY 2

Cucumber with feta and herb plate of mixed greens

- Breakfast: ½ cup nonfat Greek yogurt bested with crisp berries
- Lunch: Cucumber with Feta and Herb Salad
- Supper: Slow Cooker Spinach Artichoke Chicken [Save a segment for lunch on Day 3.]

DAY 3: NUTTY SPREAD AND FRESH RASPBERRIES ON TOAST

- Breakfast: Peanut Butter and Fresh Raspberries on Toast
- Lunch: Slow Cooker Spinach Artichoke Chicken [Leftover from supper on Day 2.]
- Supper: Simply Sautéed Lemon Tilapia with Balsamic Roasted Carrots

DAY 4

Most advantageous greek serving of mixed greens formula

- Breakfast: ½ cup nonfat Greek yogurt bested with crisp berries

- Lunch: Healthiest Greek Salad
- Supper: Quinoa Chicken Nuggets with Rosemary Fries with Low-Fat Aioli

DAY 5: TACO PLATE OF MIXED GREENS

- Breakfast: Lean, Green Protein Smoothie Bowl
- Lunch: Skinny Taco Salad in a Jar
- Supper: Chicken, Broccoli, and Asparagus Stir Fry with Crockpot Cauliflower Fried Rice [Save a segment for lunch on Day 6.]

DAY 6: OPEN-FACE GRILLED TURKEY BURGERS

- Breakfast: Skinny Protein Breakfast Frittatas
- Lunch: Chicken, Broccoli, and Asparagus Stir Fry with Crockpot Cauliflower Fried Rice [Leftover from supper on Day 5.]
- Supper: Open-Face Grilled Turkey Burger with Baked Sweet Potato Fries

DAY 7: STOVE FRESH FISH TACOS

- Breakfast: Protein Quinoa Pancakes [Save a segment for breakfast on Day 8.]
- Lunch: Salad with Clean-Eating Buttermilk Dressing
- Supper: Oven-Crisp Fish Tacos

DAY 8: CHICKEN CAESAR WRAP FORMULA

- Breakfast: Protein Quinoa Pancakes [Leftover from breakfast on Day 7.]
- Lunch: Strawberry Quinoa Salad with Poppyseed Yogurt Dressing
- Supper: Chicken Caesar Wrap with Sweet Potato Fries

DAY 9: CHICKEN PESTO PITA

- Breakfast: ½ cup nonfat Greek yogurt beat with new berries
- Lunch: Chicken Pesto Pita
- Supper: Black Pepper Salmon with Avocado Salad

Day 10
Clean eating Cobb serving of mixed greens

- Breakfast: Peanut Butter and Fresh Raspberries on Toast
- Lunch: Clean-Eating Cobb Salad
- Supper: Steak Fajita Sandwich with Baked Potatoes with Clementine Butter

DAY 11: SLOW COOKER SESAME CHICKEN

- Breakfast: ½ cup nonfat Greek yogurt beat with new berries
- Lunch: Avocado, Tomato, and Cucumber Salad
- Supper: Slow Cooker Sesame Chicken with Garlicky Sautéed Bok Choy [Save a bit for lunch on Day 12.]

DAY 12: THIN BURRITO BOWL

- Breakfast: Clean-Eating Refrigerator Oatmeal
- Lunch: Slow Cooker Sesame Chicken with Garlicky Sautéed Bok Choy [Leftover from supper on Day 11.]
- Supper: Skinny Burrito Bowls

DAY 13: AVOCADO BREAKFAST PIZZA

Breakfast: Avocado Breakfast Pizza

- Lunch: Skinny Taco Salad in a Jar
- Supper: Quick-Prep Parmesan-Crusted Chicken with Mashed Cauliflower [Save a bit of chicken for lunch on Day 14.]

DAY 14: BUCKWHEAT HOTCAKES WITH BERRY SAUCE

- Breakfast: Buckwheat Pancakes with Berry Sauce [Save a bit for breakfast on Day 15.]
- Lunch: Parmesan-Crusted Chicken Wrap [Roll extra chicken from Day 13 into an entire wheat wrap with veggies.]
- Supper: Zucchini Lasagna with a Pasta Salad with Cucumbers and Tomatoes

DAY 15: JALAPENO LIME FISH SERVING OF MIXED GREENS

- Breakfast: Buckwheat Pancakes with Berry Sauce [Leftover from breakfast on Day 14.]
- Lunch: Jalapeno Lime Tuna Salad
- Supper: Slow Cooker Caramelized Chicken with Spinach Saute with Pine Nuts and Golden Raisins [Save a bit for lunch on Day 16.]

DAY 16: BERRY AND CHIA YOGURT PARFAIT

- Breakfast: ½ cup nonfat Greek yogurt beat with new berries
- Lunch: Slow Cooker Caramelized Chicken with Spinach Sauté with Pine Nuts and Golden Raisins [Leftover from supper on Day 15.]
- Supper: Quinoa Salad with Fresh Vegetables

DAY 17: ONE-POT MEXICAN STYLE QUINOA

- Breakfast: Clean-Eating Refrigerator Oatmeal
- Lunch: Chicken and Crisp Veggie Sandwich
- Supper: Skinny Taco Lettuce Boats with One-Pot Skinny Mexican Quinoa

DAY 18: ONE-POT INDIAN DARK PEPPER CHICKEN FORMULA

- Breakfast: Bagel with Sun-Dried Tomatoes and Provolone
- Lunch: Sprouts, Veggie, and Cheese Wrap
- Supper: One-Pot Black Pepper Chicken with Lentils and Pea Risotto [Save a bit for lunch on Day 19.]

DAY 19: SWEET MORNING BREAKFAST QUINOA

- Breakfast: Sweet Morning Breakfast Quinoa [Save a bit for breakfast on Day 20.]
- Lunch: One-Pot Black Pepper Chicken with Lentils and Pea Risotto [Leftover from supper on Day 18.]
- Supper: Chicken and Black Bean Chili [Save a bit for lunch on Day 20.]

DAY 20: PISTACHIO CRUSTED HEATED WHITE FISH FILET

- Breakfast: Sweet Morning Breakfast Quinoa [Leftover from breakfast on Day 19.]
- Lunch: Chicken and Black Bean Chili [Leftover from supper on Day 19.]
- Supper: Pistachio-Crusted White Fish Filet with Twice-Baked Veggie-Stuffed Potato

DAY 21

Cucumber dill and cream cheddar sandwiches on wheat toast

- Breakfast: ½ cup nonfat Greek yogurt beat with new berries
- Lunch: Cucumber and Cheese Sandwich with a green serving of mixed greens
- Supper: Chickpea and Tomato Salad with Grilled Chicken

Chapter Four

SALADS, SOUPS, AND SANDWICHES

For me, soups and stews are always best for winter. Perfect meals for lunch are those low in fat and calories naturally. That is why I love soups and stews; when I want to make it more of a main dish for dinner, it's best to add protein.

The hearty ingredients are so satisfying, and that makes eating them more deliberate. Opt for any of these deliciously prepared recipes of lean protein and savor the flavors.

Easy Egg Salad

There are different ways to prepare eggs as a snack. They are all fabulous, especially since they are Zero Smart Points. I adore my easy egg salad recipe because it's simple, and you can prepare it with just a handful of ingredients. You must have noticed that I like easy-to-cook recipes.

This egg salad doesn't need mayonnaise! Just a few ingredients make a healthy snack. Savor the flavors.

SmartPoints value: Green plan - 2SP, Blue plan - 2SP, Purple plan - 2SP
Total time: 5 min, **Prep time**: 5 min, **Serves**: 2
Nutritional value: Calories - 229, Carbs - 3g, Fat - 17g, Protein - 12g
Ingredients

- Hard-boiled eggs - 4 pieces
- Olive oil - 1 tbsp
- Onions (diced) - 1/3 cup
- Paprika - ½ tsp
- Pepper and salt to taste

Instructions

1. Grate the peeled egg using a cheese grater
2. Mix the eggs, olive oil, onion, pepper and salt in a bowl
3. Feel free to try several combinations and find your favorite. You could try toppings like tomatoes, dill, parsley, chives, relish, pickles, olives, bell peppers, or avocados.

Summer Green Bean Salad

I've seen some people cook their green beans until they are limp as a dish-cloth. However, I like it when my green beans are just a little crispy. To keep them crispy, I blanch them in boiling water for about 3 minutes and then immediately put them in an ice bath; if I don't do that, the beans will get overcooked.

This salad is a sure hit regardless of where you got the green beans, either from your garden or from the grocery store. I usually end up eating most of all of this salad the very first night. I'm not sure you'll be lucky to have some left-overs. Often, salads get gross in the fridge overnight. The greens become unappealing. But, since I made this salad with fresh, crisp veggies, it's still as good the next day.

SmartPoints value: Green plan - 1SP, Blue plan - 1SP, Purple plan - 1SP

Total time: 18 min, Prep time: 15 min, Cooking time: 3 min, Serves:

Nutritional value: Calories - 69, Carbs – 9.1g, Fat – 3.7g, Protein - 2g

Ingredients

- Green beans (fresh, cut into pieces) - (1 lb)
- Red onion (thinly sliced) - 1/2
- Cherry tomatoes (halved) - 1 1/2 cups
- Basil (finely chopped, fresh) - 1/2 cup
- Garlic (minced) - 2 cloves
- Olive oil - 1 1/2 tbsp
- Lemon juice - 1 cup
- Pepper and salt to taste

Instructions

1. Boil a pot of water and blanch the green beans in the water for about 3 minutes. Drain the beans and transfer to an ice bath for about 2-3 minutes, then place the dried green beans in a large bowl.
2. Put the remaining ingredients and toss thoroughly.
3. Enjoy!

Chopped Greek Salad with Creamy Yogurt Dressing

This refreshingly cDashchy salad has the ingredients of a Greek salad, but it is deliciously different as it contains creamy yogurt.

SmartPoints value: Green plan - 4SP, Blue plan - 4SP, Purple plan - 4SP

Total Time: 20 min, **Prep time**: 2 min, **Cooking time**: 18 min, **Serves**: 6

Nutritional value: Calories - 29.0, Carbs - 0.5g Fat - 2.7g, Protein - 0.8g

Ingredients

- Black pepper (freshly ground) - ¼ tsp (or to taste)
- Low-fat yogurt (plain) - ¾ cup(s), (not Greek)
- Crumbled feta cheese - ½ cup(s)
- Dill (fresh, chopped) - 1 Tbsp
- Water - 3 Tbsp
- Olive oil (extra virgin) - 2 Tbsp
- Lemon zest - 1 tsp
- Lemon juice (fresh) - 1 Tbsp, (or to taste)
- Garlic cloves (very finely minced) - 1 small clove(s)
- Oregano (dried) - 1 tsp
- Table salt - ½ tsp (or to taste)
- Cucumber(s) (English variety, diced) - 1 medium
- Yellow pepper(s) (diced) - 2 medium
- Grape tomatoes - 2 cup(s), halved
- Mint leaves (fresh) - ¾ cup(s), leaves, torn
- Uncooked red onion(s) - ⅓ cup(s), chopped
- Olive(s) (pitted, sliced) - 12 medium, Kalamata

Instructions

1. Cut the tomatoes in half, and dice the cucumber, peppers, and onion. Set it aside.
2. Whip yogurt, oil, water, lemon zest, and juice together in a clean small bowl, then add garlic, dill, oregano, salt, and pepper.
3. Combine the remaining ingredients inside a large bowl and toss them together. Add the mixture to the dressing, then toss to coat.

Roasted Beet and Wheat Berry Salad

Wheat berries are grains that are rich in fibre, with a chewy texture. They're delicious when paired with roasted beets and creamy goat cheese, but you can use feta if you prefer. For added convenience, you can cook both beets and wheatberries several days in advance of serving this salad. Simply heat them again and add to the remaining ingredients when you want to assemble the salad. You can decide to serve this salad warm, at room temperature, or chilled.

SmartPoints value: Green plan: 6SP, Blue plan: 6SP, Purple plan: 3SP

Total Time: 60 min, **Prep time**: 20 min, **Cooking time**: 40 min, **Serves**: 6

Nutritional value: Calories - 141.4, Carbs - 22.8g Fat - 5.0g, Protein - 6.4g

Ingredients

- Cooking spray - 3 spray(s)
- Beets (uncooked) - 2 pound(s), red or golden (scrubbed)
- Kosher salt - 2½ tsp, divided
- Wheat berries (uncooked) - 1 cup(s)
- Orange juice (unsweetened) - 2 Tbsp
- Orange marmalade - 1 Tbsp
- Olive oil (extra-virgin) - 1 Tbsp
- Apple cider vinegar - 1 Tbsp
- Scallion(s)(uncooked) - ½ cup(s), sliced (white and light green parts), or to taste
- Parsley (fresh) - ⅓ cup(s), flat-leaf, chopped, or to taste
- Goat cheese (semisoft) - ⅓ cup(s), crumbled
- Table salt - ¼ tsp (or to taste)
- Black pepper - ¼ tsp (or to taste)

Instructions

1. Prepare the oven by heating to 400°F. Coat a clean baking pan with cooking spray.
2. Place beets on the prepared baking pan and lightly coat with cooking spray. Sprinkle the beets with a half teaspoon of salt and tightly cover with foil, then roast until tender; about 40 min.
3. Remove the pan from the oven and allow beets to cool slightly, then gently remove the skin with a knife.
4. Dice the beets or cut into thick matchsticks and set aside.
5. Cover wheatberries with two inches of water in a small saucepan and stir in one teaspoon of salt, then bring it to a boil.
6. Reduce the heat to low, cover it, and simmer until the wheat berries are tender; about 50 - 60 minutes. Drain the saucepan and set aside.
7. To make a vinaigrette, mix orange juice, marmalade, oil, vinegar and remaining teaspoon salt in a small bowl, while the beets and wheatberries cook.
8. Use a clean spoon to put the wheat berries into a serving bowl and gently toss them with the beets, vinaigrette, scallions and parsley, then season to taste with salt and pepper.
9. Garnish the dish with goat cheese and serve.

Italian Pasta Salad with Tomatoes and Artichoke Hearts

SmartPoints value: Green plan - 5SP, Blue plan - 5SP, Purple plan - 5SP
Total Time: 28 min, **Prep time:** 18 min, **Cooking time:** 10 min,
Serves: 6
Nutritional value: Calories - 296.2, Carbs - 47.3g Fat - 8.2g, Protein - 8.7g

The best time to make this pasta salad is at the height of summer when fresh tomatoes are at their glorious, unrivalled peak. Make sure you use the ripest, juiciest tomatoes you can find. Tomato juices will add a delicious flavour to the dressing.

The chopped artichoke hearts will add a briny taste to every bite. Cellentani pasta is the macaroni formed into a spiral shape, also known as cavatappi. If you can't find that variety, feel free to use whatever type you can get, although short kinds of pasta like penne, rotini, and macaroni would work best. Turn this into a meal by adding some grilled or sautéed chicken or shrimp.

Ingredients

- Tomato(es) (fresh) - 1 pound(s), ripe beefsteak or Campari, chopped (3 cups)
- Bell pepper(s) (uncooked) - 2 item(s), small, yellow and orange, diced (1 ½ cups)
- Artichoke hearts without oil (canned) - 14 oz, drained, roughly chopped
- Basil (torn or coarsely chopped) - 1 cup(s)
- Red wine vinegar - 2 Tbsp
- Olive oil (extra virgin) - 2 Tbsp
- Table salt - ½ tsp, with extra for cooking pasta
- Black pepper - ½ tsp, freshly ground
- Garlic powder - ¼ tsp, or more to taste
- Pasta (uncooked) - 6 oz, cellentani recommended (2 cups)
- Parmesan cheese (shredded) - ⅓ cup(s), or shaved, divided

Instructions

1. Combine artichoke hearts, basil, tomatoes, peppers, vinegar, oil, salt, pepper, and garlic powder in a large bowl, then toss to coat. Allow the pasta to stand while cooking, occasionally tossing.
2. Boil a pot of well-salted water and cook the pasta according to package directions. Drain and rinse it with cold water, then drain again.
3. Add the pasta to the bowl with tomato mixture and toss to coat. Add all but two Tbsp Parmesan and toss again.
4. Serve the pasta salad with the remaining cheese sprinkled over to the top.

Tofu-veggie Kebabs with Peanut-sriracha Sauce

SmartPoints value: Green plan: 7SP, Blue plan - 3SP, Purple plan - 3SP

Total Time: 41 min, **Prep time**: 35 min, **Cooking time**: 6 min, **Serves**: 4

Nutritional value: Calories - 144.7, Carbs - 9.5g Fat - 8.9g, Protein - 8.8g

Are you planning to go meatless at your next barbecue? Veggie kebabs are your perfect companion. These broccoli, tofu, and radish favorites offer a delicious option for a vegetarian, vegan, or someone who demands a fresher take on the usual cookout. Put the kebabs together quickly in the kitchen.

Then, brush them with an easy-to-make savory sauce before placing them on the grill. Powdered peanut butter makes this nutritious sauce that adds loads of flavor to the favorites.

Cooking them takes about six minutes, and they are perfect for your next picnic. You can pair them with a fresh side salad to increase the vegetable tally.

Ingredients

- Broccoli (uncooked) - 10 oz, florets (about 4 cups)
- Cooking spray - 4 spray(s)
- Firm tofu (rinsed and drained) - 28 oz
- Table salt - ½ tsp
- Radish(es) (fresh, trimmed and halved) - 8 medium
- Lime juice (fresh) - 1½ Tbsp
- Peanut butter (powdered) - 6 Tbsp
- Water - 4½ Tbsp
- Ketchup - 3 Tbsp
- White miso - 3 Tbsp, (low-sodium)
- Soy sauce (low-sodium) - 1½ Tbsp
- Sriracha hot sauce - 1½ tsp
- Sesame oil (toasted) - 1½ tsp
- Sesame seeds (unsalted toasted) - 1 Tbsp

Instructions

1. Soak up to eight 10-inches bamboo skewers in a shallow dish containing water for at least 20 minutes (or use metal skewers).
2. Put water in a large saucepan and bring it to a boil over high heat. Add salt and radishes to the pan and cook for 5 minutes.
3. Add broccoli and cook for 1 minute more. Drain a colander into the saucepan and its content, then Dash the vegetables under cold water until it is cool to the touch. Drain it properly; Pat it dry with paper towels.
4. Dry out the tofu blocks with paper towels and cut each block into 12 even cubes.

5. To prepare the sauce, stir the water and powdered peanut butter together in a medium bowl to form a smooth, loose paste.
6. Add lime juice, ketchup, miso, Sriracha, soy sauce, and oil, then stir to mix.
7. To prepare kebabs, thread two broccoli florets, two radish halves, and three tofu cubes on each skewer.
8. Apply medium-high heat to a grill. Brush the kebabs with sauce on one side and lightly coat with cooking spray off the heat.
9. Place the kebabs on the grill, sauce side down and cook for 2-3 minutes.
10. Brush the other side with the sauce, flip it and cook for another 2-3 minutes.
11. Remove the kebabs from the grill and brush them with extra sauce, then sprinkle them with sesame seeds before serving.

Crockpot Beef Stew

Using a crockpot for stew is not just comfortable but also guarantees that I don't burn it to the bottom of the pot. I love the fact that I can refrigerate my stew in the crockpot overnight, and the next morning, all I need to do is put it in the crockpot base and turn it on.

If you are thinking of a fitting meal for a cold winter evening, give this beef stew a try. It is one of the highly-rated meals over time. I believe the taste will leave you wanting more.

SmartPoints value: Green plan - 6SP, Blue plan - 6SP, Purple plan - 6SP
SmartPoints value: Green plan - 6SP, Blue plan - 6SP, Purple plan - 6SP
Total Time: 1hr 15min, **Prep time**: 15 min, **Cooking time**: 1hr, **Serves**: 8
Nutritional value: Calories – 343, Carbs – 23.5g, Fat – 17.3g, Protein – 22.2g

Ingredients

- Beef chuck roast - 2 lb
- Russet potatoes (2-in diameter) - 4 medium
- Carrots - 4 medium
- Onion - 1 large
- Garlic - 4 cloves
- Onion soup mix - 1 packet
- Fat-free beef broth - 8 cups
- Celery stalks (chopped) - 4 medium
- Add salt and pepper (to taste)

Instructions

1. Chop the roast into pieces (1 inch)

2. Cut peeled potatoes into slices (1/2 inch)
3. Cut peeled carrots into equal chunks (1/2 inch)
4. Cut onion into large pieces
5. Mix the beef, celery, carrots, potatoes, onion, garlic, onion soup mix and beef broth inside the crockpot
6. Add seasoning to taste (salt and pepper)
7. Cook till it's ready
8. This meal is easy to prepare. All you need to do is give it a try and enjoy it.

Chicken, Lentil, and Spinach Soup

SmartPoints value: Green plan - 1SP, Blue plan - 1SP, Purple plan - 1SP
Total Time: 1hr 10min, **Prep time**: 10 min, **Cooking time**: 1hr, **Serves**: 6

Nutritional value: Calories – 254, Carbs – 27g, Fat – 4.8g, Protein – 26g

As I said earlier, soups and stews are great for me during fall and winter, but this chicken, lentil, and spinach could also serve as spring meals. Though not as rich and heavy as other soups, it is quite substantial.

Ingredients

- Chicken breast - 1 lb
- French dried (green lentils) - 1 cup
- Fresh spinach - One 6 oz package
- Finely chopped onion (1 piece)
- Carrots (chopped) - 2 pieces
- Stalk of celery (chopped) - 2 pieces
- Garlic (chopped) - 6 cloves
- Olive oil (1 tbsp)
- Tomato paste - 2 tbsp
- Paprika - 1 tsp
- Chicken broth or water - 6 cups (fat-free)
- Fresh lemon juice – Half a cup
- Add salt and pepper to taste

Instructions

1. Use medium heat to heat olive oil in a large pot or Dutch oven
2. Put carrots, celery, onions, and garlic and cook till about minutes when vegetables begin to soften
3. Coat the vegetables with the tomato paste and cover till about 2-3 minutes when the paste begins to darken.
4. Stir lentils, paprika, salt, and pepper in the broth or water and bring to a boil and add in the chicken, then cook for about 5 minutes.

5. Cover and cook for about 35 – 45 minutes on medium-low heat until chicken cooks and lentil are tender but not mushy. Make sure the soup is not bubbling or boiling much as you stir periodically.
6. Shred the chicken breasts using two forks. Stir in spinach and lemon juice and cook for about 2 minutes until the spinach wilts. Turn off the heat and add additional salt and pepper to taste.
7. To enjoy the chicken stew and leave it in mind as your best, do not overcook the lentils. Keep an eye on it and make sure they are tender but firm.

Roasted Tomato Basil Soup
SmartPoints value: Green plan - 4SP, Blue plan - 4SP, Purple plan - 4SP
Total Time: 1hr 20min, **Prep time**: 10 min, **Cooking time**: 1hr 10mins, **Serves**: 4
Nutritional value: Calories – 238, Carbs – 26.1g, Fat – 3g, Protein – 5g
Most tomato soups are creamy but unfortunately has lots of fat, but this roasted tomato basil soup makes the difference. You might just say goodbye to canned tomato soup after enjoying the fresh flavors of roasted tomato basil soup.

Ingredients

- Plum tomatoes (halved) - 2 lbs
- Plum tomatoes in their juice - One 14 oz can
- Olive oil - 1 tbsp
- Onion (diced) - 1 large
- Minced garlic (4 cloves)
- Butter (2 tbsp)
- Red pepper flakes (crushed) - 1/8 tsp
- Vegetable stock - 3 cups
- Basil (fresh) - 2 cups
- Oregano (dried) - 1 tsp
- Salt and pepper as desired

Instructions

1. Line a rimmed baking sheet with parchment paper on a 400-degree preheated oven. Before placing them on the baking sheet, toss the tomatoes and garlic cloves with olive oil. Then roast for about 35-45 minutes or until tomatoes are charred.
2. Using medium heat, heat the butter in a stockpot or Dutch, then add onions and red pepper flakes. Sauté until the onion starts to brown.
3. In the canned tomato, stir the basil, oregano, and stock or water.

Then, add in the oven-roasted tomatoes and garlic, including any juices on the baking sheet. Boil and simmer uncovered for about 25-30, then stir regularly.

4. Until you reach the desired consistency, process the soup using an immersion blender.
5. Add salt and pepper to taste.

Roasted Red Pepper and Tomato Soup

Since my favorite lunch is grilled cheese sandwiches, I had to, of course, make tomato soup as a perfect match, so I thought of making it more sumptuous by adding tomatoes and red pepper and roasting them altogether. It might not be as quick as a canned tomato, but trust me, it's worth every single minute. While the soup simmers, it's easy to put the grilled cheese sandwiches together, and you'll have your desired meal.

SmartPoints value: Green plan - 1SP, Blue plan - 1SP, Purple plan - 1SP

Total Time: 1hr 20min, **Prep time**: 10 min, **Cooking time**: 1hr 10mins, **Serves**: 6

Nutritional value: Calories – 107, Carbs – 19.4g, Fat – 0.4g, Protein – 4g

Ingredients

- Plum tomatoes - 10 pieces
- Bell peppers (red) - 3 pieces
- Onion - 1 small
- Olive oil - 1 tbsp
- Garlic - 4 cloves
- Tomato paste - 1/4 cup
- Apple cider vinegar - 3 tbsp
- Paprika - 1 tsp
- Oregano (dried) - 1 tsp
- Thyme (dried) - 1 tsp
- A small handful of basil
- Desired salt and pepper to taste

Instructions

1. With a cooking spray, line a large rimmed baking sheet and put it in an over 400 degrees preheated oven.
2. Slice each tomato into four slices, remove the seeds inside the pepper and slice into eighths. Place the peppers, garlic cloves and tomatoes onto the prepared baking sheet and mist with an olive oil mister. Evenly sprinkle the paprika, oregano, thyme, and salt and pepper on top, then place in oven and roast for 30-35 minutes.
3. In a large pot, heat the olive oil and add diced onions and sauté and leave until they begin to soften in about 2 minutes.

4. Lower the heat and add roasted vegetables and garlic cloves, able cider vinegar, tomato paste, fresh basil, and two cups of water. Blend using the immersion blender until it gets smooth.
5. Lower the heat further and add in the roasted vegetables and garlic cloves, tomato paste, able cider vinegar, fresh basil, and two cups of water, add water to achieve desired consistency.
6. Add pepper and salt to taste and cover on low heat. Stir for about 20-30 minutes regularly.
7. This homemade meal is sure to become your gateway. Savor the flavor of the roasted veggies and garlic.

Black Bean-Tomato Chili
Total Time
Prep: 10 min. Cook: 35 min.
Makes
6 servings (2-1/4 quarts)
Ingredients:

- 2 tablespoons olive oil
- 1 huge onion, cleaved
- 1 medium green pepper, cleaved
- 3 garlic cloves, minced
- 1 teaspoon ground cinnamon
- 1 teaspoon ground cumin
- 1 teaspoon bean stew powder
- 1/4 teaspoon pepper
- 3 jars (14-1/2 ounces each) diced tomatoes, undrained
- 2 jars (15 ounces each) dark beans, washed and depleted
- 1 cup squeezed orange or juice from 3 medium oranges

Directions:

1. In a Dutch broiler, heat oil over medium-high warmth. Include onion and green pepper; cook and mix 8-10 minutes or until delicate. Include garlic and seasonings; cook brief longer.
2. Mix in residual fixings; heat to the point of boiling. Lessen heat; stew, secured, 20-25 minutes to enable flavors to mix, blending incidentally.

Mushroom & Broccoli Soup
Total Time
Prep: 20 min. Cook: 45 min.
Makes
8 servings

Ingredients:

- 1 bundle broccoli (around 1-1/2 pounds)
- 1 tablespoon canola oil
- 1/2 pound cut crisp mushrooms
- 1 tablespoon diminished sodium soy sauce
- 2 medium carrots, finely slashed
- 2 celery ribs, finely slashed
- 1/4 cup finely slashed onion
- 1 garlic clove, minced
- 1 container (32 ounces) vegetable juices
- 2 cups of water
- 2 tablespoons lemon juice

Directions:

1. Cut broccoli florets into reduced down pieces. Strip and hack stalks.
2. In an enormous pot, heat oil over medium-high warmth; saute mushrooms until delicate, 4-6 minutes. Mix in soy sauce; expel from skillet.
3. In the same container, join broccoli stalks, carrots, celery, onion, garlic, soup, and water; heat to the point of boiling. Diminish heat; stew, revealed, until vegetables are relaxed, 25-30 minutes.
4. Puree soup utilizing a drenching blender. Or then again, cool marginally and puree the soup in a blender; come back to the dish. Mix in florets and mushrooms; heat to the point of boiling. Lessen warmth to medium; cook until broccoli is delicate, 8-10 minutes, blending infrequently. Mix in lemon juice.

Avocado Fruit Salad with Tangerine Vinaigrette
Total Time
Prep/Total Time: 25 min.
Makes
8 servings
Ingredients:

- 3 medium ready avocados, stripped and meagerly cut
- 3 medium mangoes, stripped and meagerly cut
- 1 cup crisp raspberries
- 1 cup crisp blackberries
- 1/4 cup minced crisp mint
- 1/4 cup cut almonds, toasted

Dressing:

- 1/2 cup olive oil
- 1 teaspoon ground tangerine or orange strip
- 1/4 cup tangerine or squeezed orange
- 2 tablespoons balsamic vinegar
- 1/2 teaspoon salt
- 1/4 teaspoon naturally ground pepper

Directions:

1. Mastermind avocados and organic product on a serving plate; sprinkle with mint and almonds. In a little bowl, whisk dressing fixings until mixed; shower over a plate of mixed greens.
2. To toast nuts, prepare in a shallow container in a 350° stove for 5-10 minutes or cook in a skillet over low warmth until softly sautéed, mixing every so often.

General Salad Cauliflower
Total Time
Prep: 25 min. Cook: 20 min.
Makes
4 servings
Ingredients:

- Oil for profound fat fricasseeing
- 1/2 cup generally useful flour
- 1/2 cup cornstarch
- 1 teaspoon salt
- 1 teaspoon preparing powder
- 3/4 cup club pop
- 1 medium head cauliflower, cut into 1-inch florets (around 6 cups)

Sauce:

- 1/4 cup squeezed orange
- 3 tablespoons sugar
- 3 tablespoons soy sauce
- 3 tablespoons vegetable stock
- 2 tablespoons rice vinegar
- 2 teaspoons sesame oil
- 2 teaspoons cornstarch
- 2 tablespoons canola oil

- 2 to 6 dried pasilla or other hot chilies, cleaved
- 3 green onions, white part minced, green part daintily cut
- 3 garlic cloves, minced
- 1 teaspoon ground new gingerroot
- 1/2 teaspoon ground orange get-up-and-go
- 4 cups hot cooked rice

Directions:

1. In an electric skillet or profound fryer, heat oil to 375°. Consolidate flour, cornstarch, salt, and heating powder. Mix in club soft drink just until mixed (hitter will be slender). Plunge florets, a couple at once, into the player and fry until cauliflower are delicate and covering is light dark colored, 8-10 minutes. Channel on paper towels.
2. For the sauce, whisk together the initial six fixings; race in cornstarch until smooth.
3. In a huge pot, heat canola oil over medium-high warmth. Include chilies; cook and mix until fragrant, 2 minutes. Include white piece of onions, garlic, ginger, and orange get-up-and-go; cook until fragrant, around 1 moment. Mix soy sauce blend; add to the pan. Heat to the point of boiling; cook and mix until thickened, 4 minutes.
4. Add cauliflower to sauce; hurl to cover. Present with rice; sprinkle with daintily cut green onions.

Salad Chickpea Mint Tabbouleh
Total Time
Prep/Total Time: 30 min.
Makes
4 servings
Ingredients:

- 1 cup bulgur
- 2 cups of water
- 1 cup new or solidified peas (around 5 ounces), defrosted
- 1 can (15 ounces) chickpeas or garbanzo beans, washed and depleted
- 1/2 cup minced new parsley
- 1/4 cup minced new mint
- 1/4 cup olive oil
- 2 tablespoons julienned delicate sun-dried tomatoes (not stuffed in oil)
- 2 tablespoons lemon juice
- 1/2 teaspoon salt

- 1/4 teaspoon pepper

Directions:

1. In a huge pot, consolidate bulgur and water; heat to the point of boiling. Decrease heat; stew, secured, 10 minutes. Mix in crisp or solidified peas; cook, secured, until bulgur and peas are delicate, around 5 minutes.
2. Move to an enormous bowl. Mix in outstanding fixings. Serve warm, or refrigerate and serve cold.

Creamy Cauliflower Pakora Soup
Total Time
Prep: 20 min. Cook: 20 min.
Makes
8 servings (3 quarts)
Ingredients:

- 1 huge head cauliflower, cut into little florets
- 5 medium potatoes, stripped and diced
- 1 huge onion, diced
- 4 medium carrots, stripped and diced
- 2 celery ribs, diced
- 1 container (32 ounces) vegetable stock
- 1 teaspoon garam masala
- 1 teaspoon garlic powder
- 1 teaspoon ground coriander
- 1 teaspoon ground turmeric
- 1 teaspoon ground cumin
- 1 teaspoon pepper
- 1 teaspoon salt
- 1/2 teaspoon squashed red pepper chips
- Water or extra vegetable stock
- New cilantro leaves
- Lime wedges, discretionary

Directions

1. In a Dutch stove over medium-high warmth, heat initial 14 fixings to the point of boiling. Cook and mix until vegetables are delicate, around 20 minutes. Expel from heat; cool marginally. Procedure in groups in a blender or nourishment processor until smooth. Modify consistency as wanted with water (or extra stock). Sprinkle with new cilantro. Serve hot, with lime wedges whenever wanted.

2. Stop alternative: Before including cilantro, solidify cooled soup in cooler compartments. To utilize, in part defrost in cooler medium-term. Warmth through in a pan, blending every so often and including a little water if fundamental. Sprinkle with cilantro. Whenever wanted, present with lime wedges.

Spice Trade Beans and Bulgur
Total Time
Prep: 30 min. Cook: 3-1/2 hours
Makes
10 servings
Ingredients:

- 3 tablespoons canola oil, isolated
- 2 medium onions, slashed
- 1 medium sweet red pepper, slashed
- 5 garlic cloves, minced
- 1 tablespoon ground cumin
- 1 tablespoon paprika
- 2 teaspoons ground ginger
- 1 teaspoon pepper
- 1/2 teaspoon ground cinnamon
- 1/2 teaspoon cayenne pepper
- 1-1/2 cups bulgur
- 1 can (28 ounces) squashed tomatoes
- 1 can (14-1/2 ounces) diced tomatoes, undrained
- 1 container (32 ounces) vegetable juices
- 2 tablespoons darker sugar
- 2 tablespoons soy sauce
- 1 can (15 ounces) garbanzo beans or chickpeas, flushed and depleted
- 1/2 cup brilliant raisins
- Minced crisp cilantro, discretionary

Directions:

1. In an enormous skillet, heat 2 tablespoons oil over medium-high warmth. Include onions and pepper; cook and mix until delicate, 3-4 minutes. Include garlic and seasonings; cook brief longer. Move to a 5-qt. slow cooker.
2. In the same skillet, heat remaining oil over medium-high warmth. Include bulgur; cook and mix until daintily caramelized, 2-3 minutes or until softly sautéed.
3. Include bulgur, tomatoes, stock, darker sugar, and soy sauce to slow cooker. Cook, secured, on low 3-4 hours or until bulgur is delicate.

Mix in beans and raisins; cook 30 minutes longer. Whenever wanted, sprinkle with cilantro.

Tofu Chow Mein
Total Time
Prep: 15 min. + standing Cook: 15 min.
Makes
4 servings
Ingredients:

- 8 ounces uncooked entire wheat holy messenger hair pasta
- 3 tablespoons sesame oil, separated
- 1 bundle (16 ounces) extra-firm tofu
- 2 cups cut new mushrooms
- 1 medium sweet red pepper, julienned
- 1/4 cup decreased sodium soy sauce
- 3 green onions daintily cut

Directions:

1. Cook pasta as per bundle headings. Channel; flush with cold water and channel once more. Hurl with 1 tablespoon oil; spread onto a preparing sheet and let remain around 60 minutes.
2. In the meantime, cut tofu into 1/2-in. 3D shapes and smudge dry. Enclose by a spotless kitchen towel; place on a plate and refrigerate until prepared to cook.
3. In an enormous skillet, heat 1 tablespoon oil over medium warmth. Include pasta, spreading equitably; cook until base is daintily caramelized, around 5 minutes. Expel from skillet.
4. In the same skillet, heat remaining oil over medium-high warmth; pan sear mushrooms, pepper, and tofu until mushrooms are delicate, 3-4 minutes. Include pasta and soy sauce; hurl and warmth through. Sprinkle with green onions.

Garden Vegetable and Herb Soup
Total Time
Prep: 20 min. Cook: 30 min.
Makes
8 servings (2 quarts)
Ingredients:

- 2 tablespoons olive oil
- 2 medium onions, hacked
- 2 huge carrots, cut

- 1 pound red potatoes (around 3 medium), cubed
- 2 cups of water
- 1 can (14-1/2 ounces) diced tomatoes in sauce
- 1-1/2 cups vegetable soup
- 1-1/2 teaspoons garlic powder
- 1 teaspoon dried basil
- 1/2 teaspoon salt
- 1/2 teaspoon paprika
- 1/4 teaspoon dill weed
- 1/4 teaspoon pepper
- 1 medium yellow summer squash, split and cut
- 1 medium zucchini, split and cut

Directions:

1. In a huge pan, heat oil over medium warmth. Include onions and carrots; cook and mix until onions are delicate, 4-6 minutes. Include potatoes and cook 2 minutes. Mix in water, tomatoes, juices, and seasonings. Heat to the point of boiling. Diminish heat; stew, revealed, until potatoes and carrots are delicate, 9 minutes.
2. Include yellow squash and zucchini; cook until vegetables are delicate, 9 minutes longer. Serve or, whenever wanted, puree blend in clusters, including extra stock until wanted consistency is accomplished.

Salad Chard and White Bean Pasta
Total Time
Prep: 20 min. Cook: 20 min.
Makes
8 servings
Ingredients:

- 1 bundle (12 ounces) uncooked entire wheat or darker rice penne pasta
- 2 tablespoons olive oil
- 4 cups cut leeks (a white bit as it were)
- 1 cup cut sweet onion
- 4 garlic cloves, cut
- 1 tablespoon minced crisp savvy or 1 teaspoon scoured sage
- 1 enormous sweet potato, stripped and cut into 1/2-inch solid shapes
- 1 medium bundle Swiss chard (around 1 pound), cut into 1-inch cuts
- 1 can (15-1/2 ounces) extraordinary northern beans, flushed and depleted

- 3/4 teaspoon salt
- 1/4 teaspoon bean stew powder
- 1/4 teaspoon squashed red pepper drops
- 1/8 teaspoon ground nutmeg
- 1/8 teaspoon pepper
- 1/3 cup finely slashed crisp basil
- 1 tablespoon balsamic vinegar
- 2 cups marinara sauce, warmed

Directions:

1. Cook pasta as indicated by bundle headings. Channel, holding 3/4 cup pasta water.
2. In a 6-qt. stockpot, heat oil over medium warmth; saute leeks and onion until delicate, 5-7 minutes. Include garlic and sage; cook and mix 2 minutes.
3. Include potato and chard; cook, secured, over medium-low warmth 5 minutes. Mix in beans, seasonings and held pasta water; cook, secured, until potato and chard are delicate, around 5 minutes.
4. Include pasta, basil, and vinegar; hurl and warmth through. Present with sauce.

Cauliflower with Roasted Almond and Pepper Dip
Ingredients:
Total Time
Prep: 40 min. Bake: 35 min.
Makes
10 servings (2-1/4 cups dip)
Ingredients:

- 10 cups water
- 1 cup olive oil, isolated
- 3/4 cup sherry or red wine vinegar, isolated
- 3 tablespoons salt
- 1 cove leaf
- 1 tablespoon squashed red pepper drops
- 1 enormous head cauliflower
- 1/2 cup entire almonds, toasted
- 1/2 cup delicate entire wheat or white bread morsels, toasted
- 1/2 cup fire-simmered squashed tomatoes
- 1 container (8 ounces) broiled sweet red peppers, depleted
- 2 tablespoons minced new parsley
- 2 garlic cloves
- 1 teaspoon sweet paprika

- 1/2 teaspoon salt
- 1/4 teaspoon newly ground pepper

Directions:

1. In a 6-qt. stockpot, bring water, 1/2 cup oil, 1/2 cup sherry, salt, sound leaf, and pepper pieces to a bubble. Include cauliflower. Diminish heat; stew, revealed, until a blade effectively embeds into focus, 15-20 minutes, turning part of the way through cooking. Evacuate with an opened spoon; channel well on paper towels.
2. Preheat broiler to 450°. Spot cauliflower on a lubed wire rack in a 15x10x1-in. heating dish. Prepare on a lower broiler rack until dim brilliant, 39 minutes.
3. In the meantime, place almonds, bread morsels, tomatoes, cooked peppers, parsley, garlic, paprika, salt, and pepper in a nourishment processor; beat until finely cleaved. Include remaining sherry; process until mixed. Keep preparing while step by step including remaining oil in a constant flow. Present with cauliflower.

Spicy Grilled Broccoli
Total Time
Prep: 20 min. + standing Grill: 10 min.
Makes
6 servings
Ingredients:

- 2 packs broccoli
- MARINADE:
- 1/2 cup olive oil
- 1/4 cup juice vinegar
- 1 teaspoon onion powder
- 1 teaspoon garlic powder
- 1 teaspoon smoked paprika
- 1/2 teaspoon salt
- 1/2 teaspoon squashed red pepper pieces
- 1/4 teaspoon pepper

Direction:

1. Cut every broccoli pack into 6 pieces. In a 6-qt. stockpot, place a steamer container more than 1 in. of water. Spot broccoli in bushel. Heat water to the point of boiling. Decrease warmth to keep up a stew; steam, secured, 4-6 minutes or until fresh delicate.

2. In an enormous bowl, whisk marinade fixings until mixed. Include broccoli; delicately hurl to cover. Let stand, secured, 15 minutes.
3. Channel broccoli, saving marinade. Flame broil broccoli, secured, over medium warmth or cook 4 in. from heat 6-8 minutes or until broccoli is delicate, turning once. Whenever wanted, present withheld marinade.

Super-easy Chicken Noodle Soup
SmartPoints value: Green plan - 3SP, Blue plan - 2SP, Purple plan - 2SP
Total Time: 32 min, **Prep time**:   12 min, **Cooking time**: 20 min, **Serves**: 8
Nutritional value: Calories - 351.3, Carbs - 37.3g, Fat - 4.5g, Protein - 39.7g
In this recipe, I will make it easy for you to prepare a hearty soup for the whole family, all with just one pot. A big cup of 1 1/2 portion has only two SmartPoints value, so it's perfect for lunch, either to take to work or for your child's lunchbox, too.

Unlike other recipes like it, this one will be ready in just 32 minutes, not hours!

Now, pick up some ZeroPoint chicken breasts, frozen vegetables, a box of pasta, chicken broth, and a few more bits and pieces, and let's get you started on this family delight.

Ingredients

- Black pepper - ¼ tsp
- Chicken breast(s) (cooked) - 6 oz, chopped (skinless, boneless)
- Salted butter - 2 tsp
- Onion(s) (uncooked)- 1 large, well chopped
- Table salt - 1½ tsp, divided
- Chicken broth (reduced-sodium) - 64 oz
- Pasta (uncooked) - 4 oz, small shape such as ditalini (about 1 cup)
- Mixed vegetables (frozen) - 10 oz, such as peas, green beans, and carrots
- Tomatoes (canned) - 15 oz, petite cut, rinsed and drained
- Parmesan cheese (grated) - 1 Tbsp
- Lemon juice (fresh) - 2 tsp
- Fresh chives - ¼ cup(s), chopped (optional)

Instructions

1. Melt two teaspoons of butter in a large stockpot over medium-low heat.
2. Add well-chopped onion and 1/2 teaspoon of salt, then cook, often stirring, until the onion is soft and translucent; about 10 minutes.

3. Add the broth in the chicken and increase the heat to high, then bring it to a boil.
4. Put in the pasta, frozen vegetables, and tomatoes, then cook until pasta is soft; about 7 minutes.
5. Stir in the chicken, lemon juice, cheese, remaining one teaspoon of salt, black pepper, and chives, then cook one more minute to heat through.

Hearty Ginger Soup

Serving: 4
Prep Time: 5 minutes
Cook Time: 5 minutes

Ingredients:

- 3 cups coconut almond milk
- 2 cups water
- ½ pound boneless chicken breast halves, cut into chunks
- 3 tablespoons fresh ginger root, minced
- 2 tablespoons fish sauce
- ¼ cup fresh lime juice
- 2 tablespoons green onions, sliced
- 1 tablespoon fresh cilantro, chopped

How To:

1. Take a saucepan and add coconut almond milk and water.
2. Bring the mixture to a boil and add the chicken strips.
3. Reduce the warmth to medium and simmer for 3 minutes.
4. Stir within the ginger, juice , and fish sauce.
5. Sprinkle a couple of green onions and cilantro.
6. Serve!

Nutrition (Per Serving)

- Calories: 415
- Fat: 39g
- Carbohydrates: 8g
- Protein: 14g

Tasty Tofu and Mushroom Soup

Serving: 8
Prep Time: 10 minutes
Cook Time: 10 minutes

Ingredients:

- 3 cups prepared dashi stock
- ¼ cup shiitake mushrooms, sliced
- 1 tablespoon miso paste
- 1 tablespoon coconut aminos
- 1/8 cup cubed soft tofu
- 1 green onion, diced

How To:

1. Take a saucepan and add stock, bring back a boil.
2. Add mushrooms, cook for 4 minutes.
3. Take a bowl and add coconut aminos, miso paste and blend well.
4. Pour the mixture into stock and let it cook for six minutes on simmer.
5. Add diced green onions and enjoy!

Nutrition (Per Serving)
Calories: 100
Fat: 4g
Carbohydrates: 5g
Protein: 11

Ingenious Eggplant Soup
Serving: 8
Prep Time: 20 minutes
Cook Time: 15 minutes

Ingredients:

- 1 large eggplant, washed and cubed
- 1 tomato, seeded and chopped
- 1 small onion, diced
- 2 tablespoons parsley, chopped
- 2 tablespoons extra virgin olive oil
- 2 tablespoons distilled white vinegar
- ½ cup parmesan cheese, crumbled Sunflower seeds as needed

How To:

1. Pre-heat your outdoor grill to medium-high.
2. Pierce the eggplant a couple of times employing a knife/fork.
3. Cook the eggplants on your grill for about quarter-hour until they're charred.
4. forgot and permit them to chill .
5. Remove the skin from the eggplant and dice the pulp.

6. Transfer the pulp to a bowl and add parsley, onion, tomato, olive oil, feta cheese and vinegar.
7. Mix well and chill for 1 hour.
8. Season with sunflower seeds and enjoy!

Nutrition (Per Serving)
Calories: 99
Fat: 7g
Carbohydrates: 7g
Protein:3.4g
Loving Cauliflower Soup
Serving: 6
Prep Time: 10 minutes
Cook Time: 10 minutes
Ingredients:

- 4 cups vegetable stock
- 1-pound cauliflower, trimmed and chopped
- 7 ounces Kite ricotta/cashew cheese
- 4 ounces almond butter
- Sunflower seeds and pepper to taste

How To:

1. Take a skillet and place it over medium heat.
2. Add almond butter and melt.
3. Add cauliflower and sauté for two minutes.
4. Add stock and convey mix to a boil.
5. Cook until cauliflower is hard .
6. Stir in cheese , sunflower seeds and pepper.
7. Puree the combination using an immersion blender.
8. Serve and enjoy!

Nutrition (Per Serving)
Calories: 143
Fat: 16g
Carbohydrates: 6g
Protein: 3.4g
Simple Garlic and Lemon Soup
Serving: 3
Prep Time: 10 minutes
Cook Time: nil
Ingredients:

- 1 avocado, pitted and chopped
- 1 cucumber, chopped
- 2 bunches spinach
- 1 ½ cups watermelon, chopped
- 1 bunch cilantro, roughly chopped
- Juice from 2 lemons
- ½ cup coconut amines
- ½ cup lime juice

How To:

1. Add cucumber, avocado to your blender and pulse well.
2. Add cilantro, spinach and watermelon and blend.
3. Add lemon, juice and coconut amino.
4. Pulse a couple of more times.
5. Transfer to bowl and enjoy!

Nutrition (Per Serving)
Calories: 100
Fat: 7g
Carbohydrates: 6g
Protein: 3g
Healthy Cucumber Soup
Serving: 4
Prep Time: 14 minutes
Cook Time: Nil
Ingredients:

- 2 tablespoons garlic, minced
- 4 cups English cucumbers, peeled and diced
- ½ cup onions, diced
- 1 tablespoon lemon juice 1 ½ cups vegetable broth
- ½ teaspoon sunflower seeds
- ¼ teaspoon red pepper flakes
- ¼ cup parsley, diced
- ½ cup Greek yogurt, plain

How To:

1. Add the listed ingredients to a blender and blend to emulsify (keep aside ½ cup of chopped cucumbers).
2. Blend until smooth.
3. Divide the soup amongst 4 servings and top with extra cucumbers.
4. Enjoy chilled!

Nutrition (Per Serving)
Calories: 371
Fat: 36g
Carbohydrates: 8g
Protein: 4g
Mushroom Cream Soup
Serving: 4
Prep Time: 5 minutes
Cook Time: 30 minutes
Ingredients:

- 1 tablespoon olive oil
- ½ large onion, diced
- 20 ounces mushrooms, sliced
- 6 garlic cloves, minced
- 2 cups vegetable broth
- 1 cup coconut cream
- ¾ teaspoon sunflower seeds
- ¼ teaspoon black pepper
- 1 cup almond milk

How To:

1. Take an outsized sized pot and place it over medium heat.
2. Add onion and mushrooms to the vegetable oil and sauté for 10-15 minutes.
3. confirm to stay stirring it from time to time until browned evenly.
4. Add garlic and sauté for 10 minutes more.
5. Add vegetable broth, coconut milk , almond milk[MOU6], black pepper and sunflower seeds.
6. Bring it to a boil and lower the temperature to low.
7. Simmer for quarter-hour .
8. Use an immersion blender to puree the mixture.
9. Enjoy!

Nutrition (Per Serving)
Calories: 200
Fat: 17g
Carbohydrates: 5g
Protein: 4g
Curious Roasted Garlic Soup
Serving: 10
Prep Time: 10 minutes
Cook Time: 60 minutes

Ingredients:

- 1 tablespoon olive oil
- 2 bulbs garlic, peeled
- 3 shallots, chopped
- 1 large head cauliflower, chopped
- 6 cups vegetable broth
- Sunflower seeds and pepper to taste

How To:

1. Pre-heat your oven to 400 degrees F.
2. Slice ¼ inch top of garlic bulb and place it in aluminum foil.
3. Grease with vegetable oil and roast in oven for 35 minutes.
4. Squeeze flesh out of the roasted garlic.
5. Heat oil in saucepan and add shallots, sauté for six minutes.
6. Add garlic and remaining ingredients.
7. Cover pan and reduce heat to low.
8. Let it cook for 15-20 minutes.
9. Use an immersion blender to puree the mixture. 10. Season soup with sunflower seeds and pepper.
10. Serve and enjoy!

Nutrition (Per Serving)
Calories: 142
Fat: 8g
Carbohydrates: 3.4g
Protein: 4g
Amazing Roasted Carrot Soup
Serving: 4
Prep Time: 10 minutes
Cook Time: 50 minutes
Ingredients:

- 8 large carrots, washed and peeled
- 6 tablespoons olive oil
- 1-quart broth
- Cayenne pepper to taste
- Sunflower seeds and pepper to taste

How To:

1. Pre-heat your oven to 425 degrees F.
2. Take a baking sheet and add carrots, drizzle vegetable oil and roast

for 30-45 minutes.
3. Put roasted carrots into blender and add broth, puree.
4. Pour into saucepan and warmth soup.
5. Season with sunflower seeds, pepper and cayenne.
6. Drizzle vegetable oil .
7. Serve and enjoy!

Nutrition (Per Serving)
Calories: 222
Fat: 18g
Net Carbohydrates: 7g
Protein: 5g
Simple Pumpkin Soup
Serving: 4
Prep Time: 5 minutes
Cook Time: 6-8 hours
Ingredients:

- 1 small pumpkin, halved, peeled, seeds removed, cubed
- 2 cups chicken broth
- 1 cup coconut milk
- Pepper and thyme to taste

How To:

1. Add all the ingredients to a crockpot.
2. Close the lid.
3. Cook for 6-8 hours on low.
4. Make a smooth puree by employing a blender.
5. Garnish with roasted seeds.
6. Serve and enjoy!

Nutrition (Per Serving)
Calories: 60
Fat: 2g
Net Carbohydrates: 10g
Protein: 3g
Coconut Avocado Soup
Serving: 4
Prep Time: 5 minutes
Cook Time: 5-10 minutes
Ingredients:

- 2 cups vegetable stock

- 2 teaspoons Thai green curry paste
- Pepper as needed
- 1 avocado, chopped
- 1 tablespoon cilantro, chopped
- Lime wedges
- 1 cup coconut milk

How To:

1. Add milk, avocado, curry paste, pepper to blender and blend.
2. Take a pan and place it over medium heat.
3. Add mixture and warmth , simmer for five minutes.
4. Stir in seasoning, cilantro and simmer for 1 minute.
5. Serve and enjoy!

Nutrition (Per Serving)
Calories: 250
Fat: 30g
Net Carbohydrates: 2g
Protein: 4g
Coconut Arugula Soup
Serving: 4
Prep Time: 5 minutes
Cook Time: 5-10 minutes
Ingredients:

- Black pepper as needed
- 1 tablespoon olive oil
- 2 tablespoons chives, chopped
- 2 garlic cloves, minced
- 10 ounces baby arugula
- 2 tablespoons tarragon, chopped
- 4 tablespoons coconut milk yogurt
- 6 cups chicken stock
- 2 tablespoons mint, chopped
- 1 onion, chopped
- ½ cup coconut milk

How To:

1. Take a saucepan and place it over medium-high heat, add oil and let it heat up.
2. Add onion and garlic and fry for five minutes.
3. Stir available and reduce the warmth , let it simmer.

4. Stir in tarragon, arugula, mint, parsley and cook for six minutes.
5. Mix in seasoning , chives, coconut yogurt and serve.
6. Enjoy!

Nutrition (Per Serving)
Calories: 180
Fat: 14g
Net Carbohydrates: 20g
Protein: 2g

Awesome Cabbage Soup
Serving: 3
Prep Time: 7 minutes
Cook Time: 25 minutes
Ingredients:

- 3 cups non-fat beef stock
- 2 garlic cloves, minced
- 1 tablespoon tomato paste
- 2 cups cabbage, chopped
- ½ yellow onion
- ½ cup carrot, chopped
- ½ cup green beans
- ½ cup zucchini, chopped
- ½ teaspoon basil
- ½ teaspoon oregano
- Sunflower seeds and pepper as needed

How To:

1. Grease a pot with non-stick cooking spray.
2. Place it over medium heat and permit the oil to heat up.
3. Add onions, carrots, and garlic and sauté for five minutes.
4. Add broth, ingredient , green beans, cabbage, basil, oregano, sunflower seeds, and pepper.
5. Bring the entire mix to a boil and reduce the warmth , simmer for 5-10 minutes until all veggies are tender.
6. Add zucchini and simmer for five minutes more.
7. Sever hot and enjoy!

Nutrition (Per Serving)
Calories: 22
Fat: 0g
Carbohydrates: 5g
Protein: 1g

Ginger Zucchini Avocado Soup
Serving: 3
Prep Time: 7 minutes
Cook Time: 25 minutes
Ingredients:

- 1 red bell pepper, chopped
- 1 big avocado
- 1 teaspoon ginger, grated
- Pepper as needed
- 2 tablespoons avocado oil
- 4 scallions, chopped
- 1 tablespoon lemon juice
- 29 ounces vegetable stock
- 1 garlic clove, minced
- 2 zucchini, chopped
- 1 cup water

How To:

1. Take a pan and place over medium heat, add onion and fry for 3 minutes.
2. Stir in ginger, garlic and cook for 1 minute.
3. Mix in seasoning, zucchini stock, water and boil for 10 minutes.
4. Remove soup from fire and let it sit, blend in avocado and blend using an immersion blender.
5. Heat over low heat for a short time .
6. Adjust your seasoning and add juice , bell pepper.
7. Serve and enjoy!

Nutrition (Per Serving)
Calories: 155
Fat: 11g
Carbohydrates: 10g
Protein: 7g

Greek Lemon and Chicken Soup
Serving: 4
Prep Time: 15 minutes
Cook Time: 30 minutes
Ingredients:

- 2 cups cooked chicken, chopped
- 2 medium carrots, chopped
- ½ cup onion, chopped ¼ cup lemon juice

- 1 clove garlic, minced
- 1 can cream of chicken soup, fat-free and low sodium
- 2 cans chicken broth, fat-free
- ¼ teaspoon ground black pepper
- 2/3 cup long-grain rice
- 2 tablespoons parsley, snipped

How To:

1. Add all of the listed ingredients to a pot (except rice and parsley).
2. Season with sunflower seeds and pepper.
3. Bring the combination to a overboil medium-high heat.
4. Stir in rice and set heat to medium.
5. Simmer for 20 minutes until rice is tender.
6. Garnish parsley and enjoy!

Nutrition (Per Serving)
Calories: 582
Fat: 33g
Carbohydrates: 35g
Protein: 32g
Morning Peach
Serving: 4
Prep Time: 10 minutes
Cook Time: 5 minutes
Ingredients:

- 6 small peaches, cored and cut into wedges
- ¼ cup coconut sugar
- 2 tablespoons almond butter
- ¼ teaspoon almond extract

How To:

1. Take alittle pan and add peaches, sugar, butter and flavor.
2. Toss well.
3. Cook over medium-high heat for five minutes, divide the combination into bowls and serve.
4. Enjoy!

Nutrition (Per Serving)
Calories: 198
Fat: 2g
Carbohydrates: 11g

Protein: 8g
Garlic and Pumpkin Soup
Serving: 4
Prep Time: 10 minutes
Cook Time: 5 hours
Ingredients:

- 1-pound pumpkin chunks
- 1 onion, diced
- 2 cups vegetable stock
- 1 2/3 cups coconut cream
- ½ stick almond butter
- 1 teaspoon garlic, crushed
- 1 teaspoon ginger, crushed
- Pepper to taste

How To:

1. Add all the ingredients into your Slow Cooker.
2. Cook for 4-6 hours on high.
3. Puree the soup by using an immersion blender.
4. Serve and enjoy!

Nutrition (Per Serving)
Calories: 235
Fat: 21g
Carbohydrates: 11g
Protein: 2g
Butternut and Garlic Soup
Serving: 4
Prep Time: 5 minutes
Cook Time: 35 minutes
Ingredients:

- 4 cups butternut squash, cubed
- 4 cups vegetable broth, stock
- ½ cup low fat cream
- 2 garlic cloves, chopped
- Pepper to taste

How To:

1. Add butternut squash, garlic cloves, broth, salt and pepper during a large pot.

2. Place the pot over medium heat and canopy with the lid.
3. Bring back boil then reduce the temperature.
4. Let it simmer for 30-35 minutes.[MOU7]
5. Blend the soup for 1-2 minutes until you get a smooth mixture.
6. Stir the cream through the soup.
7. Serve and enjoy!

Nutrition (Per Serving)
Calories: 180
Fat: 14g
Carbohydrates: 21g
Protein: 3g
Minty Avocado Soup
Serving: 4
Prep Time: 10 minutes + Chill time
Cook Time: nil
Ingredients:

- 1 avocado, ripe
- 1 cup coconut almond milk, chilled
- 2 romaine lettuce leaves
- 20 mint leaves, fresh
- 1 tablespoon lime juice
- Sunflower seeds, to taste

How To:

1. Activate your slow cooker and add all the ingredients into it.
2. Mix them during a kitchen appliance .
3. Make a smooth mixture.
4. Let it chill for 10 minutes.
5. Serve and enjoy!

Nutrition (Per Serving)
Calories: 280
Fat: 26g
Carbohydrates: 12g
Protein: 4g
Celery, Cucumber and Zucchini Soup
Serving: 2
Prep Time: 10 minutes + Chill time
Cook Time: nil
Ingredients:

- 3 celery stalks, chopped
- 7 ounces cucumber, cubed
- 1 tablespoon olive oil
- 2/5 cup fresh cream, 30%, low fat
- 1 red bell pepper, chopped
- 1 tablespoon dill, chopped
- 10 ½ ounces zucchini, cubed
- Sunflower seeds and pepper, to taste

How To:

1. Put the vegetables during a juicer and juice.
2. Then mix within the vegetable oil and fresh cream.
3. Season with sauce and pepper.
4. Garnish with dill.
5. Serve it chilled and enjoy!

Nutrition (Per Serving)
Calories: 325
Fat: 32g
Carbohydrates: 10g
Protein: 4g
Rosemary and Thyme Cucumber Soup
Serving: 3
Prep Time: 10 minutes + Chill time
Cook Time: nil
Ingredients:

- 4 cups vegetable broth
- 1 teaspoon thyme, freshly chopped
- 1 teaspoon rosemary, freshly chopped
- 2 cucumbers, sliced1 cup low fat cream
- 1 pinch of sunflower seeds

How To:

1. Take an outsized bowl and add all the ingredients.
2. Whisk well.
3. Blend until smooth by using an immersion blender.
4. Let it chill for 1 hour.
5. Serve and enjoy!

Nutrition (Per Serving)

- Calories: 111
- Fat: 8g
- Carbohydrates: 4g
- Protein: 5g

Guacamole Soup
Serving: 3
Prep Time: 10 minute + Chill time
Cook Time: nil
Ingredients:

- 3 cups vegetable broth 2 ripe avocados, pitted
- ½ cup cilantro, freshly chopped
- 1 tomato, chopped
- ½ cup low fat cream
- Sunflower seeds & black pepper, to taste

How To:

1. Add all the ingredients into a blender.
2. Blend until creamy by using an immersion blender.
3. Let it chill for 1 hour.
4. Serve and enjoy!

Nutrition (Per Serving)
Calories: 289
Fat: 26g
Carbohydrates: 5g
Protein: 10g
Cucumber and Zucchini Soup
Serving: 3
Prep Time: 10 minutes + Chill time
Cook Time: nil
Ingredients:

- 2 tablespoons olive oil
- 1 tablespoon fresh dill
- 2/5 cup fresh cream
- 7 ounces cucumber, cubed
- 10 ½ zucchini, cubed
- 1 red pepper, chopped
- 3 celery stalks, chopped
- Sunflower seeds and pepper to taste

How To:

1. Add all the veggies during a juice and make a smooth juice.
2. Mix within the fresh cream and vegetable oil .
3. Season with pepper and sunflower seeds.
4. Garnish with dill.
5. Serve chilled and enjoy!

Nutrition (Per Serving)
Calories: 100
Fat: 8g
Carbohydrates: 4g
Protein: 2g
Crockpot Pumpkin Soup
Serving: 3
Prep Time: 10 minute
Cook Time: 6-8 hours
Ingredients:

- 1 small pumpkin, halved, peeled, seeds removed, and pulp cubed
- 2 cups chicken broth
- 1 cup of coconut almond milk
- Sunflower seeds, pepper, thyme, and pepper, to taste

How To:

1. Add all the ingredients to a crockpot.
2. Close the lid.
3. Cook for 6-8 hours on LOW.
4. Make a smooth puree by employing a blender.
5. Garnish with roasted seeds.
6. Serve and enjoy!

Nutrition (Per Serving)
Calories: 60
Fat: 5g
Carbohydrates: 4g
Protein: 4g
Tomato Soup
Serving: 3
Prep Time: 10 minutes
Cook Time: 6-8 hours
Ingredients:

- 4 cups water or vegetable broth
- 7 large tomatoes, ripe
- ½ cup macadamia nuts, raw
- 1 medium onion, chopped
- Sunflower seeds and pepper to taste

How To:

1. Take a nonstick skillet and add the onion.
2. Brown the onion for five minutes.
3. Add all the ingredients to a crockpot.
4. Cook for 6-8 hours on LOW.
5. Make a smooth puree by employing a blender.
6. Serve it warm and enjoy!

Nutrition (Per Serving)
Calories: 145
Fat: 12g
Carbohydrates: 8g
Protein: 6g
Pumpkin, Coconut and Sage Soup
Serving: 3
Prep Time: 10 minute
Cook Time: 30 minutes
Ingredients:

- 1 cup pumpkin, canned
- 6 cups chicken broth
- 1 cup low fat coconut almond milk
- 1 teaspoon sage, chopped
- 3 garlic cloves, peeled
- Sunflower seeds and pepper to taste

How To:

1. Take a stockpot and add all the ingredients except coconut almond milk into it.
2. Place stockpot over medium heat.
3. Let it bring back a boil.
4. Reduce heat to simmer for half-hour .
5. Add the coconut almond milk and stir.
6. Serve bacon and enjoy!

Nutrition (Per Serving)

Calories: 145
Fat: 12g
Carbohydrates: 8g
Protein: 6g

Sweet Potato and Leek Soup

Serving: 6
Prep Time: 10 minutes
Cook Time: 8 hours

Ingredients:

- 6 cups sweet potatoes, peeled and cubed
- 2 leeks, whites and greens, sliced
- 6 cups vegetable stock
- 1 teaspoon dried thyme
- 1 teaspoon salt
- ¼ teaspoon fresh ground black pepper

How To:

1. Add sweet potatoes, leeks, thyme, stock, salt and pepper to your Slow Cooker.
2. Close lid and cook on LOW for 8 hours.
3. Mash with potato masher/ use an immersion blender to smooth the soup.
4. Serve and enjoy!

Nutrition (Per Serving)

Calories: 234
Fat: 2g
Carbohydrates: 47g
Protein: 8g

The Kale and Spinach Soup

Serving: 4
Prep Time: 5 minutes
Cook Time: 10 minutes

Ingredients:

- 3 ounces coconut oil
- 8 ounces kale, chopped
- 2 avocados, diced
- 4 1/3 cups coconut almond milk
- Sunflower seeds and pepper to taste

How To:

1. Take a skillet and place it over medium heat. 2. Add kale and sauté for 2-3 minutes
2. Add kale to blender.
3. Add water, spices, coconut almond milk and avocado to blender also .
4. Blend until smooth and pour mix into bowl.
5. Serve and enjoy!

Nutrition (Per Serving)
Calories: 124
Fat: 13g
Carbohydrates: 7g
Protein: 4.2g
Japanese Onion Soup
Serving: 4
Prep Time: 15 minutes
Cook Time: 45 minutes
Ingredients:

- ½ stalk celery, diced
- 1 small onion, diced
- ½ carrot, diced
- 1 teaspoon fresh ginger root, grated
- ¼ teaspoon fresh garlic, minced
- 2 tablespoons chicken stock
- 3 teaspoons beef bouillon granules
- 1 cup fresh shiitake, mushrooms
- 2 quarts water
- 1 cup baby Portobello mushrooms, sliced
- 1 tablespoon fresh chives

How To:

1. Take a saucepan and place it over high heat, add water, bring back a boil.
2. Add beef bouillon, celery, onion, chicken broth , carrots, half the mushrooms, ginger, garlic.
3. placed on the lid and reduce heat to medium, cook for 45 minutes.
4. Take another saucepan and add another half mushroom.
5. Once the soup is cooked, strain the soup into the pot with uncooked mushrooms.
6. Garnish with chives and enjoy!

Nutrition (Per Serving)

Calories: 25
Fat: 0.2g
Carbohydrates: 5g
Protein: 1.4g

Amazing Broccoli and Cauliflower Soup

Serving: 4
Prep Time: 10 minutes
Cooking Time: 8 hours

Ingredients:

- 3 cups broccoli florets
- 2 cups cauliflower florets
- 2 garlic cloves, minced
- ½ cup shallots, chopped
- 1 carrot, chopped
- 3 ½ cups low sodium veggie stick
- Pinch of pepper
- 1 cup fat-free milk
- 6 ounces low-fat cheddar, shredded
- 1 cup non-fat Greek yogurt

How To:

1. Add broccoli, cauliflower, garlic, shallots, carrot, stock, pepper to your Slow Cooker.
2. Stir well and place lid.
3. Cook on LOW for 8 hours.
4. Add milk and cheese.
5. Use an immersion blender to smooth the soup.
6. Add yogurt and blend another time .
7. Ladle into bowls and enjoy!

Nutrition (Per Serving)

Calories: 218
Fat: 11g
Carbohydrates: 15g
Protein: 12g

Amazing Zucchini Soup

Serving: 4
Prep Time: 10 minutes
Cook Time: 20 minutes

Ingredients:

- 1 onion, chopped

- 3 zucchini, cut into medium chunks
- 2 tablespoons coconut milk
- 2 garlic cloves, minced
- 4 cups chicken stock
- 2 tablespoons coconut oil
- Pinch of salt
- Black pepper to taste

How To:

1. Take a pot and place over medium heat.
2. Add oil and let it heat up.
3. Add zucchini, garlic, onion and stir.
4. Cook for five minutes.
5. Add stock, salt, pepper and stir.
6. bring back a boil and reduce the warmth .
7. Simmer for 20 minutes.
8. Remove from heat and add coconut milk.
9. Use an immersion blender until smooth.
10. Ladle into soup bowls and serve.
11. Enjoy!

Nutrition (Per Serving)
Calories: 160
Fat: 2g
Carbohydrates: 4g
Protein: 7g
Portuguese Kale and Sausage Soup
Serving: 4
Prep Time: 10 minutes
Cook Time: 35 minutes
Ingredients:

- 1 yellow onion, chopped
- 16 ounces sausage, chopped
- 3 sweet potatoes, chopped
- 4cups chicken stock1 pound kale, chopped pepper as needed

How To:

1. Take a pot and place it over medium heat.
2. Add sausage and brown each side .
3. Transfer to bowl.
4. Heat pot again over medium heat.

5. Add onion and stir for five minutes.
6. Add stock, sweet potatoes, stir and convey to a simmer.
7. Cook for 20 minutes.
8. Use an immersion blender to blend.
9. Add kale and pepper and simmer for two minutes over low heat.
10. Ladle soup to bowls and top with sausage with pieces.
11. Serve and enjoy!

Nutrition (Per Serving)
Calories: 200
Fat: 2g
Carbohydrates: 6g
Protein:8g
Dazzling Pizza Soup
Serving: 6
Prep Time: 5 minutes
Cook Time: 30 minutes
Ingredients:

- 12 ounces chicken meat, sliced
- 4 ounces uncured pepperoni
- 1 can 25 ounces marinara
- 1 can 14.5 ounces fire roasted tomatoes
- 1 large onion, diced
- 15 ounces mushrooms, sliced
- 1 can 3 ounce sliced black olives
- tablespoon dried oregano
- 1 teaspoon garlic powder
- ½ teaspoon salt

How To:

1. Take large sized saucepan and add within the peperoni, chicken meat, marinara, onions, tomatoes, mushroom, oregano, olives, salt and garlic powder.
2. Cook the mixture for half-hour over medium level heat and soften the mushroom and onions.
3. Serve hot.

Nutrition (Per Serving)
Calories: 90
Fat: 2g
Carbohydrates: 17g
Protein: 3g

Mesmerizing Lentil Soup

Serving: 4
Prep Time: 10 minutes
Cooking Time: 8 hours

Ingredients:

- 1 pound dried lentils, soaked overnight and rinsed
- carrots, peeled and chopped
- 1 celery stalk, chopped
- 1 onion, chopped
- 6 cups vegetables broth
- 1 ½ teaspoons garlic powder
- 1 teaspoon ground cumin
- 1 teaspoon smoked paprika
- 1 teaspoon dried thyme
- ¼ teaspoon liquid smoke
- ¼ teaspoon salt
- ¼ teaspoon ground pepper

How To:

1. Add listed ingredients to Slow Cooker and stir well.
2. Place lid and cook for 8 hours on LOW.
3. Stir and serve.
4. Enjoy!

Nutrition (Per Serving)

Calories: 307
Fat: 1g
Carbohydrates: 56g
Protein: 20g

Organically Healthy Chicken Soup

Serving: 4
Prep Time: 10 minutes
Cook Time: 12-15 minutes

Ingredients:

- cans (14 ounces each) low sodium chicken broth
- 2 cups water
- 1 cup twisted spaghetti
- ¼ teaspoon pepper
- cups mixed vegetables (such as broccoli, carrots etc.)
- 1 and ½ cups chicken, cooked and cubed
- 1 tablespoon fresh basil, snipped

- ¼ cup parmesan, finely shredded

How To:

1. Take a Dutch Oven and add broth, water, pepper and bring the mixture to a boil. 2. Gently stir in pasta and wait until the mixture reaches boiling point again,
2. Lower down the heat and let the mixture simmer for 5 minutes (covered).
3. Remove lid and stir in the vegetables, return the mixture boil and lower down heat once again.
4. Cover and let it simmer over low heat for 5-8 minutes until the pasta and veggies and tender and cooked.
5. Stir in cooked chicken and garnish with basil.
6. Serve with a topping of parmesan.
7. Enjoy!

Nutrition Values (Per Serving)
Calories: 400
Fat: 9g
Carbohydrates: 37g
Protein: 45g
Potato and Asparagus Bisque
Serving: 4
Prep Time: 5 minutes
Cook Time: 6 minutes
Ingredients:

- 1 ½ pound asparagus
- 2 pounds sweet potatoes
- cups vegetable broth
- 1 large sized onion
- 8 cloves garlic
- 2 tablespoons dried dill
- 2 tablespoons flavored vinegar
- 3-4 cups almond milk
- 4 tablespoons Dijon mustard
- 4 tablespoons yeast

How To:

1. Add the listed ingredients (except milk, mustard and yeast) to your pot.
2. Lock the lid and cook on HIGH pressure for 6 minutes.

3. Release the pressure naturally.
4. Open the lid and add almond milk, yeast and mustard.
5. Puree using immersion blender.
6. Serve over rice.
7. Enjoy!

Nutrition (Per Serving)
Calories: 430
Fat: 12g
Carbohydrates: 77g
Protein: 6g
Cabbage and Leek Soup
Serving: 4
Prep Time: 10 minutes
Cook Time: 25 minutes
Ingredients:

- 2 tablespoons coconut oil
- ½ head chopped up cabbage
- 3-4 diced ribs celery
- 2-3 carefully cleaned and chopped leeks
- 1 diced bell pepper
- 2-3 diced carrots
- 2/3 cloves minced garlic
- 4 cups chicken broth
- 1 teaspoon Italian seasoning
- 1 teaspoon Creole seasoning
- Black pepper as needed
- 2-3 cups mixed salad greens

How To:

1. Set your pot to Sauté mode and add coconut oil.
2. Allow the oil to heat up.
3. Add the veggies (except salad greens) starting from the carrot, making sure to stir well after each vegetable addition.
4. Make sure to add the garlic last.
5. Season with Italian seasoning, black pepper and Creole seasoning.
6. Add broth and lock the lid.
7. Cook on SOUP mode for 20 minutes.
8. Release the pressure naturally and add salad greens, stir well and allow to sit for a while.
9. Allow for a few minutes to wilt the veggies.
10. Season with a bit of flavored vinegar and pepper and enjoy!

Nutrition (Per Serving)
Calories: 32
Fat: 0g
Carbohydrates: 4g
Protein: 2g
Onion Soup
Serving: 4
Prep Time: 10 minutes
Cook Time: 3 hours
Ingredients:

- 2 tablespoons avocado oil
- yellow onions, cut into halved and sliced
- Black pepper to taste
- 5 cups beef stock
- 3 thyme sprigs
- 1 tablespoon tomato paste

How To:

1. Take a pot and place it over medium high heat.
2. Add onion and thyme and stir.
3. Reduce heat to low and cook for 30 minutes.
4. Uncover pot and cook onions for 1 hour and 30 minutes more, stirring often.
5. Add tomato paste, stock and stir.
6. Simmer for 1 hour more.
7. Ladle soup into bowls and enjoy!

Nutrition (Per Serving)
Calories: 200
Fat: 4g
Carbohydrates: 6g
Protein: 8g
Carrot, Ginger and Turmeric Soup
Serving: 4
Prep Time: 15 minutes
Cook Time: 40 minutes
Ingredients:

- cups chicken broth
- ¼ cup full fat coconut milk, unsweetened
- ¾ pound carrots, peeled and chopped
- 1 teaspoon turmeric, ground

- 2 teaspoons ginger, grated
- 1 yellow onion, chopped
- 2 garlic cloves, peeled
- Pinch of pepper

How To:

1. Take a stockpot and add all the ingredients except coconut milk into it.
2. Place stockpot over medium heat.
3. Bring to a boil.
4. Reduce heat to simmer for 40 minutes.
5. Remove the bay leaf.
6. Blend the soup until smooth by using an immersion blender.
7. Add the coconut milk and stir.
8. Serve immediately and enjoy!

Nutrition (Per Serving)
Calories: 79
Fat: 4g
Carbohydrates: 7g
Protein: 4g
Offbeat Squash Soup
Serving: 4
Prep Time: 10 minutes
Cook Time: 50 minutes
Ingredients:

- 1 butternut squash, cut in halve lengthwise and deseeded
- 14 ounces coconut milk
- Pinch of salt
- Black pepper to taste
- Handful of parsley, chopped
- Pinch of nutmeg, ground

How To:

1. Add butternut squash halves on a lined baking sheet.
2. Place in oven and bake for 45 minutes at 350 degrees F.
3. Leave squash to cool down and scoop out the flesh to a pot.
4. Add half of the coconut milk to the pot and blend using immersion blender.
5. Heat soup over medium-low heat and add remaining coconut milk.
6. Add a pinch of salt, black pepper to taste.

7. Add nutmeg, parsley and blend using an immersion blender once again for a few seconds.
8. Cook for 4 minutes.
9. Serve and enjoy!

Nutrition (Per Serving)
Calories: 144
Fat: 10g
Carbohydrates: 7g
Protein: 2g
Leek and Cauliflower Soup
Serving: 6
Prep Time: 10 minutes
Cook Time: 40 minutes
Ingredients:

- 3 cups cauliflower, riced
- 1 bay leaf
- 1 teaspoon herbs de Provence
- 2 garlic cloves, peeled and diced
- ½ cup coconut milk
- 2 ½ cups vegetable stock
- 1 tablespoon coconut oil
- ½ teaspoon cracked pepper
- 1 leek, chopped

How To:

1. Take a pot, heat oil into it.
2. Sauté the leeks in the oil for 5 minutes.
3. Add the garlic and then stir-cook for another minute.
4. Add all the remaining ingredients and mix them well.
5. Cook for 30 minutes.
6. Stir occasionally.
7. Blend the soup until smooth by using an immersion blender.
8. Serve hot and enjoy!

Nutrition (Per Serving)
Calories: 90
Fat: 7g
Carbohydrates: 4g
Protein: 2g
Dreamy Zucchini Bowl
Serving: 4

Prep Time: 10 minutes
Cook Time: 20 minutes
Ingredients:

- 1 onion, chopped
- 3 zucchini, cut into medium chunks
- 2 tablespoons coconut almond milk
- 2 garlic cloves, minced
- 4 cups vegetable stock
- 2 tablespoons coconut oil
- Pinch of sunflower seeds
- Black pepper to taste

How To:

1. Take a pot and place it over medium heat.
2. Add oil and let it heat up.
3. Add zucchini, garlic, onion and stir.
4. Cook for 5 minutes.
5. Add stock, sunflower seeds, pepper and stir.
6. Bring to a boil and reduce heat.
7. Simmer for 20 minutes.
8. Remove from heat and add coconut almond milk.
9. Use an immersion blender until smooth.
10. Ladle into soup bowls and serve.
11. Enjoy!

Nutrition (Per Serving)
Calories: 160
Fat: 2g
Carbohydrates: 4g
Protein: 7g
Cold Crab and Watermelon Soup
Serving: 4
Prep Time: 10 minutes + chill time
Cook Time: nil
Ingredients:

- ¼ cup basil, chopped
- 2 pounds tomatoes
- 5 cups watermelon, cubed
- ¼ cup wine vinegar
- 2 garlic cloves, minced
- 1 zucchini, chopped

- Pepper to taste
- 1 cup crabmeat

How To:

1. Take your blender and add tomatoes, basil, vinegar, 4 cups watermelon, garlic, 1/3 cup oil, pepper and pulse well.
2. Transfer to fridge and chill for 1 hour.
3. Divide into bowls and add zucchini, crab and remaining watermelon.
4. Serve and enjoy!

Nutrition (Per Serving)

- Calories: 121
- Fat: 3g
- Carbohydrates: 4g
- Protein: 8g

Paleo Lemon and Garlic Soup
Serving: 4
Prep Time: 10 minutes
Cook Time: 10 minutes
Ingredients:

- 6 cups shellfish stock
- 1 tablespoon garlic, minced
- 1 tablespoon coconut oil, melted
- 2 whole eggs
- ½ cup lemon juice
- Pinch of salt
- White pepper to taste
- 1 tablespoon arrowroot powder
- Finely chopped cilantro for serving

How To:

1. Heat up a pot with oil over medium high heat.
2. Add garlic, stir cook for 2 minutes.
3. Add stock (reserve ½ cup for later use).
4. Stir and bring mix to a simmer.
5. Take a bowl and add eggs, sea salt, pepper, reserved stock, lemon juice and arrowroot.
6. Whisk well.

7. Pour in to the soup and cook for a few minutes.
8. Ladle soup into bowls and serve with chopped cilantro.
9. Enjoy!

Nutrition (Per Serving)
Calories: 135
Fat: 3g
Carbohydrates: 12g
Protein: 8
Brussels Soup
Serving: 4
Prep Time: 10 minutes
Cook Time: 20 minutes
Ingredients:

- 2 tablespoons olive oil
- 1 yellow onion, chopped
- 2 pounds Brussels sprouts, trimmed and halved
- 4 cups chicken stock
- ¼ cup coconut cream

How To:

1. Take a pot and place it over medium heat.
2. Add oil and let it heat up.
3. Add onion and stir-cook for 3 minutes.
4. Add Brussels sprouts and stir, cook for 2 minutes.
5. Add stock and black pepper, stir and bring to a simmer.
6. Cook for 20 minutes more.
7. Use an immersion blender to make the soup creamy.
8. Add coconut cream and stir well.
9. Ladle into soup bowls and serve.
10. Enjoy!

Nutrition (Per Serving)

- Calories: 200
- Fat: 11g
- Carbohydrates: 6g
- Protein: 11g

Spring Soup and Poached Egg
Serving: 4
Prep Time: 5 minutes

Cook Time: 15 minutes
Ingredients:

- 2 whole eggs
- 32 ounces chicken broth
- 1 head romaine lettuce, chopped

How To:

1. Bring the chicken broth to a boil.
2. Reduce the heat and poach the 2 eggs in the broth for 5 minutes.
3. Take two bowls and transfer the eggs into a separate bowl.
4. Add chopped romaine lettuce into the broth and cook for a few minutes.
5. Serve the broth with lettuce into the bowls.
6. Enjoy!

Nutrition (Per Serving)
Calories: 150
Fat: 5g
Carbohydrates: 6g
Protein: 16g
Lobster Bisque
Serving: 4
Prep Time: 10 minutes
Cook Time: 15 minutes
Ingredients:

- ¾ pound lobster, cooked and lobster
- 4 cups chicken broth
- 2 garlic cloves, chopped
- ¼ teaspoon pepper
- ½ teaspoon paprika
- 1 yellow onion, chopped
- ½ teaspoon salt
- 14 ½ ounces tomatoes, diced
- 1 tablespoon coconut oil
- 1 cup low fat cream

How To:

1. Take a stockpot and add the coconut oil over medium heat.
2. Then sauté the garlic and onion for 3 to 5 minutes.
3. Add diced tomatoes, spices and chicken broth and bring to a boil.

4. Reduce to a simmer, then simmer for about 10 minutes.
5. Add the warmed heavy cream to the soup.
6. Blend the soup till creamy by using an immersion blender.
7. Stir in cooked lobster.
8. Serve and enjoy!

Nutrition (Per Serving)
Calories: 180
Fat: 11g
Carbohydrates: 6g
Protein: 16g
Tomato Bisque
Serving: 4
Prep Time: 10 minutes
Cook Time: 40 minutes
Ingredients:

- 4 cups chicken broth
- 1 cup low fat cream
- 1 teaspoon thyme dried
- 3 cups canned whole, peeled tomatoes
- 2 tablespoons almond butter
- 3 garlic cloves, peeled
- Pepper as needed

How To:

1. Take a stockpot and first add the butter to the bottom of a stockpot.
2. Then add all the ingredients except heavy cream into it.
3. Bring to a boil.
4. Simmer for 40 minutes.
5. Warm the heavy cream and stir into the soup.
6. Serve and enjoy!

Nutrition (Per Serving)
Calories: 141
Fat: 12g
Carbohydrates: 4g
Protein: 4g
Chipotle Chicken Chowder
Serving: 4
Prep Time: 10 minutes
Cook Time: 23 minutes

Ingredients:

- 1 medium onion, chopped
- 2 garlic cloves, minced
- 6 bacon slices, chopped
- 4 cups jicama, cubed
- 3 cups chicken stock
- 1 teaspoon salt
- 2 cups low-fat, cream1 tablespoon olive oil
- 2 tablespoons fresh cilantro, chopped
- 1 ¼ pounds chicken, thigh boneless, cut into 1 inch chunks
- ½ teaspoon pepper
- 1 chipotle pepper, minced

How To:

1. Heat olive oil over medium heat in a large sized saucepan, add bacon.
2. Cook until crispy, add onion, garlic, and jicama.
3. Cook for 7 minutes, add chicken stock and chicken.
4. Bring to a boil and reduce temperature to low.
5. Simmer for 10 minutes
6. Season with salt and pepper.
7. Add heavy cream and chipotle, simmer for 5 minutes.
8. Sprinkle chopped cilantro and serve, enjoy!

Nutrition (Per Serving)
Calories: 350
Fat: 22g
Carbohydrates: 8g
Protein: 22g
Bay Scallop Chowder
Serving: 4
Prep Time: 10 minutes
Cook Time: 18 minutes
Ingredients:

- 1 medium onion, chopped
- 2 ½ cups chicken stock
- 4 slices bacon, chopped
- 3 cups daikon radish, chopped
- ½ teaspoon dried thyme
- 2 cups low-fat cream
- 1 tablespoon almond butter

- Pepper to taste
- 1 pound bay scallops

How To:

1. Heat olive over medium heat in a large sized saucepan, add bacon and cook until crisp, add onion and daikon radish.
2. Cook for 5 minutes, add chicken stock.
3. Simmer for 8 minutes, season with salt and pepper, thyme. 4. Add heavy cream, bay scallops, simmer for 4 minutes
4. Serve and enjoy!

Nutrition (Per Serving)
Calories: 307
Fat: 22g
Carbohydrates: 7g
Protein: 22g
Salmon and Vegetable Soup
Serving: 4
Prep Time: 10 minutes
Cook Time: 22 minutes
Ingredients:

- 2 tablespoons extra-virgin olive oil
- 1 leek, chopped
- 1 red onion, chopped
- Pepper to taste
- 2 carrots, chopped
- 4 cups low stock vegetable stock
- 4 ounces salmon, skinless and boneless, cubed
- ½ cup coconut cream
- 1 tablespoon dill, chopped

How To:

1. Take a pan and place it over medium heat, add leek, onion, stir and cook for 7 minutes.
2. Add pepper, carrots, stock and stir.
3. Boil for 10 minutes.
4. Add salmon, cream, dill and stir.
5. Boil for 5-6 minutes.
6. Ladle into bowls and serve.
7. Enjoy!

Nutrition (Per Serving)
Calories: 240
Fat: 4g
Carbohydrates: 7g
Protein: 12g
Garlic Tomato Soup
Serving: 4
Prep Time: 15 minutes
Cook Time: 15 minutes
Ingredients:

- Roma tomatoes, chopped
- 1 cup tomatoes, sundried
- 2 tablespoons coconut oil
- 5 garlic cloves, chopped
- 14 ounces coconut milk
- 1 cup vegetable broth
- Pepper to taste
- Basil, for garnish

How To:

1. Take a pot, heat oil into it.
2. Sauté the garlic in it for ½ minute.
3. Mix in the Roma tomatoes and cook for 8-10 minutes.
4. Stir occasionally.
5. Add in the rest of the ingredients, except the basil, and stir well.
6. Cover the lid and cook for 5 minutes.
7. Let it cool.
8. Blend the soup until smooth by using an immersion blender.
9. Garnish with basil.
10. Serve and enjoy!

Nutrition (Per Serving)
Calories: 240
Fat: 23g
Carbohydrates: 16g
Protein: 7g
Melon Soup
Serving: 4
Prep Time:6 minutes
Cook Time: Nil
Ingredients:

- 4 cups casaba melon, seeded and cubed
- 1 tablespoon fresh ginger, grated
- ¾ cup coconut milk Juice of 2 limes

How To:
Add the lime juice, coconut milk, casaba melon, ginger and salt into your blender.

Blend for 1-2 minutes until you get a smooth mixture.

Serve and enjoy!

Nutrition (Per Serving)
Calories: 134
Fat: 9g
Carbohydrates: 13g
Protein: 2g

Spring Salad
Serving: 2
Prep Time: 10-15 minutes
Cook Time: 0 minutes

Ingredients:

- 2 ounces mixed green vegetables
- 3 tablespoons roasted pine nuts
- 2 tablespoons 5-minute 5 Keto Raspberry Vinaigrette
- 2 tablespoons shaved Parmesan
- 2 slices bacon
- Pepper as required

How To:

1. Take a cooking pan and add bacon, cook the bacon until crispy.
2. Take a bowl and add the salad ingredients and mix well, add crumbled bacon into the salad.
3. Mix well.
4. Dress it with your favorite dressing.
5. Enjoy!

Nutrition (Per Serving)
Calories: 209
Fat: 17g
Net Carbohydrates: 10g
Protein: 4g

Hearty Orange and Onion Salad
Serving: 2
Prep Time: 10 minutes

Cook Time: nil
Ingredients:

- 6 large oranges
- 3 tablespoons red wine vinegar
- 6 tablespoons olive oil
- 1 teaspoon dried oregano
- 1 red onion, thinly sliced
- 1 cup olive oil
- ¼ cup fresh chives, chopped Ground black pepper

How To:

1. Peel orange and cut into 4-5 crosswise slices.
2. Transfer orange to shallow dish.
3. Drizzle vinegar, olive oil on top.
4. Sprinkle oregano.
5. Toss well to mix.
6. Chill for 30 minutes and arrange sliced onion and black olives on top.
7. Sprinkle more chives and pepper.
8. Serve and enjoy!

Nutrition (Per Serving)
Calories: 120
Fat: 6g
Carbohydrates: 20g
Protein: 2g
Ground Beef Bell Peppers
Serving: 3
Prep Time: 10 minutes
Cook Time: 10 minutes
Ingredients:

- 1 onion, chopped
- 2 tablespoons coconut oil
- 1 pound ground beef
- 1 red bell pepper, diced
- 2 cups spinach, chopped
- Pepper to taste

How To:

1. Take a skillet and place it over medium heat.

2. Add onion and cook until slightly browned.
3. Add spinach and ground beef.
4. Stir fry until done.
5. Take the mixture and fill up the bell peppers.
6. Serve and enjoy!

Nutrition (Per Serving)
Calories: 350
Fat: 23g
Carbohydrates: 4g
Protein: 28g
Healthy Mediterranean Lamb Chops
Serving: 4
Prep Time: 10 minutes
Cook Time: 10-minute
Ingredients:

- 4 lamb shoulder chops, 8 ounces each
- 2 tablespoons Dijon mustard
- 2 tablespoons Balsamic vinegar
- ½ cup olive oil
- 2 tablespoons shredded fresh basil

How To:

1. Pat your lamb chops dry using a kitchen towel and arrange them on a shallow glass baking dish.
2. Take a bowl and whisk in Dijon mustard, balsamic vinegar, pepper and mix them well.
3. Whisk in the oil very slowly into the marinade until the mixture is smooth.
4. Stir in basil.
5. Pour the marinade over the lamb chops and stir to coat both sides well .
6. Cover the chops and allow them to marinate for 1-4 hours (chilled).
7. Take the chops out and let them rest for 30 minutes to allow the temperature to reach a normal level.
8. Pre-heat your grill to medium heat and add oil to the grate.
9. Grill the lamb chops for 5-10 minutes per side until both sides are browned.
10. Once the center reads 145 degrees F, the chops are ready, serve and enjoy!

Nutrition (Per Serving)

Calories: 521
Fat: 45g
Carbohydrates: 3.5g
Protein: 22g
A Turtle Friend Salad
Serving: 6
Prep Time: 5 minutes
Cook Time: 5 minutes
Ingredients:

- 1 Romaine lettuce, chopped
- 3 Roma tomatoes, diced
- 1 English cucumber, diced
- 1 small red onion, diced
- ½ cup parsley, chopped
- 2 tablespoons virgin olive oil
- ½ large lemon, juice
- 1 teaspoon garlic powder
- Sunflower seeds and pepper to taste

How To:

1. Wash the vegetables thoroughly under cold water.
2. Prepare them by chopping, dicing or mincing as needed.
3. Take a large salad bowl and transfer the prepped veggies.
4. Add vegetable oil, olive oil, lemon juice, and spice.
5. Toss well to coat.
6. Serve chilled if preferred.
7. Enjoy!

Nutrition (Per Serving)
Calories: 200
Fat: 8g
Carbohydrates: 18g
Protein: 10g
Avocado and Cilantro Mix
Serving: 2
Prep Time: 10 minutes
Cook Time: nil
Ingredients:

- 2 avocados, peeled, pitted and diced
- 1 sweet onion, chopped
- 1 green bell pepper, chopped

- 1 large ripe tomato, chopped
- ¼ cup of fresh cilantro, chopped
- ½ lime, juiced
- Sunflower seeds and pepper as needed

How To:

1. Take a medium sized bowl and add onion, tomato, avocados, bell pepper, lime and cilantro.
2. Give the whole mixture a toss.
3. Season accordingly and serve chilled.
4. Enjoy!

Nutrition (Per Serving)
Calories: 126
Fat: 10g
Carbohydrates: 10g
Protein: 2g
Exceptional Watercress and Melon Salad
Serving: 4
Prep Time: 15 minutes
Cook Time: 20 minutes
Ingredients:

- 3 tablespoons lime juice
- 1 teaspoon date paste
- 1 teaspoon fresh ginger root, minced
- ¼ cup vegetable oil
- 2 bunch watercress, chopped
- 2 ½ cups watermelon, cubed
- 2 ½ cups cantaloupe, cubed
- 1/3 cup almonds, toasted and sliced

How To:

1. Take a large sized bowl and add lime juice, ginger, date paste.
2. Whisk well and add oil.
3. Season with pepper and sunflower seeds.
4. Add watercress, watermelon.
5. Toss well
6. Transfer to a serving bowl and garnish with sliced almonds.
7. Enjoy!

Nutrition (Per Serving)

Calories: 274
Fat: 20g
Carbohydrates: 21g
Protein: 7g

Zucchini and Onions Platter

Serving: 4
Prep Time: 15 minutes
Cook Time: 45 minutes

Ingredients:

- 3 large zucchini, julienned
- 1 cup cherry tomatoes, halved
- ½ cup basil
- 2 red onions, thinly sliced
- ¼ teaspoon sunflower seeds
- 1 teaspoon cayenne pepper
- 2 tablespoons lemon juice

How To:

1. Create zucchini Zoodles by using a vegetable peeler and shaving the zucchini with peeler lengthwise until you get to the core and seeds.
2. Turn zucchini and repeat until you have long strips.
3. Discard seeds.
4. Lay strips in cutting board and slice lengthwise to your desired thickness.
5. Mix Zoodles in a bowl alongside onion, basil, tomatoes and toss.
6. Sprinkle sunflower seeds and cayenne pepper on top.
7. Drizzle lemon juice.
8. Serve and enjoy!

Nutrition (Per Serving)
Calories: 156
Fat: 8g
Carbohydrates: 6g
Protein: 7g

Tender Watermelon and Radish Salad

Serving: 4
Prep Time: 15 minutes
Cook Time: 25 minutes

Ingredients:

- medium beets, peeled and cut into 1-inch chunks
- 1 teaspoon extra virgin olive oil

- 4 cups seedless watermelon, diced
- 1 tablespoon fresh thyme, chopped
- 1 lemon, juiced
- 2 cups kale, torn
- 3 cups radish, diced
- Sunflower seeds, to taste
- Pepper, to taste

How To:

1. Pre-heat your oven to 350 degrees F.
2. Take a small bowl and add beets, olive oil and toss well to coat the beets.
3. Roast beets for 25 minutes until tender.
4. Transfer to large bowl and cool them.
5. Add watermelon, kale, radishes, thyme, lemon juice, and toss.
6. Season sea sunflower seeds and pepper.
7. Serve and enjoy!

Nutrition (Per Serving)
Calories: 178
Fat: 2g
Carbohydrates: 39g
Protein: 6g
Fiery Tomato Salad
Serving: 4
Prep Time: 10 minutes
Cook Time: 25 minutes
Ingredients:

- ½ cup scallions, chopped
- 1 pound cherry tomatoes
- 3 teaspoons olive oil
- Sea sunflower seeds and freshly ground black pepper, to taste
- 1 tablespoon red wine vinegar

How To:

1. Season tomatoes with spices and oil.
2. Heat your oven to 450 degrees F.
3. Take a baking sheet and spread the tomatoes.
4. Bake for 15 minutes.
5. Stir and turn the tomatoes.
6. Then, bake again for 10 minutes.

7. Take a bowl and mix the roasted tomatoes with all the remaining ingredients.
8. Serve and enjoy!

Nutrition (Per Serving)
Calories: 115
Fat: 10.4g
Carbohydrates: 5.4g
Protein: 12g
Healthy Cauliflower Salad
Serving: 4
Prep Time: 10 minutes
Cook Time: nil
Ingredients:

- 1 head cauliflower, broken into florets
- 1 small onion, chopped
- 1/8 cup extra virgin olive oil
- ¼ cup apple cider vinegar
- ½ teaspoon sea salt
- ½ teaspoon black pepper
- ¼ cup dried cranberries
- ¼ cup pumpkin seeds

How To:

1. Wash the cauliflower thoroughly and break down into florets.
2. Transfer the florets to a bowl.
3. Take another bowl and whisk in oil, salt, pepper and vinegar.
4. Add pumpkin seeds, cranberries to the bowl with dressing.
5. Mix well and pour dressing over cauliflower florets.
6. Toss well.
7. Add onions and toss.
8. Chill and serve.
9. Enjoy!

Nutrition (Per Serving)
Calories: 163
Fat: 11g
Carbohydrates: 16g
Protein: 3g
Chickpea Salad
Serving: 4
Prep Time: 6 minutes

Cook Time: Nil
Ingredients:

- 1 cup canned chickpeas, drained and rinsed.
- 2 spring onions, thinly sliced.
- 1 small cucumber, diced.
- 2 green bell peppers, chopped.
- 2 tomatoes, diced.
- 2 tablespoons fresh parsley, chopped.
- 1 teaspoon capers, drained and rinsed.
- Half a lemon, juiced.
- 2 tablespoons sunflower oil.
- 1 tablespoon red wine vinegar.
- Pinch of dried oregano.
- Sunflower seeds and pepper to taste

How To:

1. Take a medium sized bowl and add chickpeas, spring onions, cucumber, bell pepper, tomato, parsley and capers.
2. Take another bowl and mix in the rest of the ingredients, pour mixture over chickpea salad and toss well.
3. Coat and serve, enjoy!

Nutrition (Per Serving)
Calories: 74
Fat: 0.7g
Carbohydrates: 16g
Protein: 2g
Dashing Bok Choy Samba
Serving: 3
Prep Time: 5 minutes
Cook Time: 15 minutes
Ingredients:

- 4 bok choy, sliced
- 1 onion, sliced
- ½ cup Parmesan cheese, grated
- 4 teaspoons coconut cream
- Sunflower seeds and freshly ground black pepper, to taste

How To:

1. Mix bok choy with black pepper and sunflower seeds.

2. Take a cooking pan, heat the oil and to sauté sliced onion for 5 minutes.
3. Then add cream and seasoned bok choy.
4. Cook for 6 minutes.
5. Stir in Parmesan cheese and cover with a lid.
6. Reduce the heat to low and cook for 3 minutes.
7. Serve warm and enjoy!

Nutrition (Per Serving)
Calories: 112
Fat: 4.9g
Carbohydrates: 1.9g
Protein: 3g
Simple Avocado Caprese Salad
Serving: 6
Prep Time: 15 minutes
Cook Time: 29 minutes
Ingredients:

- 2 avocados, cubed
- 1 cup cherry tomatoes, halved
- 8 ounces mozzarella balls, halved
- 2 tablespoons finely chopped fresh basil
- 2 tablespoons olive oil
- 2 tablespoons balsamic vinegar
- 1 tablespoon sunflower seeds Fresh ground black pepper

How To:

1. Take a bowl and add the listed ingredients, toss them well until thoroughly mixed.
2. Season with pepper according to your taste.
3. Serve and enjoy!

Nutrition (Per Serving)
Calories: 358
Fat: 30g
Carbohydrates: 9g
Protein: 14g
The Rutabaga Wedge Dish
Serving: 4
Prep Time: 15 minutes
Cook Time: 45 minutes
Ingredients:

- 2 medium rutabagas, medium, cleaned and peeled
- 4 tablespoons almond butter
- ½ teaspoon sunflower seeds
- ½ teaspoon onion powder
- 1/8 teaspoon black pepper
- ½ cup buffalo wing sauce
- ¼ cup blue cheese dressing, low fat and low sodium
- 2 green onions, chopped

How To:

1. Pre-heat your oven to 400 degrees F.
2. Line a baking sheet with parchment paper.
3. Wash and peel rutabagas, clean and peel them, and cut into wedge shapes.
4. Take a skillet and place it over low heat, add almond butter and melt.
5. Stir in onion powder, sunflower seeds, onion, black pepper.
6. Use seasoned almond butter to coat wedges.
7. Arrange wedges in a single layer on the baking sheet.
8. Bake for 30 minutes.
9. Remove and coat in buffalo sauce and return to oven.
10. Bake for 15 minutes more.
11. Place wedges on serving plate and trickle with blue cheese dressing.
12. Garnish with chopped green onion and enjoy!

Nutrition (Per Serving)
Calories: 235
Fat: 15g
Carbohydrates: 10g
Protein: 2.5g
Red Coleslaw
Serving: 4
Prep Time: 10 minutes
Cook Time: 0 minutes
Ingredients:

- 1 2/3 pounds red cabbage
- 2 tablespoons ground caraway seeds
- 1 tablespoon whole grain mustard
- 1 1/4 cups mayonnaise
- Sunflower seeds and black pepper

How To:

1. Take a large bowl and all the remaining ingredients.
2. Mix it well and let it sit for 10 minutes.
3. Serve and enjoy!

Nutrition (Per Serving)
Calories: 406
Fat: 40.8g
Carbohydrates: 10g
Protein: 2.2g
Classic Tuna Salad
Serving: 4
Prep Time: 10 minutes
Cook Time: Nil
Ingredients:

- 12 ounces white tuna, in water
- ½ cup celery, diced
- 2 tablespoons fresh parsley, chopped
- 2 tablespoons low-calorie mayonnaise, low fat and low sodium
- ½ teaspoon Dijon mustard
- ½ teaspoon sunflower seeds
- ¼ teaspoon fresh ground black pepper

Direction

1. Take a medium sized bowl and add tuna, parsley, and celery.
2. Mix well and add mayonnaise and mustard.
3. Season with pepper and sunflower seeds.
4. Stir and add olives, relish, chopped pickle, onion and mix well.
5. Serve and enjoy

Nutrition (Per Serving)
Calories: 137
Fat: 5g
Carbohydrates: 1g
Protein: 20g
Greek Salad
Serving: 4
Prep Time: 6 minutes
Cook Time: Nil
Ingredients:

- 2 cucumbers, diced
- 2 tomatoes, sliced

- 1 green lettuce, cut into thin strips
- 2 red bell peppers, cut
- ½ cup black olives pitted
- 3 ½ ounces feta cheese, cut
- 1 red onion, sliced
- 2 tablespoons olive oil
- 2 tablespoons lemon juice
- Sunflower seeds and pepper to taste

Direction

1. Dice cucumbers and slice up the tomatoes.
2. Tear the lettuce and cut it into thin strips.
3. De-seed and cut the peppers into strips.
4. Take a salad bowl and mix in all the listed vegetables, add olives and feta cheese (cut into cubes).
5. Take a small cup and mix in olive oil and lemon juice, season with sunflower seeds and pepper.
6. Pour mixture into the salad and toss well, enjoy!

Nutrition (Per Serving)
Calories: 132
Fat: 4g
Carbohydrates: 3g
Protein: 5g
Fancy Greek Orzo Salad
Serving: 4
Prep Time: 5 minutes and 24 hours chill time
Cook Time: 10 minutes
Ingredients:

- 1 cup orzo pasta, uncooked
- ½ cup fresh parsley, minced
- 6 teaspoons olive oil
- 1 onion, chopped
- 1 ½ teaspoons oregano

How To:

1. Cook the orzo and drain them.
2. Add to a serving dish.
3. Add 2 teaspoons of oil.
4. Take another dish and add parsley, onion, remaining oil and oregano.

5. Season with sunflower seeds, pepper according to your taste.
6. Pour the mixture over the orzo and let it chill for 24 hours.
7. Serve and enjoy at lunch!

Nutrition (Per Serving)
Calories: 399
Fat: 12g
Carbohydrates: 55g
Protein:16g
Homely Tuscan Tuna Salad
Serving: 4
Prep Time: 5-10 minutes
Cook Time: Nil
Ingredients:

- 15 ounces small white beans
- 6 ounces drained chunks of light tuna
- cherry tomatoes, quartered
- 4 scallions, trimmed and sliced
- 2 tablespoons lemon juice

How To:
Add all of the listed ingredients to a bowl and gently stir.
Season with sunflower seeds and pepper accordingly, enjoy!
Nutrition (Per Serving)
Calories: 322
Fat: 8g
Carbohydrates: 32g
Protein:30g
Asparagus Loaded Lobster Salad
Serving: 4
Prep Time: 10 minutes
Cook Time: Nil
Ingredients:

- 8 ounces lobster, cooked and chopped
- 3 ½ cups asparagus, chopped and steamed
- 2 tablespoons lemon juice
- 4 teaspoons extra virgin olive oil
- ¼ teaspoon kosher sunflower seeds
- Pepper
- ½ cup cherry tomatoes halved
- 1 basil leaf, chopped
- 2 tablespoons red onion, diced

How To:

1. Whisk in lemon juice, sunflower seeds, pepper in a bowl and mix with oil.
2. Take a bowl and add the rest of the ingredients.
3. Toss well and pour dressing on top.

Serve and enjoy!
Nutrition (Per Serving)
Calories: 247
Fat: 10g
Carbohydrates: 14g
Protein: 27g
Tasty Yogurt and Cucumber Salad
Serving: 4
Prep Time: 10 minutes
Cook Time: Nil
Ingredients:

- 5-6 small cucumbers, peeled and diced
- 1 (8 ounces) container plain Greek yogurt
- 2 garlic cloves, minced
- 1 tablespoon fresh mint, minced
- Sea sunflower seeds and fresh black pepper
- **How To:**
- Take a large bowl and add cucumbers, garlic, yogurt, mint.
- Season with sunflower seeds and pepper.
- Refrigerate the salad for 1 hour and serve.
- Enjoy!

Nutrition (Per Serving)
Calories: 74
Fat: 0.7g
Carbohydrates: 16g
Protein: 2g
Unique Eggplant Salad
Serving: 3
Prep Time: 10 minutes
Cook Time: 30 minutes
Ingredients:

- 2 eggplants, peeled and sliced
- 2 garlic cloves
- 2 green bell pepper, sliced, seeds removed

- ½ cup fresh parsley
- ½ cup mayonnaise, low fat, low sodium Sunflower seeds and black pepper

How To:

1. Preheat your oven to 480 degrees F.
2. Take a baking pan and add eggplant, bell peppers and season with black [MOU15][F16]pepper to it.
3. Bake for about 30 minutes.
4. Flip the vegetables after 20 minutes.
5. Then, take a bowl, add baked vegetables and all the remaining ingredients.
6. Mix well.
7. Serve and enjoy!

Nutrition (Per Serving)
Calories: 196
Fat: 108.g
Carbohydrates: 13.4g
Protein: 14.6g
Zucchini Pesto Salad
Serving: 4
Prep Time: 10 minutes
Cook Time: 10 minutes
Ingredients:

- 2 cups spiral pasta
- 2 zucchini, sliced and halved
- 4 tomatoes, cut
- 1 cup white mushrooms, cut
- 1 small red onion, chopped
- 2 tablespoons fresh basil leaves, chopped
- 2 tablespoons sunflower oil
- 1 tablespoon lemon juice
- Pepper and sunflower seeds to taste

How To:

1. Cook the pasta according to the package instructions, drain and rinse under cold water.
2. Take a large bowl and add zucchini, tomatoes, mushrooms, onion, and pasta.
3. Mix well,

4. In a food processor, add oil, lemon juice, basil, blue cheese, black, and process well.
5. Pour the mixture over the salad and toss well.
6. Serve and enjoy!

Nutrition (Per Serving)
Calories: 301
Fat: 25g
Net Carbohydrates: 7g
Protein: 10g

Wholesome Potato and Tuna Salad
Serving: 4
Prep Time: 10 minutes
Cook Time: nil

Ingredients:

- 1 pound baby potatoes, scrubbed, boiled
- 1 cup tuna chunks, drained
- 1 cup cherry tomatoes, halved
- 1 cup medium onion, thinly sliced
- 8 pitted black olives
- 2 medium hard-boiled eggs, sliced
- 1 head Romaine lettuce
- ¼ cup olive oil
- 2 tablespoons lemon juice
- 1 tablespoon Dijon mustard
- 1 teaspoon dill weed, chopped Pepper as needed

How To:

1. Take a small glass bowl and mix in your olive oil, lemon juice, Dijon mustard and dill.
2. Season the mix with pepper and salt.
3. Add in the tuna, baby potatoes, cherry tomatoes, red onion, green beans, black olives and toss everything nicely.
4. Arrange your lettuce leaves on a beautiful serving dish to make the base of your salad.
5. Top them with your salad mixture and place the egg slices.
6. Drizzle with the previously prepared Salad Dressing.
7. Serve hot

Nutrition (Per Serving)
Calories: 406
Fat: 22g

Carbohydrates: 28g
Protein: 26g
Baby Spinach Salad
Serving: 2
Prep Time: 10 minutes
Cook Time: nil
Ingredients:

- 1 bag baby spinach, washed and dried
- 1 red bell pepper, cut in slices
- 1 cup cherry tomatoes, cut in halves
- 1 small red onion, finely chopped
- 1 cup black olives, pitted
- For dressing:
- 1 teaspoon dried oregano
- 1 large garlic clove
- 3 tablespoons red wine vinegar
- 4 tablespoons olive oil
- Sunflower seeds and pepper to taste

How To:

1. Prepare the dressing by blending in garlic, olive oil, vinegar in a food processor.
2. Take a large salad bowl and add spinach leaves, toss well with the dressing.
3. Add remaining ingredients and toss again, season with sunflower seeds and pepper and enjoy!

Nutrition (Per Serving)
Calories: 126
Fat: 10g
Carbohydrates: 10g
Protein: 2g
Elegant Corn Salad
Serving: 6
Prep Time: 10 minutes
Cooking Time: 2 hours
Ingredients:

- 2 ounces prosciutto, cut into strips
- 1 teaspoon olive oil
- 2 cups corn
- 1/2 cup salt-free tomato sauce

- 1 teaspoon garlic, minced
- 1 green bell pepper, chopped

How To:

1. Grease your Slow Cooker with oil.
2. Add corn, prosciutto, garlic, tomato sauce, bell pepper to your Slow Cooker.
3. Stir and place lid.
4. Cook on HIGH for 2 hours.
5. Divide between serving platters and enjoy!

Nutrition (Per Serving)
Calories: 109
Fat: 2g
Carbohydrates: 10g
Protein: 5g
Arabic Fattoush Salad
Serving: 4
Prep Time: 15 minutes
Cook Time: 2-3 minutes
Ingredients:

- 1 whole wheat pita bread
- 1 large English cucumber, diced
- 2 cup grape tomatoes, halved
- ½ medium red onion, finely diced
- ¾ cup fresh parsley, chopped
- ¾ cup mint leaves, chopped
- 1 clove garlic, minced
- ¼ cup fat free feta cheese, crumbled
- 1 tablespoon olive oil
- 1 teaspoon ground sumac
- Juice from ½ a lemon
- Salt and pepper as needed

How To:

1. Mist pita bread with cooking spray.
2. Season with salt.
3. Toast until the breads are crispy.
4. Take a large bowl and add the remaining ingredients and mix (except feta).
5. Top the mix with diced toasted pita and feta.

6. Serve and enjoy!

Nutrition (Per Serving)
Calories: 86
Fat: 3g
Carbohydrates: 9g
Protein: 9g

Heart Warming Cauliflower Salad
Serving: 3
Prep Time: 8 minutes
Cook Time: nil

Ingredients:

- 1 head cauliflower, broken into florets
- 1 small onion, chopped
- 1/8 cup extra virgin olive oil
- ¼ cup apple cider vinegar
- ½ teaspoon of sea salt
- ½ teaspoon of black pepper
- ¼ cup dried cranberries
- ¼ cup pumpkin seeds

How To:

1. Wash the cauliflower and break it up into small florets.
2. Transfer to a bowl.
3. Whisk oil, vinegar, salt and pepper in another bowl
4. Add pumpkin seeds, cranberries to the bowl with dressing.
5. Mix well and pour the dressing over the cauliflower.
6. Add onions and toss.
7. Chill and serve.
8. Enjoy!

Nutrition (Per Serving)
Calories: 163
Fat: 11g
Carbohydrates: 16g
Protein: 3g

Great Greek Sardine Salad
Serving: 2
Prep Time: 10 minutes
Cook Time: 10 minutes

Ingredients:

- 2 tablespoons extra virgin olive oil
- 1 garlic clove, minced
- 2 teaspoons dried oregano
- ½ teaspoon freshly ground pepper
- 3 medium tomatoes, cut into large sized chunks
- 1 can (15 ounces) rinsed chickpeas
- 1/3 cup feta cheese, crumbled
- ¼ cup red onion, sliced
- 2 tablespoons Kalamata olives, sliced
- 2 cans 4-ounce drained sardines, with bones and packed in either oil or water

How To:

1. Take a large bowl and whisk in lemon juice, oregano, garlic, oil, pepper and mix well.
2. Add tomatoes, chickpeas, cucumber, olives, feta and mix.
3. Divide the salad amongst serving platter and top with sardines.
4. Enjoy!

Nutrition (Per Serving)
Calories: 347
Fat: 18g
Carbohydrates: 29g
Protein: 17g
Shrimp and Egg Medley
Serving: 4
Prep Time: 15 minutes
Cook Time: nil
Ingredients:

- 4 hard boiled eggs, peeled and chopped
- 1 pound cooked shrimp, peeled and deveined, chopped
- 1 sprig fresh dill, chopped
- ¼ cup mayonnaise
- 1 teaspoon Dijon mustard
- 4 fresh lettuce leaves

How To:

1. Take a large serving bowl and add the listed ingredients (except lettuce).
2. Stir well.
3. Serve over bed of lettuce leaves.

4. Enjoy!

Nutrition (Per Serving)
Calories: 292
Fat: 17g
Carbohydrates: 1.6g
Protein: 30g

Creamy Shrimp Salad
Serving: 4
Prep Time: 20 minutes
Cook Time: 5 minutes

Ingredients:

- 4 pounds large shrimp
- 1 lemon, quartered
- 3 cups celery stalks, chopped
- 1 red onion, chopped
- 2 cups mayonnaise
- 2 tablespoons white wine vinegar
- 1 teaspoon Dijon mustard
- Salt and pepper as needed

How To:

1. Take a large pan and place it over medium heat.
2. Add water (salted) and bring water to boil.
3. Add shrimp and lemon, cook for 3 minutes.
4. Let them cool.
5. Peel and de-vein the shrimps.
6. Take a large bowl and add cooked shrimp alongside remaining ingredients.
7. Stir well.
8. Serve immediately or chilled!

Nutrition (Per Serving)
Calories: 153
Fat: 5g
Carbohydrates: 8g
Protein: 19g

Passionate Quinoa and Black Bean Salad
Serving: 6
Prep Time: 5 minutes
Cook Time: 15 minutes

Ingredients:

- 1 cup uncooked quinoa
- 1 can 15 ounce black beans, drained and rinsed
- 1/3 cup cilantro, chopped
- 1 tablespoon olive oil
- 1 clove garlic, minced
- Juice from 1 lime
- Salt and pepper as needed

How To:

1. Cook quinoa according to the package instructions.
2. Transfer quinoa to a medium bowl and let it cool for 10 minutes.
3. Add remaining ingredients and toss well.
4. Serve and enjoy!

Nutrition (Per Serving)
Calories: 188
Fat: 4g
Carbohydrates: 29g
Protein: 8g

Zucchini Noodle Salad
Serving: 3
Prep Time: 15 minutes
Cook Time: nil

Ingredients:

- 2 large zucchini, spiralized/peeled into thin strips
- 1 small tomato, diced
- ¼ red onion, sliced thinly
- 1 large avocado, diced
- ½ cup olive oil
- ¼ cup balsamic vinegar
- 1 garlic clove, minced
- 2 teaspoons Dijon mustard
- Salt and pepper to taste
- ¼ cup blue cheese, crumbles

How To:

1. Take a large bowl and add zucchini noodles, onion, tomato, avocado.
2. Take a small bowl and whisk in olive oil, vinegar, mustard, garlic, salt and pepper.
3. Drizzle over salad and toss.

4. Divide into serving bowls and top with blue cheese crumbles.
5. Enjoy!

Nutrition (Per Serving)
Calories: 770
Fat: 74g
Carbohydrates: 12g
Protein: 8g
Onion and Orange Healthy Salad
Serving: 3
Prep Time: 10 minutes
Cook Time: nil
Ingredients:

- 6 large oranges
- 3 tablespoons red wine vinegar
- 6 tablespoons olive oil
- 1 teaspoon dried oregano
- 1 red onion, thinly sliced
- 1 cup olive oil
- ¼ cup fresh chives, chopped Ground black pepper

How To:

1. Peel the oranges and cut each of them in 4-5 crosswise slices.
2. Transfer the oranges to a shallow dish.
3. Drizzle vinegar, olive oil and sprinkle oregano.
4. Toss.
5. Chill for 30 minutes.
6. Arrange sliced onion and black olives on top.
7. Decorate with additional sprinkle of chives and fresh grind of pepper.
8. Serve and enjoy!

Nutrition (Per Serving)
Calories: 120
Fat: 6g
Carbohydrates: 20g
Protein: 2g
Stir Fried Almond and Spinach
Serving: 2
Prep Time: 10 minutes
Cook Time: 15 minutes
Ingredients:

- 34 pounds spinach
- 3 tablespoons almonds
- Salt to taste
- 1 tablespoon coconut oil

How To:

1. Add oil to a large pot and place on high heat.
2. Add spinach and let it cook, stirring frequently.
3. Once the spinach is cooked and tender, season with salt and stir.
4. Add almonds and enjoy!

Nutrition (Per Serving)
Calories: 150
Fat: 12g
Carbohydrates: 10g
Protein: 8g
Cilantro and Avocado Platter
Serving: 6
Prep Time: 10 minutes
Cook Time: nil
Ingredients:

- 2 avocados, peeled , pitted and diced
- 1 sweet onion, chopped
- 1 green bell pepper, chopped
- 1 large ripe tomato, chopped
- ¼ cup fresh cilantro, chopped
- ½ lime, juiced
- Salt and pepper as needed

How To:

1. Take a medium sized owl and add onion, bell pepper, tomato, avocados, lime and cilantro.
2. Mix well and give it a toss.
3. Season with salt and pepper according to your taste.
4. Serve and enjoy!

Nutrition (Per Serving)
Calories: 126
Fat: 10g
Carbohydrates: 10g
Protein: 2g

Chicken Breast Salad
Serving: 4
Prep Time: 25 minutes
Cook Time: 30-55 minutes
Ingredients:

- 3 ½ ounces chicken breast
- 2 tablespoons spinach
- 1 ¾ ounces lettuces
- 1 bell pepper
- 2 tablespoons olive oil
- Lemon juice to taste

How To:

1. Boil chicken breast without adding salt, cut the meat into small strips.
2. Put the spinach in boiling water for a few minutes, cut into small strips .
3. Cut pepper in strips as well.
4. Add everything to a bowl and mix with juice and oil.
5. Serve!

Nutrition (Per Serving)
Calories: 100
Fat: 11g
Carbohydrates: 3g
Protein: 6g

Broccoli Salad
Serving: 1
Prep Time: 5 minutes
Cook Time: 10 minutes
Ingredients:

- broccoli florets
- 2 red onions, sliced
- 1-ounce bacon, chopped into small pieces
- 1 cup coconut cream
- 1 teaspoon sesame seeds Salt

How To:

1. Cook bacon in hot oil until crispy.
2. Cook onions in fat left from the bacon.

3. Take a pan of boiling water and add broccoli florets, boil for a few minutes.
4. Take a salad bowl and add bacon pieces, onions, broccoli florets, coconut cream and salt.
5. Toss well and top with sesame seeds.
6. Enjoy!

Nutrition (Per Serving)
Calories: 280
Fat: 26g
Carbohydrates: 8g
Protein: 10g

Hearty Quinoa and Fruit Salad
Serving: 5
Prep Time: 5 minutes
Cook Time: 10 minutes

Ingredients:

- 3 ½ ounces Quinoa
- 3 peaches, diced
- 1 ½ ounces toasted hazelnuts, chopped
- Handful of mint, chopped
- Handful of parsley, chopped
- 2 tablespoons olive oil
- Zest of 1 lemon
- Juice of 1 lemon

How To:

1. Take medium sized saucepan and add quinoa.
2. Add 1 ¼ cups of water and bring it to a boil over medium-high heat.
3. Reduce the heat to low and simmer for 20 minutes.
4. Drain any excess liquid.
5. Add fruits, herbs, hazelnuts to the quinoa.
6. Allow it to cool and season.
7. Take a bowl and add olive oil, lemon zest and lemon juice.
8. Pour the mixture over the salad and give it a mix.
9. Enjoy!

Nutrition (Per Serving)
Calories: 148
Fat: 8g
Carbohydrates: 16g
Protein: 5g

Amazing Quinoa and Black Bean Salad
Serving: 4
Prep Time: 5 minutes
Cook Time: 2-3 minutes
Ingredients:

- 1 cup uncooked quinoa
- 1 can 15 ounce black beans, drained and rinsed
- 1/3 cup cilantro, chopped
- 1 tablespoon olive oil
- 1 clove garlic, minced
- Juice from 1 lime
- Salt and pepper as needed

How To:

1. Cook quinoa according to package instructions.
2. Transfer quinoa to a medium bowl and allow it to cool for 10 minutes.
3. Add the rest of the ingredients and toss.
4. Serve and enjoy!
5. Enjoy!

Nutrition (Per Serving)
Calories: 188
Fat: 4g
Carbohydrates: 29g
Protein: 8g

Authentic Mediterranean Pearl and Couscous
Serving: 4
Prep Time: 15 minutes
Cook Time: 10 minutes
Ingredients:

- For The Vinaigrette
- 1 large lemon, juiced
- 1/3 cup extra virgin olive oil
- 1 teaspoon dill weed
- 1 teaspoon garlic powder
- Salt and pepper as needed
- For Israeli Couscous
- 2 cups Pearl Couscous
- Extra virgin olive oil
- 2 cups grape tomatoes, halved

- Water as needed
- 1/3 cup red onions, chopped
- ½ English Cucumber, chopped
- 15 ounces chickpeas
- 14 ounce (can) fresh artichoke hearts, chopped
- ½ cup kalamata olives, pitted
- 15-20 pieces fresh basil leaves, torn and chopped
- 3 ounces fresh baby mozzarella cheese

How To:

1. Start by preparing the vinaigrette. Take a bowl and add the ingredients listed under vinaigrette.
2. Mix them well and keep it on the side.
3. Take a medium sized heavy pot and place it over medium heat.
4. Add 2 tablespoons of olive oil and allow it to heat up.
5. Add couscous and keep cooking until golden brown.
6. Add 3 cups of boiling water and cook the couscous according to package instructions.
7. Once done, drain in a colander and keep on the side.
8. Take another large sized mixing bowl and add the rest of the ingredients, except cheese and basil.
9. Add the cooked couscous and basil to the mix and mix everything well.
10. Give the vinaigrette a nice stir and whisk it into the couscous salad.
11. Mix well.
12. Adjust the seasoning as required.
13. Add mozzarella cheese.
14. Garnish with some basil.
15. Enjoy!

Nutrition (Per Serving)
Calories: 393
Fat: 13g
Carbohydrates: 57g
Protein: 13g
Mesmerizing Fruit Bowl
Serving: 1
Prep Time: 30 minutes
Cook Time: nil
Ingredients:

- 2 fresh ripe mangoes
- 2 cups pineapple chunks

- Fresh pineapple tips
- 1 banana, sliced
- 1-2 cups fresh papaya, cubed
- 1 kiwi fruit, cubed
- 2 cups seedless grapes, halved
- ¼ cup coconut milk
- 2 tablespoons lime juice
- 3-4 tablespoons sugar
- Strawberries, cranberries or raspberries as topping

How To:

1. Slice the fruits above, except the contrasting red ones such as dried cranberries, raspberries and strawberries.
2. Add them to your mixing bowl and drizzle a bit of lime juice on top.
3. Stir well and sprinkle a bit of sugar on top, give it a nice stir.
4. Allow it to chill for 30 minutes and serve the salad with a bit of coconut milk.
5. Season the sweetness accordingly and top it with some cranberries, raspberries and strawberries.
6. Enjoy!

Nutrition (Per Serving)
Calories: 209
Fat: 0g
Carbohydrates: 43g
Protein: 2g
Tangy Strawberry Salad
Serving: 4
Prep Time: 15 minutes
Cook Time: nil
Ingredients:

- 4 slices bacon, cooked and crumbled
- 10 large strawberries, stem removed and sliced
- 4 cups baby spinach
- 1 avocado, chopped

For Dressing

- Zest of 1 lemon
- ¼ red onion, minced
- ¼ cup red wine vinegar
- 1 tablespoon Dijon mustard

- 1 lemon, juiced
- 1 teaspoon poppy seed
- ½ cup extra light olive oil

How To:

1. Add all the dressing ingredients to a blender and blend until you have a smooth mixture (except poppy seeds).
2. Stir in poppy seeds after blending.
3. Take a large bowl and toss strawberries, bacon, spinach and avocado.
4. Mix well and drizzle the dressing on top.
5. Serve and enjoy!

Nutrition (Per Serving)
Calories: 96
Fat: 1g
Carbohydrates: 22g
Protein: 3g
Peachful Applesauce Salad
Serving: 6
Prep Time: 15 minutes
Cook Time: nil
Ingredients:

- 1 cup diet lemon lime-soda
- 1 pack sugar-free fruit mixed peach gelatin
- 1 cup unsweetened applesauce
- 2 cups coconut whip cream
- 1/8 teaspoon ground nutmeg
- 1/8 teaspoon vanilla extract
- 1 fresh peach, peeled and chopped

How To:

1. Take a saucepan and bring the soda to a boil over medium heat.
2. Remove heat.
3. Stir in sugar-free peach gelatin until dissolved.
4. Add applesauce and stir.
5. Let it chill until partially set.
6. Fold in whipped topping and vanilla extract.
7. Fold in the peach and wait until firm.
8. Serve and enjoy!

Nutrition (Per Serving)
Calories: 354
Fat: 17g
Carbohydrates: 37g
Protein: 15g
The Citrus Lover's Salad
Serving: 16
Prep Time: 10 minutes
Cook Time: nil
Ingredients:

- 1 medium zucchini, julienned
- ½ cup olive oil
- 1 medium red onion, sliced
- 1 cup fresh broccoli, cut into florets
- 1 cup fresh cauliflower florets
- 1/8 teaspoon pepper
- 1 medium cucumber, halved and sliced
- ¼ cup white wine vinegar
- 1 teaspoon dried oregano
- 1 medium carrot, julienned
- ½ teaspoon ground mustard
- ¼ teaspoon garlic powder
- 1/8 teaspoon celery salt

How To:

1. Add olives and veggies to a small bowl.
2. Take another bowl and whisk in vinegar, seasoning, oil.
3. Pour the mixture over veggies and toss.
4. Let sit for 3 hours.
5. Serve and enjoy!

Nutrition (Per Serving)
Calories: 72
Fat: 7g
Carbohydrates: 2g
Protein: 2g
Wicked Vanilla Fruit Salad
Serving: 5
Prep Time: 10 minutes
Cook Time: nil
Ingredients:

- 8 cans mandarin orange, drained
- 4 packs instant vanilla pudding mix
- 6 cans pineapple chunks
- 10 medium red apples, chopped

How To:

1. Drain pineapples, making sure to reserve the liquid.
2. Keep them on the side.
3. Add cold water to the juice to make 6 cups liquid in total.
4. Whisk the juice mix and pudding mix into a large bowl for about 2 minutes.
5. Let it stand for 2 minutes until soft-set.
6. Stir in apples, oranges and reserved pineapple.
7. Chill in fridge and serve.
8. Enjoy!

Nutrition (Per Serving)
Calories: 33
Fat: 0g
Carbohydrates: 8g
Protein: 0g
Green Papaya Salad
Serving: 6
Prep Time: 10 minutes
Cook Time: nil
Ingredients:

- 10 small shrimps, dried
- 2 small red Thai Chilies
- 1 garlic clove, peeled
- ¼ cup tamarind juice
- 1 tablespoon palm sugar
- 1 tablespoon Thai fish sauce, low sodium
- 1 lime, cut into 1-inch pieces
- 4 cherry tomatoes, halved
- 3 long beans, trimmed into 1-inch pieces
- 1 carrot, coarsely shredded
- ½ English cucumber, coarsely chopped and seeded
- 1/6 small green cabbage, cored and thinly sliced
- 1 pound unripe green papaya, quartered, seeded and shredded using a mandolin
- 3 tablespoons unsalted roasted peanuts

How To:

1. Take a mortar and pestle and crush your shrimp alongside garlic, chilies.
2. Add tamarind juice, fish sauce and palm sugar.
3. Squeeze the juice from the lime pieces and pour 3 quarts over the mortar.
4. Grind [MOU17][F18]the mixture in the mortar to make a dressing, keep the dressing on the side.
5. Take a bowl, add the remaining ingredients (excluding the peanut), making sure to add the papaya last.
6. Use a spoon and stir in the dressing.
7. Mix the vegetables and fruit and coat them well.
8. Transfer to your serving dish.
9. Garnish with some peanuts and lime pieces.
10. Enjoy!

Nutrition (Per Serving)
Calories: 316
Fat: 13g
Carbohydrates: 5g
Protein: 11g
Pineapple, Papaya and Mango Delight
Serving: 2
Prep Time: 20 minutes
Cook Time: nil
Ingredients:

- 1 pound fresh pineapple, peeled and cut into chunks
- mango, peeled, pitted and cubed
- papayas, peeled, seeded and cubed
- tablespoons fresh lime juice
- ¼ cup fresh mint leaves, chopped

How To:

1. Take a large bowl and add the listed ingredients.
2. Toss well to coat.
3. Put in fridge and chill.

Serve and enjoy!
Nutrition (Per Serving)
Calories: 292
Fat: 11g

Carbohydrates: 42g

Protein: 8g

Cashew and Green Apple Salad

Serving: 2

Prep Time: 15 minutes

Cook Time: nil

Ingredients:

- ½ large apple, cored and sliced
- 2 cups mixed fresh greens
- 1 tablespoon unsalted cashews
- 1 tablespoon apple cider vinegar

How To:

1. Take a serving bowl and add apple, cashews and greens.
2. Drizzle apple cider vinegar on top.
3. Serve immediately!

Nutrition (Per Serving)

Calories: 118

Fat: 4g

Carbohydrates: 19g

Protein: 3g

Watermelon and Tomato Mix

Serving: 2

Prep Time: 20 minutes

Cook Time: nil

Ingredients:

- 1 large red tomato, cubed
- 1 large yellow tomato, cubed
- 2 cups fresh watermelon, peeled, seeded and cubed

Dressing

- ¼ cup olive oil
- ¼ cup rice wine vinegar
- 2 teaspoons honey
- 2 tablespoons chili garlic sauce
- 1 tablespoon fresh lemon basil, chopped Salt and pepper as needed

How To:

1. Take a large bowl and add all the salad ingredients.
2. Take another bowl and add the dressing ingredients.
3. Beat well until combined.
4. Pour dressing over salad and toss.
5. Serve and enjoy!

Nutrition (Per Serving)
Calories: 87
Fat: 7g
Carbohydrates: 7g
Protein: 0.6g

Chapter Five

FISH AND SEAFOOD RECIPES

Seafood-Stuffed Salmon Fillets

All out Time

Prep: 25 min. Heat: 20 min.

Makes

12 servings

Nutritional Facts

1 stuffed filet: 454 calories, 27g fat (6g immersed fat), 123mg cholesterol, 537mg sodium, 9g starch (0 sugars, 0 filaments), and 41g protein.

Ingredients

- 1-1/2 cups cooked long-grain rice
- 1 bundle (8 ounces) impersonation crabmeat
- 2 tablespoons cream cheddar, relaxed
- 2 tablespoons margarine, dissolved
- 2 garlic cloves, minced
- 1/2 teaspoon each dried basil, marjoram, oregano, thyme, and rosemary, squashed
- 1/2 teaspoon celery seed, squashed
- 12 salmon filets (8 ounces each and 1-1/2 inches thick)
- 3 tablespoons olive oil
- 2 teaspoons dill weed
- 1-1/2 teaspoons salt

Direction

1. Preheat stove to 400°. In an enormous bowl, join rice, crab, cream

cheddar, spread, garlic, basil, marjoram, oregano, thyme, rosemary, and celery seed.

2. Cut a pocket on a level plane in each filet to inside 1/2 in. of the inverse side. Load up with stuffing blend; secure with toothpicks. Spot salmon on 2 lubed 15x10x1-in. heating skillet. Brush with oil; sprinkle with dill and salt.

3. Bake 18-22 minutes or until fish just starts to chip effectively with a fork. Dispose of toothpicks before serving.

Classic Crab Boil
All out Time
Prep: 10 min. Cook: 30 min.
Makes
2 servings
Nutritional Facts
1 crab: 245 calories, 3g fat (o immersed fats), 169mg cholesterol, 956mg sodium, 2g starch (o sugars, o fiber), 50g protein.
Ingredients

- 2 tablespoons mustard seed
- 2 tablespoons celery seed
- 1 tablespoon dill seed
- 1 tablespoon coriander seeds
- 1 tablespoon entire allspice
- 1/2 teaspoon entire cloves
- 4 cove leaves
- Cheesecloth
- 8 quarts water
- 1/4 cup salt
- 1/4 cup lemon juice
- 1 teaspoon cayenne pepper
- 2 entire live Dungeness crab (2 pounds each)
- Melted margarine and lemon wedges

Directions

1. Place the initial seven fixings on a twofold thickness of cheesecloth. Assemble corners of fabric to encase seasonings; tie safely with string.

2. In an enormous stockpot, bring water, salt, lemon juice, cayenne and flavor sack to a bubble. Utilizing tongs add crab to stockpot; come back to a bubble. Decrease heat; stew, secured, until shells turn splendid red, around 15 minutes.

3. Using tongs, expel crab from the pot. Dash under virus water or

dive into ice water. Present with dissolved margarine and lemon wedges.

Foil-Packet Shrimp and Sausage Jambalaya
All out Time
Prep: 20 min. Heat: 20 min.
Makes
6 servings
1 parcel: 287 calories, 12g fat (4g immersed fat), 143mg cholesterol, 1068mg sodium, 23g starch (3g sugars, 2g fiber), 23g protein.

Ingredients

- 12 ounces completely cooked andouille wiener joins, cut into 1/2-inch cuts
- 12 ounces uncooked shrimp (31-40 for every pound), stripped and deveined
- 1 medium green pepper, slashed
- 1 medium onion, slashed
- 2 celery ribs, slashed
- 3 garlic cloves, minced
- 2 teaspoons Creole flavoring
- 1 can (14-1/2 ounces) fire-simmered diced tomatoes, depleted
- 1 cup uncooked moment rice
- 1 can (8 ounces) tomato sauce
- 1/2 cup chicken juices

Directions

1. Preheat broiler to 425°. In an enormous bowl, join all fixings. Partition blend among 6 lubed 18x12-in. Bits of substantial foil. Crease foil around blend and pleat edges to seal, framing bundles; place on a heating sheet. Prepare until shrimp turn pink and rice is delicate, 20-25 minutes.

Lemony Scallops with Angel Hair Pasta
Complete Time
Prep/Total Time: 25 min.
Makes
4 servings
Nourishment Facts
1-1/2 cups: 404 calories, 13g fat (2g soaked fat), 27mg cholesterol, 737mg sodium, 48g starch (4g sugars, 6g fiber), and 25g protein.

Ingredients

- 8 ounces uncooked multigrain holy messenger hair pasta
- 3 tablespoons olive oil, separated
- 1 pound ocean scallops, tapped dry
- 2 cups cut radishes (around 1 pack)
- 2 garlic cloves, cut
- 1/2 teaspoon squashed red pepper chips
- 6 green onions, daintily cut
- 1/2 teaspoon legitimate salt
- 1 tablespoon ground lemon get-up-and-go
- 1/4 cup lemon juice

Directions

1. In a 6-qt. stockpot, cook pasta as per bundle bearings; channel and come back to the pot.
2. Meanwhile, in a huge skillet, heat 2 tablespoons oil over medium-high warmth; singe scallops in clusters until misty and edges are brilliant darker, around 2 minutes for every side. Expel from skillet; keep warm.
3. In a similar skillet, saute radishes, garlic and pepper chips in residual oil until radishes are delicate, 2-3 minutes. Mix in green onions and salt; cook 1 moment. Add to pasta; hurl to consolidate. Sprinkle with lemon pizzazz and juice. Top with scallops to serve.

Pan-Seared Salmon with Dill Sauce
Complete Time
Prep/Total Time: 25 min.
Makes
4 servings
Nourishment Facts
1 salmon filet with 1/4 cup sauce: 366 calories, 25g fat (4g soaked fat), 92mg cholesterol, 349mg sodium, 4g starch (3g sugars, 0 fibers), 31g protein. Diabetic trades: 4 lean meat, 2-1/2 fat.
Ingredients:

- 1 tablespoon canola oil
- 4 salmon filets (6 ounces each)
- 1 teaspoon Italian flavoring
- 1/4 teaspoon salt
- 1/2 cup decreased fat plain yogurt
- 1/4 cup decreased fat mayonnaise
- 1/4 cup finely hacked cucumber
- 1 teaspoon cut crisp dill

Directions

1. In a huge skillet, heat oil over medium-high warmth. Sprinkle salmon with Italian flavoring and salt. A spot in skillet, skin side down. Lessen warmth to medium. Cook until fish just starts to drop effectively with a fork, around 5 minutes on each side.
2. Meanwhile, in a little bowl, join yogurt, mayonnaise, cucumber, and dill. Present with salmon.

Broiled Tilapia
SmartPoints value: Green plan - 2SP, Blue plan - 0SP, Purple plan - 0SP
Total Time: 13 min, **Prep time**: 8 min, **Cooking time**: 5 min, **Serves**: 4
Nutritional value: Cal - 154.8, Carbs - 1.5g, Fat - 6.4g, Protein - 22.8g
You can apply this recipe with other types of fish, such as sole, halibut, flounder, and even shellfish. You also swap lime juice for lemon juice.

Ingredients

- Black pepper - ¼ tsp, freshly ground
- Cooking spray - 1 spray(s)
- Garlic (herb seasoning) - 2 tsp
- Lemon juice (fresh) - 1 Tbsp
- Table salt - ½ tsp (or to taste)
- Tilapia fillet(s) (uncooked) - 20 oz, four 5 oz fillets

Instructions

1. Prepare your grill by preheating. Coat a skillet with cooking spray.
2. Apply seasoning to both sides of the fish with salt and pepper.
3. Transfer the fish to the prepared skillet and drizzle it with lemon juice, then sprinkle garlic herb seasoning over the top.
4. Broil the fish until it is fork-tender; about 5 minutes.

Grilled Miso-Glazed Cod
SmartPoints value: Green plan - 3SP, Blue plan - 2SP, Purple plan - 2SP
Total Time: 35 min, **Prep time**: 10 min, **Cooking time**: 15 min, **Serves**: 4
Nutritional value: Cal - 227.2, Carbs - 15.0g, Fat - 3.1g, Protein - 30.0g
This marinade produces a fantastic glaze for grilled cod. You can pair it with grilled scallions, drizzled with low-sodium soy sauce, and sesame oil to make a complete meal. If you don't have a fish basket, put foil on one area of your grill to prevent the fish from sticking out below it. Alternatively, you can broil the fish instead. Cod makes a perfect choice for grilling. Flip the fish when it starts to flake and turn opaque. Use a spatula with a broader mouth when turning the fish to help prevent the fish from breaking apart

when turning. It is preferable to serve this dish with roasted carrots or broccoli.

Ingredients

- White miso - 3 Tbsp
- Sugar (dark brown) - 1½ Tbsp
- Sake - 1 Tbsp
- Mirin - ½ fl oz, (1 Tbsp)
- Atlantic cod (uncooked) - 20 oz, (fillets, skin removed
- Cooking spray - 1 spray(s)
- Uncooked scallion(s) (chopped) - 2 Tbsp

Instructions

1. Whisk together miso, sugar, sake, and mirin in a small bowl and spread the mixture over the cod. Cover the cod and refrigerate for at least 2 hours or up to 24 hours.
2. Coat a grill pan off the heat with cooking spray and preheat to medium heat.
3. Remove the cod from marinade (reserve marinade). Place it in a fish grilling basket and grill until the cod is opaque and flakes easily with a fork.
4. Grill each side for about 5 to 7 min (brush the cod with the remaining marinade half-way through the grilling phase to create a thicker glaze). Serve the cod garnished with scallions.

Grilled Tuna with Herb Butter
SmartPoints value: Green plan - 4SP, Blue plan - 3SP, Purple plan - 3SP
Total Time: 18 min, **Prep time**: 12 min, **Cooking time**: 6 min,
Serves: 4
Nutritional value: Calories - 192.0, Carbs - 8.3g, Fat - 2.5g, Protein - 38.3g
You can prepare this grilled tuna recipe in under 20 minutes. Drizzle some olive oil and lime over the tuna before you start cooking it for a unique flavor. You can nicely substitute with a lemon if you don't have a lime. I will recommend that you use salted butter for the sauce instead of unsalted butter to enhance the flavor of the dish. The secret ingredient in this grilled fish recipe is the freshly made herb butter. It also tastes great when drizzled over the spinach.

Ingredients

- Olive oil - 1 tsp
- Lime juice (fresh) - 1 tsp
- Black pepper - ⅛ tsp, or to taste
- Cooking spray - 1 spray(s)

- Salted butter – 2 Tbsp, softened
- Chives (finely chopped) – 1 Tbsp, fresh
- Parsley (fresh) – 1 Tbsp, finely chopped
- Tarragon (fresh) – 1 Tbsp, finely chopped
- Lime zest (fresh, minced) – 1 tsp
- Table salt – ¼ tsp, or to taste
- Spinach (fresh) – 1 pound(s), baby-variety, steamed
- Yellowfin tuna (uncooked) – 1 pound(s), one steak cut 1- to 1-1/2 inches thick

Instructions

1. Drizzle oil and lime juice on both sides of the fish and set it aside.
2. Coat your grill with cooking spray off heat, and preheat the grill on high heat.
3. Combine softened butter, chives, parsley, tarragon, lime zest, salt, and pepper in a small metal bowl and then set aside.
4. Grill the tuna on one side for three minutes, then carefully turn it and cook on the other side for another three minutes or longer until you have achieved the desired degree of cooking.
5. Place the bowl containing butter mixture on the grill just until it melts. Don't let it cook.
6. Slice the tuna thinly and serve it over spinach, then drizzle melted herb butter over the top.

Notes: If you prefer, you can broil the tuna on a grill pan. In this recipe, you will prepare the tuna like a steak. In case you prefer your tuna to be more well done, add about 1 minute to your total cooking time. However, tuna cooks rapidly, so make sure you do not overcook it. The herb butter is excellent on both the tuna and the spinach.

Lemon-Herb Roasted Salmon

SmartPoints value: Green plan - 5SP, Blue plan - 2SP, Purple plan - 2SP

Total Time: 31 min, **Prep time**: 16 min, **Cooking time**: 15 min, **Serves**: 4

Nutritional value: Calories - 118.1, Carbs - 1.0g, Fat - 6.8g, Protein - 12.9g

Give your family a fabulous salmon flavor with lemon juice, lemon zest, and fresh herbs in this easy entrée that will be ready in about 30 minutes. I have used pink salmon fillets because they are less fatty compared to some other salmon varieties like sockeye and Coho salmon.

The salmon should flake when pierced with a fork. That's an excellent indicator that it is ready. Ensure that you zest the lemon before juicing it.

To produce enough zest and juice for this recipe, you will need about two lemons. The mix of fresh herbs in this dish is lovely. However, you can use whatever combination you like; this recipe is versatile. Stir a few red pepper flakes into the herb mixture to add a little heat.

Ingredients

- Black pepper (coarsely ground) - ⅛ tsp (or to taste)
- Cooking spray - 1 spray(s)
- Lemon juice (fresh) - 4 Tbsp, divided
- Lemon zest (finely grated) - 1 tsp (with extra for garnish, if you like)
- Minced garlic - 1 tsp
- Oregano (fresh) - 1 tsp
- Parsley (fresh, chopped) - 1 Tbsp (with extra for garnish, if you like)
- Uncooked wild pink salmon fillet(s) (also known as humpback salmon) - 1½ pound(s), four 6-oz pieces about 1-inch-thick each
- Table salt - ⅛ tsp (or to taste)
- Sugar - 1½ Tbsp
- Thyme (fresh, chopped) - 1 Tbsp (with extra for garnish, if you like)

Instructions

1. Heat your oven to 400°F before using it. Get a small, shallow baking dish and coat it with cooking spray.
2. Apply seasoning to both sides of the salmon with salt and pepper, then place the salmon in the prepared baking dish and drizzle on it with two tablespoons of lemon juice.
3. Whisk the remaining two tablespoons of lemon juice, sugar, parsley, thyme, lemon zest, garlic, and oregano together in a small bowl, then continue whisking until the sugar dissolves in the mixture and set it aside.
4. Roast the salmon until it is close to being ready; about 13 minutes, then remove it from the oven and top it with the lemon-herb mixture.
5. Return it to the oven and allow it to roast until the salmon is fork-tender, about 2 minutes more. Garnish the dish with fresh herbs that you chopped and the grated zest, if you like.

Grilled Tuna Provencal
SmartPoints value: Green plan - 3SP, Blue plan - 2SP, Purple plan - 2SP
Total Time: 20 min, **Prep time**: 10 min, **Cooking time**: 10 min, **Serves**: 4
Nutritional value: Calories - 335, Carbs - 14.6g, Fat - 15.5g, Protein - 36.1g
This one-dish meal is usually ready in just 20 minutes, oozing with a delicious French flavor. You can make the whole meal in one pan, aiding clean up after cooking. To cook with a grill pan and get the best result, you need to preheat the pan for at least five minutes to ensure that you distribute the heat

evenly. That will help you avoid overcooking parts of the meat while not cooking other parts. If you're not sure about the hotness of the grill pan, drop a half teaspoon of water on there to see if it evaporates.

With steamed spinach or a bed of rice, this dish tastes lovely.

Ingredients

- Black pepper (freshly ground, divided) - ¾ tsp
- Cooking spray - 3 spray(s)
- Uncooked tuna (about 1- to 1 1/2-in thick) - 1 pound(s)
- Olive(s) (pitted and chopped)- 6 large
- Olive oil - 1 Tbsp
- Rosemary (fresh, minced) - 1 Tbsp
- Red wine - 2 fl oz
- Sea salt - ¾ tsp, divided
- Tomato(es) (fresh, diced) - 2½ cup(s)
- Garlic clove(s) (minced) - 2 medium clove(s)
- Parsley (fresh, minced) - 2 Tbsp
- Sugar - ⅛ tsp

Instructions

1. Wash the tuna thoroughly and pat it dry. Rub 1/4 teaspoon each of salt and pepper over it, then set it aside.
2. Combine tomatoes, parsley, rosemary, garlic, olives, oil, and the remaining 1/2 teaspoon each of salt and pepper in a separate bowl, then set it aside.
3. Get a reasonably large grill pan and coat it with cooking spray, then set it over medium-high heat. When the pan is visibly hot, cook the tuna for 2 to 3 minutes (or longer) per side for a rare cook (or thorough cook). As soon as you have prepared the tuna, remove it to a serving plate and wrap it with aluminum foil to keep it warm.
4. Add the red wine, tomato mixture, and sugar to the hot grill pan and cook, scraping the bottom of the pan frequently, until the tomato mixture reduces to about two cups. The alcohol must have cooked off.
5. Remove foil from the tuna, slice it thinly, and serve with tomato mixture over the top.

Grilled Cod Fillets with Lemon Dill Butter

SmartPoints value: Green plan - 3SP, Blue plan - 2SP, Purple plan - 2SP

Total Time: 25 min, **Prep time**: 15 min, **Cooking time**: 10 min, **Serves**: 4

Nutritional value: Calories - 318.7g, Carbs - 6.7g, Fat - 13.0g, Protein - 41.7g

Grill the fish on slices of lemon topped with dill to add a delicious flavor to this dish. Become confident at grilling fish. With the layer of lemon slices, you can easily prevent the fish from sticking to the grate. To make use of a stove-top, prepare a grill pan by preheating it over medium-high heat until it is almost smoking, then continue with the recipe. The mixture of lemon, butter, and dill creates a robust sauce that becomes ready in minutes, even though it tastes like you spent hours preparing it. It is preferable to serve this dish with grilled asparagus.

Ingredients

- Olive oil -2 tsp
- Uncooked Atlantic cod - 24 oz, or another firm white fish like tilapia (four 6-oz fillets)
- Table salt - ½ tsp
- Lemon(s) (sliced 1/4-in thick) - 2 medium (you'll need 12 slices total)
- Dill - 2 tsp, chopped
- Dill - 4 sprig(s)
- Light butter - 4 tsp (at room temp.)
- Lemon zest - 1 tsp

Instructions

1. Get your grill ready by preheating to medium-high heat. Continue the heating for at least 10 minutes after it reaches the desired temperature, then scrape the grate clean with a steel brush and coat it lightly with oil.
2. While the grill heats up, pat the fish dry and sprinkle salt on it.
3. Place three lemon slices on the grill carefully, overlapping slightly, and top it with a dill sprig and fish fillet.
4. Repeat the same with the remaining lemon, dill, and fish. Cover the grill and cook without turning for 8-10 minutes until the fish is opaque all the way through and yields easily to a thin-bladed knife.
5. While the cooking is on-going, mix the butter, chopped dill, and zest in a small shallow bowl.
6. Transfer each lemon-dill-fish portion to a plate using two thin-bladed spatulas and top them with 1 1/2 tsp of lemon-dill butter and serve (serving the lemon slices is optional).

Spicy Baked Shrimp
Serving: 4
Prep Time: 10 minutes
Cook Time: 25 minutes + 2-4 hours
Ingredients:

- ½ ounce large shrimp, peeled and deveined
- Cooking spray as needed
- 1 teaspoon low sodium coconut amines
- 1 teaspoon parsley
- ½ teaspoon olive oil
- ½ tablespoon honey
- 1 tablespoon lemon juice

How To:

1. Pre-heat your oven to 450 degrees F.
2. Take a baking dish and grease it well.
3. Mix altogether the ingredients and toss.
4. Transfer to oven and bake for 8 minutes until shrimp turns pink.
5. Serve and enjoy!

Nutrition (Per Serving)
Calories: 321
Fat: 9g
Carbohydrates: 44g
Protein: 22g
Shrimp and Cilantro Meal
Serving: 4
Prep Time: 10 minutes
Cook Time: 5 minutes
Ingredients:

- ¾ pounds shrimp, deveined and peeled
- tablespoons fresh lime juice
- ¼ teaspoon cloves, minced
- ½ teaspoon ground cumin
- 1 tablespoon olive oil
- 1 ¼ cups fresh cilantro, chopped
- 1 teaspoon lime zest
- ½ teaspoon sunflower seeds
- ¼ teaspoon pepper

Direction

1. Take an outsized sized bowl and add shrimp, cumin, garlic, juice , ginger and toss well.
2. Take an outsized sized non-stick skillet and add oil, allow the oil to heat up over medium-high heat.
3. Add shrimp mixture and sauté for 4 minutes.

4. Remove the warmth and add cilantro, lime zest, sunflower seeds, and pepper.
5. Mix well and serve hot!

Nutrition (Per Serving)
Calories: 177
Fat: 6g
Carbohydrates: 2g
Protein: 27g
The Original Dijon Fish
Serving: 2
Prep Time: 3 minutes
Cook Time: 12 minutes
Ingredients:

- 1 perch, flounder or sole fish florets
- 1 tablespoon Dijon mustard
- 1 ½ teaspoons lemon juice
- teaspoon low sodium Worcestershire sauce, low sodium
- tablespoons Italian seasoned bread crumbs
- 1 almond butter flavored cooking spray

How To:

1. Preheat your oven to 450 degrees F.
2. Take an 11 x 7-inch baking dish and arrange your fillets carefully.
3. Take a little sized bowl and add juice, Worcester sauce, mustard and blend it well.
4. Pour the combination over your fillet.
5. Sprinkle an honest amount of breadcrumbs.
6. Bake for 12 minutes until fish flakes off easily.
7. Cut the fillet in half portions and enjoy!

Nutrition (Per Serving)
Calories: 125
Fat: 2g
Carbohydrates: 6g
Protein: 21g
Lemony Garlic Shrimp
Serving: 4
Prep Time: 5-10 minutes
Cook Time: 10-15 minutes
Ingredients:

- 1 ¼ pounds shrimp, boiled or steamed
- tablespoons garlic, minced
- ¼ cup lemon juice
- tablespoons olive oil
- ¼ cup parsley

How To:

1. Take alittle skillet and place over medium heat, add garlic and oil and stir-cook for 1 minute.
2. Add parsley, juice and season with sunflower seeds and pepper accordingly.
3. Add shrimp during a large bowl and transfer the mixture from the skillet over the shrimp.
4. Chill and serve.
5. Enjoy!

Nutrition (Per Serving)
Calories: 130
Fat: 3g
Carbohydrates:2g
Protein:22g

Baked Zucchini Wrapped Fish
Serving: 2
Prep Time: 15 minutes
Cook Time: 15 minutes

Ingredients:

- 24-ounce cod fillets, skin removed
- tablespoon of blackening spices
- zucchini, sliced lengthwise to form ribbon
- ½ tablespoon of olive oil

How To:

1. Season the fish fillets with blackening spice.
2. Wrap each fillet with zucchini ribbons.
3. Place fish on a plate.
4. Take a skillet and place over medium heat.
5. Pour oil and permit the oil to heat up.
6. Add wrapped fish to the skillet and cook all sides for 4 minutes.
7. Serve and enjoy!

Nutrition (Per Serving)

Calories: 397

Fat: 23g

Carbohydrates: 2g

Protein: 46g

Heart-Warming Medi Tilapia

Serving: 4

Prep Time: 15 minutes

Cook Time: 15 minute

Ingredients:

- tablespoons sun-dried tomatoes, packed in oil, drained and chopped
- tablespoon capers, drained
- tilapia fillets
- tablespoon oil from sun-dried tomatoes
- tablespoons kalamata olives, chopped and pitted

How To:

1. Pre-heat your oven to 372 degrees F.
2. Take alittle sized bowl and add sun-dried tomatoes, olives, capers and stir well.
3. Keep the mixture on the side.
4. Take a baking sheet and transfer the tilapia fillets and arrange them side by side.
5. Drizzle vegetable oil everywhere them.
6. Bake in your oven for 10-15 minutes.
7. After 10 minutes, check the fish for a "Flaky" texture.
8. Once cooked, top the fish with the tomato mixture and serve!

Nutrition (Per Serving)

Calories: 183

Fat: 8g

Carbohydrates: 18g

Protein:83g

Baked Salmon and Orange Juice

Serving: 2

Prep Time: 10 minutes

Cook Time: 10 minutes

Ingredients:

- ½ pound salmon steak
- Juice of 1 orange
- Pinch ginger powder, black pepper, and sunflower seeds

- Juice of ½ lemon
- 1-ounce coconut almond milk

How To:

1. Preheat oven to 350 degrees F.
2. Rub salmon steak with spices and let it sit for quarter-hour .
3. Take a bowl and squeeze an orange.
4. Squeeze juice also and blend .
5. Pour almond milk into the mixture and stir.
6. Take a baking dish and line with aluminium foil .
7. Place steak thereon and pour the sauce over steak.
8. Cover with another sheet and bake for 10 minutes.
9. Serve and enjoy!

Nutrition (Per Serving)
Calories: 300
Fat: 3g
Carbohydrates: 1g
Protein: 7g
Lemon and Almond butter Cod
Serving: 2
Prep Time: 5 minutes
Cook Time: 20 minutes
Ingredients:

- tablespoons almond butter, divided
- thyme sprigs, fresh and divided
- teaspoons lemon juice, fresh and divided
- cod fillets, 6 ounces each Sunflower seeds to taste

How To:

1. Pre-heat your oven to 400 degrees F.
2. Season cod fillets with sunflower seeds on each side .
3. Take four pieces of foil, each foil should be 3 times bigger than the fillets.
4. Divide fillets between the foil and top with almond butter, juice , thyme.
5. Fold to make a pouch and transfer pouches to the baking sheet.
6. Bake for 20 minutes.
7. Open and let the steam out.
8. Serve and enjoy!

Nutrition (Per Serving)
Calories: 284
Fat: 18g
Carbohydrates: 2g
Protein: 32g
Shrimp Scampi
Serving: 4
Prep Time: 25 minutes
Cook Time: Nil
Ingredients:

- teaspoons olive oil
- 1 ¼ pounds medium shrimp
- 6-8 garlic cloves, minced
- ½ cup low sodium chicken broth
- ½ cup dry white wine
- ¼ cup fresh lemon juice
- ¼ cup fresh parsley + 1 tablespoon extra, minced
- ¼ teaspoon sunflower seeds
- ¼ teaspoon fresh ground pepper
- slices lemon

How To:

1. Take an outsized sized bowl and place it over medium-high heat.
2. Add oil and permit the oil to heat up.
3. Add shrimp and cook for 2-3 minutes.
4. Add garlic and cook for 30 seconds.
5. Take a slotted spoon and transfer the cooked shrimp to a serving platter.
6. Add broth, juice , wine, ¼ cup of parsley, pepper, and sunflower seeds to the skillet.
7. Bring the entire mix to a boil.
8. Keep boiling until the sauce has been reduced to half.
9. Spoon the sauce over the cooked shrimp.
10. Garnish with parsley and lemon.
11. Serve and enjoy!

Nutrition (Per Serving)
Calories: 184
Fat: 6g
Carbohydrates: 6g
Protein: 15g
Lemon and Garlic Scallops

Serving: 4
Prep Time: 10 minutes
Cook Time: 5 minutes
Ingredients:

- 1 tablespoon olive oil
- ¼ pounds dried scallops
- tablespoons all-purpose flour
- ¼ teaspoon sunflower seeds
- 4-5 garlic cloves, minced
- 1 scallion, chopped
- 1 pinch of ground sage
- lemon juice
- tablespoons parsley, chopped

Direction

1. Take a non-stick skillet and place over medium-high heat.
2. Add oil and permit the oil to heat up.
3. Take a medium sized bowl and add scallops alongside sunflower seeds and flour.
4. Place the scallops within the skillet and add scallions, garlic, and sage.
5. Sauté for 3-4 minutes until they show an opaque texture.
6. Stir in juice and parsley.
7. Remove heat and serve hot!

Nutrition (Per Serving)
Calories: 151
Fat: 4g
Carbohydrates: 10g
Protein: 18g
Walnut Encrusted Salmon
Serving: 34
Prep Time: 10 minutes
Cook Time: 14 minutes
Ingredients:

- ½ cup walnuts
- tablespoons stevia
- ½ tablespoon Dijon mustard
- ¼ teaspoon dill
- salmon fillets (3 ounces each)
- 1 tablespoon olive oil

- Sunflower seeds and pepper to taste

How To:

1. Pre-heat your oven to 350 degrees F.
2. Add walnuts, mustard, stevia to kitchen appliance and process until your required consistency is achieved.
3. Take a frypan and place it over medium heat.
4. Add oil and let it heat up.
5. Add salmon and sear for 3 minutes.
6. Add walnut mix and coat well.
7. Transfer coated salmon to baking sheet, bake in oven for 8 minutes.
8. Serve and enjoy!

Nutrition (Per Serving)
Calories: 373
Fat: 43g
Carbohydrates: 4g
Protein: 20g

Roasted Lemon Swordfish
Serving: 4
Prep Time: 10 minutes
Cook Time: 70-80 minutes
Ingredients:

- ¼ cup parsley, chopped
- ½ teaspoon garlic, chopped
- ½ teaspoon canola oil
- swordfish fillets, 6 ounces each
- ¼ teaspoon sunflower seeds
- tablespoon sugar
- lemons, quartered and seeds removed

How To:

1. Preheat your oven to 375 degrees F.
2. Take a small-sized bowl and add sugar, sunflower seeds, lemon wedges.
3. Toss well to coat them.
4. Take a shallow baking dish and add lemons, cover with aluminum foil .
5. Roast for about hour until lemons are tender and browned (Slightly).

6. Heat your grill and place the rack about 4 inches far away from the source of warmth .
7. Take a baking pan and coat it with cooking spray.
8. Transfer fish fillets to the pan and brush with oil on top spread garlic on top.
9. Grill for about 5 minutes all sides until fillet turns opaque.
10. Transfer fish to a serving platter, squeeze roasted lemon on top.
11. Sprinkle parsley, serve with a lemon wedge on the side.
12. Enjoy!

Nutrition (Per Serving)
Calories: 280
Fat: 12g
Net Carbohydrates: 4g
Protein: 34g
Especial Glazed Salmon
Serving: 4
Prep Time: 45 minutes
Cook Time: 10 minutes
Ingredients:

- Pieces of salmon fillets, 5 ounces each
- tablespoons coconut aminos
- Teaspoon olive oil
- 2 teaspoons ginger, minced
- teaspoons garlic, minced
- 2 tablespoons sugar-free ketchup
- tablespoons dry white wine
- 2 tablespoons red boat fish sauce, low sodium

How To:

1. Take a bowl and blend in coconut aminos, garlic, ginger, fish sauce and blend .
2. Add salmon and let it marinate for 15-20 minutes.
3. Take a skillet/pan and place it over medium heat.
4. Add oil and let it heat up.
5. Add salmon fillets and cook on high heat for 3-4 minutes per side.
6. Remove dish once crispy.
7. Add sauce and wine.
8. Simmer for five minutes on low heat.
9. Return salmon to the glaze and flip until each side are glazed.
10. Serve and enjoy!

Nutrition (Per Serving)
Calories: 372
Fat: 24g
Carbohydrates: 3g
Protein: 35g
Generous Stuffed Salmon Avocado
Serving: 2
Prep Time: 10 minutes
Cook Time: 30 minutes
Ingredients:

- ripe organic avocado
- ounces wild caught smoked salmon
- ounce cashew cheese
- tablespoons extra virgin olive oil
- Sunflower seeds as needed

How To:

1. Cut avocado in half and deseed.
2. Add the rest of the ingredients to a food processor and process until coarsely chopped.
3. Place mixture into avocado.
4. Serve and enjoy!

Nutrition (Per Serving)
Calories: 525
Fat: 48g
Carbohydrates: 4g
Protein: 19g
Spanish Mussels
Serving: 4
Prep Time: 10 minutes
Cook Time: 23 minutes
Ingredients:

- tablespoons olive oil
- pounds mussels, scrubbed
- Pepper to taste
- cups canned tomatoes, crushed
- shallot, chopped
- garlic cloves, minced
- cups low sodium vegetable stock
- 1/3 cup cilantro, chopped

How To:

1. Take a pan and place it over medium-high heat, add shallot and stir-cook for 3 minutes.
2. Add garlic, stock, tomatoes, pepper, stir and reduce heat, simmer for 10 minutes.
3. Add mussels, cilantro, and toss.
4. Cover and cook for 10 minutes more.
5. Serve and enjoy!

Nutrition (Per Serving)
Calories: 210
Fat: 2g
Carbohydrates: 5g
Protein: 8g
Tilapia Broccoli Platter
Serving: 2
Prep Time: 4 minutes
Cook Time: 14 minutes
Ingredients:

- Ounce tilapia, frozen
- 1 tablespoon almond butter
- 1 tablespoon garlic, minced
- 1 teaspoon lemon pepper seasoning
- 1 cup broccoli florets, fresh

How To:

1. Pre-heat your oven to 350 degrees F.
2. Add fish in aluminum foil packets.
3. Arrange broccoli around fish.
4. Sprinkle lemon pepper on top.
5. Close the packets and seal.
6. Bake for 14 minutes.
7. Take a bowl and add garlic and almond butter, mix well and keep the mixture on the side.
8. Remove the packet from oven and transfer to platter.
9. Place almond butter on top of the fish and broccoli, serve and enjoy!

Nutrition (Per Serving)
Calories: 362
Fat: 25g

Carbohydrates: 2g
Protein: 29g
Salmon with Peas and Parsley Dressing
Serving: 4
Prep Time: 15 minutes
Cook Time: 15 minutes
Ingredients:

- 16 ounces salmon fillets, boneless and skin-on
- 1 tablespoon parsley, chopped
- 10 ounces peas
- 9 ounces vegetable stock, low sodium
- 2 cups water
- ½ teaspoon oregano, dried
- ½ teaspoon sweet paprika
- 2 garlic cloves, minced
- A pinch of black pepper

How To:

1. Add garlic, parsley, paprika, oregano and stock to a kitchen appliance and blend.
2. Add water to your Instant Pot.
3. Add steam basket.
4. Add fish fillets inside the steamer basket.
5. Season with pepper.
6. Lock the lid and cook on high for 10 minutes.
7. Release the pressure naturally over 10 minutes .
8. Divide the fish amongst plates.
9. Add peas to the steamer basket and lock the lid again, cook on high for five minutes.
10. Quick release the pressure.
11. Divide the peas next to your fillets and serve with the parsley dressing drizzled
12. on top
13. Enjoy!

Nutrition (Per Serving)
Calories: 315
Fat: 5g
Carbohydrates: 14g
Protein: 16g
Mackerel and Orange Medley
Serving: 4

Prep Time: 10 minutes
Cook Time: 10 minutes
Ingredients:

- mackerel fillets, skinless and boneless
- spring onion, chopped
- 1 teaspoon olive oil
- 1-inch ginger piece, grated
- Black pepper as needed
- Juice and zest of 1 whole orange
- 1 cup low sodium fish stock

How To:

1. Season the fillets with black pepper and rub vegetable oil .
2. Add stock, fruit juice , ginger, orange peel and onion to Instant Pot.
3. Place a steamer basket and add the fillets.
4. Lock the lid and cook on high for 10 minutes.
5. Release the pressure naturally over 10 minutes.
6. Divide the fillets amongst plates and drizzle the orange sauce from the pot over the fish.
7. Enjoy!

Nutrition (Per Serving)
Calories: 200
Fat: 4g
Carbohydrates: 19g
Protein: 14g
Spicy Chili Salmon
Serving: 4
Prep Time: 10 minutes
Cook Time: 7 minutes
Ingredients:

- salmon fillets, boneless and skin-on
- 2 tablespoons assorted chili peppers, chopped
- Juice of 1 lemon
- 1 lemon, sliced
- 1 cup water
- Black pepper

How To:

1. Add water to the moment Pot.

2. Add steamer basket and add salmon fillets, season the fillets with salt and pepper.
3. Drizzle juice on top.
4. Top with lemon slices.
5. Lock the lid and cook on high for 7 minutes.
6. Release the pressure naturally over 10 minutes.
7. Divide the salmon and lemon slices between serving plates.
8. Enjoy!

Nutrition (Per Serving)
Calories: 281
Fats: 8g
Carbs: 19g
Protein:7g

Simple One Pot Mussels
Serving: 4
Prep Time: 10 minutes
Cook Time: 5 minutes

Ingredients:

- 2 tablespoons butter
- 2 chopped shallots
- minced garlic cloves
- ½ cup broth
- ½ cup white wine
- 2 pounds cleaned mussels
- Lemon and parsley for serving

How To:

1. Clean the mussels and take away the beard.
2. Discard any mussels that don't close when tapped against a tough surface.
3. Set your pot to Sauté mode and add chopped onion and butter.
4. Stir and sauté onions.
5. Add garlic and cook for 1 minute.
6. Add broth and wine.
7. Lock the lid and cook for five minutes on high .
8. Release the pressure naturally over 10 minutes.
9. Serve with a sprinkle of parsley and enjoy!

Nutrition (Per Serving)
Calories: 286
Fats: 14g

Carbs: 12g
Protein: 28g

Lemon Pepper and Salmon

Serving: 3
Prep Time: 5 minute
Cook Time: 6 minutes

Ingredients:

- ¾ cup water
- Few sprigs of parsley, basil, tarragon, basil
- 1 pound of salmon, skin on
- teaspoons ghee
- ¼ teaspoon salt
- ½ teaspoon pepper
- ½ lemon, thinly sliced
- 1 whole carrot, julienned

How To:

1. Set your pot to Sauté mode and water and herbs.
2. Place a steamer rack inside your pot and place salmon.
3. Drizzle the ghee on top of the salmon and season with salt and pepper.
4. Cover lemon slices.
5. Lock the lid and cook on high for 3 minutes.
6. Release the pressure naturally over 10 minutes.
7. Transfer the salmon to a serving platter.
8. Set your pot to Sauté mode and add vegetables.
9. Cook for 1-2 minutes.
10. Serve with vegetables and salmon.
11. Enjoy!

Nutrition (Per Serving)

Calories: 464
Fat: 34g
Carbohydrates: 3g
Protein: 34g

Simple Sautéed Garlic and Parsley Scallops

Serving: 4
Prep Time: 5 minutes
Cook Time: 25 minutes

Ingredients:

- 8 tablespoons almond butter

- 2 garlic cloves, minced
- 16 large sea scallops
- Sunflower seeds and pepper to taste
- 1 ½ tablespoons olive oil

How To:

1. Seasons scallops with sunflower seeds and pepper.
2. Take a skillet, place it over medium heat, add oil and let it heat up.
3. Sauté scallops for two minutes per side, repeat until all scallops are cooked.
4. Add almond butter to the skillet and let it melt.
5. Stir in garlic and cook for quarter-hour .
6. Return scallops to skillet and stir to coat.
7. Serve and enjoy!

Nutrition (Per Serving)
Calories: 417
Fat: 31g
Net Carbohydrates: 5g
Protein: 29g
Salmon and Cucumber Platter
Serving: 4
Prep Time: 10 minutes
Cook Time: nil
Ingredients:

- 2 cucumbers, cubed
- 2 teaspoons fresh squeezed lemon juice
- ounces non-fat yogurt
- teaspoon lemon zest, grated
- Pepper to taste
- teaspoons dill, chopped
- 8 ounces smoked salmon, flaked

How To:

1. Take a bowl and add cucumbers, juice , lemon peel , pepper, dill, salmon, yogurt and toss well.
2. Serve cold.
3. Enjoy!

Nutrition (Per Serving)
Calories: 242

Fat: 3g
Carbohydrates: 3g
Protein: 3g

Tuna Paté

Serving: 4
Prep Time: 10 minutes
Cook Time: nil

Ingredients:

- ounces canned tuna, drained and flaked
- teaspoons fresh lemon juice
- 1 teaspoon onion, minced
- ounces low-fat cream cheese
- ¼ cup parsley, chopped

How To:

1. Take a bowl and blend in tuna, cheese , juice , parsley, onion and stir well.
2. Serve cold and enjoy!

Nutrition (Per Serving)

Calories: 172
Fat: 2g
Carbohydrates: 8g
Protein: 4g

Cinnamon Salmon

Serving: 4
Prep Time: 10 minutes
Cook Time: 10 minutes

Ingredients:

- 2 salmon fillets, boneless and skin on
- Pepper to taste
- 1 tablespoon cinnamon powder
- 1 tablespoon organic olive oil

How To:

1. Take a pan and place it over medium heat, add oil and let it heat up.
2. Add pepper, cinnamon and stir.
3. Add salmon, skin side up and cook for five minutes on each side .
4. Divide between plates and serve.
5. Enjoy!

Nutrition (Per Serving)
Calories: 220
Fat: 8g
Carbohydrates: 11g
Protein: 8g
Scallop and Strawberry Mix
Serving: 4
Prep Time: 10 minutes
Cook Time: 6 minutes
Ingredients:

- ounces scallops
- ½ cup Pico De Gallo
- ½ cup strawberries, chopped
- 1 tablespoon lime juice
- Pepper to taste

How To:

1. Take a pan and place it over medium heat, add scallops and cook for 3 minutes on each side .
2. Remove heat.
3. Take a bowl and add strawberries, juice , Pico De Gallo, scallops, pepper and toss well.
4. Serve and enjoy!

Nutrition (Per Serving)
Calories: 169
Fat: 2g
Carbohydrates: 8g
Protein: 13g
Salmon and Orange Dish
Serving: 4
Prep Time: 10 minute
Cook Time: 15 minutes
Ingredients:

- salmon fillets
- cup orange juice
- tablespoons arrowroot and water mixture
- 1 teaspoon orange peel, grated
- 1 teaspoon black pepper

How To:

1. Add the listed ingredients to your pot.
2. Lock the lid and cook on high for 12 minutes.
3. Release the pressure naturally.
4. Serve and enjoy!

Nutrition (Per Serving)
Calories:583
Fat: 20g
Carbohydrates: 71g
Protein: 33g
Mesmerizing Coconut Haddock
Serving: 3
Prep Time: 10 minutes
Cook Time: 12 minutes
Ingredients:

- Haddock fillets, 5 ounces each, boneless
- 2 tablespoons coconut oil, melted
- 1 cup coconut, shredded and unsweetened
- ¼ cup hazelnuts, ground Sunflower seeds to taste

How To:

1. Pre-heat your oven to 400 degrees F.
2. Line a baking sheet with parchment paper.
3. Keep it on the side.
4. Pat fish fillets with towel and season with sunflower seeds.
5. Take a bowl and stir in hazelnuts and shredded coconut.
6. Drag fish fillets through the coconut mix until each side are coated well.
7. Transfer to baking dish.
8. Brush with copra oil .
9. Bake for about 12 minutes until flaky.
10. Serve and enjoy!

Nutrition (Per Serving)
Calories: 299
Fat: 24g
Carbohydrates: 1g
Protein: 20g
Asparagus and Lemon Salmon Dish
Serving: 3
Prep Time: 5 minutes
Cook Time: 15 minutes

Ingredients:

- 2 salmon fillets, 6 ounces each, skin on
- Sunflower seeds to taste
- 1-pound asparagus, trimmed 2 cloves garlic, minced
- tablespoons almond butter
- ¼ cup cashew cheese

How To:
Pre-heat your oven to 400 degrees F.
Line a baking sheet with oil.
Take a kitchen towel and pat your salmon dry, season as needed.

1. Put salmon onto the baking sheet and arrange asparagus around it.
2. Place a pan over medium heat and melt almond butter.
3. Add garlic and cook for 3 minutes until garlic browns slightly.
4. Drizzle sauce over salmon.
5. Sprinkle salmon with cheese and bake for 12 minutes until salmon looks cooked all the way and is flaky.
6. Serve and enjoy!

Nutrition (Per Serving)
Calories: 434
Fat: 26g
Carbohydrates: 6g
Protein: 42g
Ecstatic "Foiled" Fish
Serving: 4
Prep Time: 20 minutes
Cook Time: 40 minutes
Ingredients:

- 2 rainbow trout fillets
- tablespoon olive oil
- teaspoon garlic salt
- 1 teaspoon ground black pepper
- 1 fresh jalapeno pepper, sliced
- 1 lemon, sliced

How To:

1. Pre-heat your oven to 400 degrees F.
2. Rinse your fish and pat them dry.

3. Rub the fillets with olive oil, season with some garlic salt and black pepper.
4. Place each of your seasoned fillets on a large sized sheet of aluminum foil.
5. Top it with some jalapeno slices and squeeze the juice from your lemons over your fish.
6. Arrange the lemon slices on top of your fillets.
7. Carefully seal up the edges of your foil and form a nice enclosed packet.
8. Place your packets on your baking sheet.
9. Bake them for about 20 minutes.
10. Once the flakes start to flake off with a fork, the fish is ready!

Nutrition (Per Serving)
Calories: 213
Fat: 10g
Carbohydrates: 8g
Protein: 24g
Brazilian Shrimp Stew
Serving: 4
Prep Time: 20 minutes
Cook Time: 25 minutes
Ingredients:

- Tablespoons lime juice
- 1 ½ tablespoons cumin, ground
- ½ tablespoons paprika
- ½ teaspoons garlic, minced
- ½ teaspoons pepper
- Pounds tilapia fillets, cut into bits
- 1 large onion, chopped
- Large bell peppers, cut into strips
- 1 can (14 ounces) tomato, drained
- 1 can (14 ounces) coconut milk handful of cilantros, chopped

How To:

1. Take a large sized bowl and add lime juice, cumin, paprika, garlic, pepper and mix well.
2. Add tilapia and coat it up.
3. Cover and allow to marinate for 20 minutes.
4. Set your Instant Pot to Sauté mode and add olive oil.
5. Add onions and cook for 3 minutes until tender.
6. Add pepper strips, tilapia, and tomatoes to a skillet.

7. Pour coconut milk and cover, simmer for 20 minutes.
8. Add cilantro during the final few minutes.
9. Serve and enjoy!

Nutrition (Per Serving)
Calories: 471
Fat: 44g
Carbohydrates: 13g
Protein: 12g
Inspiring Cajun Snow Crab
Serving: 2
Prep Time: 10 minutes
Cook Time: 10 minutes
Ingredients:

- 1 lemon, fresh and quartered tablespoons
- Cajun seasoning
- Bay leaves
- Snow crab legs, precooked and defrosted Golden ghee

How To:

1. Take a large pot and fill it about halfway with sunflower seeds and water.
2. Bring the water to a boil.
3. Squeeze lemon juice into the pot and toss in remaining lemon quarters.
4. Add bay leaves and Cajun seasoning.
5. Season for 1 minute.
6. Add crab legs and boil for 8 minutes (make sure to keep them submerged the whole time).
7. Melt ghee in microwave and use as dipping sauce, enjoy!

Nutrition (Per Serving)
Calories: 643
Fat: 51g
Carbohydrates: 3g
Protein: 41g
Grilled Lime Shrimp
Serving: 8
Prep Time: 25 minutes
Cook Time: 5 minutes
Ingredients:

- 1-pound medium shrimp, peeled and deveined
- 1 lime, juiced
- ½ cup olive oil
- Cajun seasoning

How To:

1. Take a re-sealable zip bag and add lime juice, Cajun seasoning, olive oil.
2. Add shrimp and shake it well, let it marinate for 20 minutes.
3. Pre-heat your outdoor grill to medium heat.
4. Lightly grease the grate.
5. Remove shrimp from marinade and cook for 2 minutes per side.
6. Serve and enjoy!

Nutrition (Per Serving)
Calories: 188
Fat: 3g
Net Carbohydrates: 1.2g
Protein: 13g
Calamari Citrus
Serving: 4
Prep Time: 10 minutes
Cook Time: 5 minutes
Ingredients:

- 1 lime, sliced
- lemon, sliced
- Pounds calamari tubes and tentacles, sliced
- Pepper to taste
- ¼ cup olive oil
- garlic cloves, minced
- tablespoons lemon juice
- orange, peeled and cut into segments
- tablespoons cilantro, chopped

How To:

1. Take a bowl and add calamari, pepper, lime slices, lemon slices, orange slices, garlic, oil, cilantro, lemon juice and toss well.
2. Take a pan and place it over medium-high heat.
3. Add calamari mix and cook for 5 minutes.
4. Divide into bowls and serve.
5. Enjoy!

Nutrition (Per Serving)
Calories: 190
Fat: 2g
Net Carbohydrates: 11g
Protein: 14g
Spiced Up Salmon
Serving: 4
Prep Time: 10 minutes
Cook Time: 10 minutes
Ingredients:

- Salmon fillets
- 2 tablespoons olive oil
- 1 teaspoon cumin, ground
- 1 teaspoon sweet paprika
- 1 teaspoon chili powder
- ½ teaspoon garlic powder
- Pinch of pepper

How To:

1. Take a bowl and add cumin, paprika, onion, chili powder, garlic powder, pepper and toss well.
2. Rub the salmon in the mixture.
3. Take a pan and place it over medium heat, add oil and let it heat up.
4. Add salmon and cook for 5 minutes, both sides.
5. Divide between plates and serve.
6. Enjoy!

Nutrition (Per Serving)
Calories: 220
Fat: 10g
Net Carbohydrates: 8g
Protein: 10g
Coconut Cream Shrimp
Serving: 4
Prep Time: 10 minutes
Cook Time: nil
Ingredients:

- 1 pound shrimp, cooked , peeled and deveined
- 1 tablespoon coconut cream
- ¼ teaspoon jalapeno, chopped ½ teaspoon lime juice
- 1 tablespoon parsley, chopped Pinch of pepper

How To:

1. Take a bowl and add shrimp, cream, jalapeno, lime juice, parsley, pepper.
2. Toss well and divide into small bowls.
3. Serve and enjoy!

Nutrition (Per Serving)
Calories: 183
Fat: 5g
Net Carbohydrates: 12g
Protein: 8g
Shrimp and Avocado Platter
Serving: 8
Prep Time: 10 minutes
Cook Time: nil
Ingredients:

- 2 green onions, chopped
- 2 avocados, pitted, peeled and cut into chunks
- 2 tablespoons cilantro, chopped
- 1 cup shrimp, cooked, peeled and deveined Pinch of pepper

How To:

1. Take a bowl and add cooked shrimp, avocado, green onions, cilantro, pepper.
2. Toss well and serve.
3. Enjoy!

Nutrition (Per Serving)
Calories: 160
Fat: 2g
Net Carbohydrates: 5g
Protein: 6g
Calamari
Serving: 4
Prep Time: 10 minutes +1-hour marinating
Cook Time: 8 minutes
Ingredients:

- 2 tablespoons extra virgin olive oil
- 1 teaspoon chili powder
- ½ teaspoon ground cumin

- Zest of 1 lime
- Juice of 1 lime
- Dash of sea sunflower seeds
- ½ pounds squid, cleaned and split open, with tentacles cut into ½ inch rounds
- tablespoons cilantro, chopped
- tablespoons red bell pepper, minced

How To:

1. Take a medium bowl and stir in olive oil, chili powder, cumin, lime zest, sea sunflower seeds, lime juice and pepper.
2. Add squid and let it marinade and stir to coat, coat and let it refrigerate for 1 hour
3. Pre-heat your oven to broil.
4. Arrange squid on a baking sheet, broil for 8 minutes turn once until tender.
5. Garnish the broiled calamari with cilantro and red bell pepper.
6. Serve and enjoy!

Nutrition (Per Serving)
Calories: 159
Fat: 13g
Carbohydrates: 12g
Protein: 3g
Hearty Deep-Fried Prawn and Rice Croquettes
Serving: 8
Prep Time: 25 minute
Cook Time: 13 minutes
Ingredients:

- 2 tablespoons almond butter
- ½ onion, chopped
- ounces shrimp, peeled and chopped
- 2 tablespoons all-purpose flour
- tablespoon white wine
- ½ cup almond milk
- tablespoons almond milk
- cups cooked rice
- 1 tablespoon parmesan, grated
- 1 teaspoon fresh dill, chopped
- 1 teaspoon sunflower seeds
- Ground pepper as needed
- Vegetable oil for frying

- tablespoons all-purpose flour
- 1 whole egg
- ½ cup breadcrumbs

How To:

1. Take a large skillet and place it over medium heat, add almond butter and let it melt.
2. Add onion, cook and stir for 5 minutes.
3. Add shrimp and cook for 1-2 minutes.
4. Stir in 2 tablespoons flour, white wine, pour in almond milk gradually and cook for 3-5 minutes until the sauce thickens.
5. Remove white sauce from heat and stir in rice, mix evenly.
6. Add parmesan, cheese, dill, sunflower seeds, pepper and let it cool for 15 minutes.
7. Heat oil in large saucepan and bring it to 350 degrees F.
8. Take a bowl and whisk in egg, spread breadcrumbs on a plate.
9. Form rice mixture into 8 balls and roll 1 ball in flour, dip in egg and coat with crumbs, repeat with all balls.
10. Deep fry balls for 3 minutes.
11. Enjoy!

Nutrition (Per Serving)
Calories: 182
Fat: 7g
Carbohydrates: 21g
Protein: 7g
Easy Garlic Almond butter Shrimp
Serving: 4
Prep Time: 15 minutes
Cook Time: 30 minutes
Ingredients:

- pounds shrimp
- 1-2 tablespoons garlic, minced
- ½ cup almond butter
- 1 tablespoon lemon pepper seasoning
- ½ teaspoon garlic powder

How To:

1. Pre-heat your oven to 300 degrees F.
2. Take a bowl and mix in garlic and almond butter.
3. Place shrimp in a pan and dot with almond butter garlic mix.

4. Sprinkle garlic powder and lemon pepper.
5. Bake for 30 minutes.
6. Enjoy!

Nutrition (Per Serving)
Calories: 749
Fat: 30g
Net Carbohydrates: 7g
Protein: 74g
Blackened Tilapia
Serving: 2
Prep Time: 9 minutes
Cook Time: 9 minutes
Ingredients:

- 1 cup cauliflower, chopped
- 1 teaspoon red pepper flakes
- 1 tablespoon Italian seasoning
- 1 tablespoon garlic, minced
- ounces tilapia
- cup English cucumber, chopped with peel
- tablespoons olive oil
- 1 sprig dill, chopped
- 1 teaspoon stevia
- tablespoons lime juice
- 2 tablespoons Cajun blackened seasoning

How To:

1. Take a bowl and add the seasoning ingredients (except Cajun).
2. Add a tablespoon of oil and whip.
3. Pour dressing over cauliflower and cucumber.
4. Brush the fish with olive oil on both sides.
5. Take a skillet and grease it well with 1 tablespoon of olive oil.
6. Press Cajun seasoning on both sides of fish.
7. Cook fish for 3 minutes per side.
8. Serve with vegetables and enjoy!

Nutrition (Per Serving)
Calories: 530
Fat: 33g
Net Carbohydrates: 4g
Protein: 32g
Light Lobster Bisque

Serving: 4
Prep Time: 10 minutes 400
Cook Time: 6 minutes

Ingredients:

- 1 cup diced carrots
- 1 cup diced celery
- 29 ounces diced tomatoes
- 2 minced whole shallots 1 clove of minced garlic
- 1 tablespoon butter
- 32-ounce chicken broth, low-sodium
- 1 teaspoon dill, dried
- 1 teaspoon freshly ground black pepper
- ½ teaspoon paprika
- lobster tails
- 1-pint heavy whipping cream

How To:

1. Add butter, garlic and minced shallots to a microwave safe bowl.
2. Microwave for 2-3 minutes on HIGH.
3. Add tomatoes, celery, carrot, minced shallots, garlic to your Instant Pot.
4. Add chicken broth and spices to the Pot.
5. Use a knife to cut the lobster tails if you prefer and add them to the Instant Pot.
6. Lock the lid and cook on HIGH pressure for 4 minutes.
7. Release the pressure naturally over 10 minutes.
8. Use an immersion blender to puree to your desired chunkiness.
9. Serve and enjoy!

Nutrition (Per Serving)
Calories: 437
Fats: 17g
Carbs: 21g
Protein: 38g

Herbal Shrimp Risotto
Serving: 4
Prep Time: 10 minutes
Cook Time: 8 minutes

Ingredients:

- 2 pounds shrimp with their tails removed
- cup instant rice

- cups vegetable broth
- 1 chopped up onion
- 1 cup chicken breast cut into fine strips
- ¼ cup lemon juice
- 1 teaspoon crushed red pepper
- ¼ cup parsley
- ¼ cup fresh dill
- pieces chopped up garlic cloves
- 1 tablespoon black pepper
- ½ cup parmesan
- 1 cup mozzarella cheese

How To:

1. Add the listed ingredients to your Instant Pot and stir.
2. Lock the lid and cook on HIGH pressure for 8 minutes.
3. Release the pressure naturally over 10 minutes.
4. Open lid and top with cheese.
5. Serve hot and enjoy!

Nutrition (Per Serving)
Calories: 463
Fat: 8g
Carbohydrates: 63g
Protein: 29g
Thai Pumpkin Seafood Stew
Serving: 4
Prep Time: 5 minutes
Cook Time: 35 minutes
Ingredients:

- 1 ½ tablespoons fresh galangal, chopped
- 1 teaspoon lime zest
- 1 small kabocha squash
- 32 medium sized mussels, fresh
- 1 pound shrimp
- 16 thai leaves
- 1 can coconut milk
- 1 tablespoon lemongrass, minced
- garlic cloves, roughly chopped
- 32 medium clams, fresh
- ½ pounds fresh salmon
- tablespoons coconut oil
- Pepper to taste

How To:

1. Add coconut milk, lemongrass, galangal, garlic, lime leaves in a small-sized saucepan, bring to a boil.
2. Let it simmer for 25 minutes.
3. Strain mixture through a fine sieve into the large soup pot and bring to a simmer.
4. Add oil to a pan and heat up, add Kabocha squash.
5. Season with salt and pepper, sauté for 5 minutes.
6. Add mix to coconut mix.
7. Heat oil in a pan and add fish shrimp, season with salt and pepper, cook for 4 minutes.
8. Add mixture to coconut milk, mix alongside clams and mussels.
9. Simmer for 8 minutes, garnish with basil and enjoy!

Nutrition (Per Serving)
Calories: 370
Fat: 16g
Net Carbohydrates: 10g
Protein: 16g
Pistachio Sole Fish
Serving: 4
Prep Time: 5 minutes
Cook Time: 10 minutes
Ingredients:

- (5 ounces) boneless sole fillets
- Sunflower seeds and pepper as needed
- ½ cup pistachios, finely chopped
- Juice of 1 lemon
- 1 teaspoon extra virgin olive oil

How To:

1. Pre-heat your oven to 350 degrees F.
2. Line a baking sheet with parchment paper and keep it on the side.
3. Pat fish dry with kitchen towels and lightly season with sunflower seeds and pepper.
4. Take a small bowl and stir in pistachios.
5. Place sole on the prepared baking sheet and press 2 tablespoons of pistachio mixture on top of each fillet.
6. Drizzle fish with lemon juice and olive oil.
7. Bake for 10 minutes until the top is golden and fish flakes with a fork.

8. Serve and enjoy!

Nutrition (Per Serving)
Calories: 166
Fat: 6g
Carbohydrates: 2g
Protein: 26g
Panko-Crusted Cod
Prep time: 10 minutes
Cook time: 15 minutes
Servings: 2
Ingredients

- Panko-style breadcrumbs – ¼ cup
- Garlic - 1 clove, minced Extra-virgin olive oil – 1 Tbsp.
- Nonfat Greek yogurt – 3 Tbsp.
- Mayonnaise – 1 Tbsp.
- Lemon juice – 1 ½ tsp.
- Tarragon – ½ tsp.
- Pinch of salt
- Cod – 10 ounces, cut into two portions

Method

1. Preheat the oven to 425F.
2. Coat a baking pan with cooking spray.
3. In a bowl, combine olive oil, garlic, and breadcrumbs.
4. In another bowl, combine lemon juice, mayonnaise, yogurt, tarragon, and salt.
5. Place fish in the baking pan. Top each piece with one-half yogurt mixture then 1/3 breadcrumb mixture.
6. Bake in the oven for 15 minutes.
7. Serve.

Nutritional Facts Per Serving
Calories: 225
Fat: 10g
Carb: 13g
Protein: 18g
Sodium 270mg
Grilled Salmon And Asparagus With Lemon Butter
Prep time: 10 minutes
Cook time: 20 minutes
Servings: 4

Ingredients

- Salmon – 1 ¼ pound, cut into 4 portions
- Asparagus – 2 bunches, ends trimmed
- Olive oil cooking spray Salt – ½ tsp.
- Freshly ground black pepper – ¼ tsp.
- Garlic powder – ¼ tsp.
- Olive oil – 1 Tbsp.
- Butter – 1 Tbsp.
- Lemon juice – 3 Tbsp.

Method

1. On a baking sheet, place the salmon and asparagus. Spray lightly with cooking spray. Season with salt, pepper, and garlic powder.
2. Grease and preheat grill. Place salmon and asparagus on it.
3. Grill total 6 minutes, 3 mintues per side, or until opaque, turning once.
4. Grill the asparagus for 5 to 7 minutes, or until tender, turning occasionally.
5. In a bowl, place butter, olive oil, and lemon juice. Microwave to melt.
6. Drizzle fish with this mixture.
7. Serve.

Nutritional Facts Per Serving
Calories: 190
Fat: 8g
Carb: 6g
Protein: 24g
Sodium 445mg
Pan-Roasted Fish Fillets With Herb Butter
Prep time: 10 minutes
Cook time: 5 minutes
Servings: 2
Ingredients

- Fish fillets – 2 (5-ounce each) ½ to 1 inch thick Salt – ¼ tsp. Ground black pepper Olive oil – 3 Tbsp.
- Unsalted butter -1 Tbsp. divided
- Fresh thyme – 2 sprigs
- Chopped flat-leaf parsley - 1 Tbsp. Lemon wedges

Method

1. Rub the fish with pepper and salt.
2. Heat oil in a skillet.
3. Place fillets and cook until around the edges, about 2 to 3 minutes. Then flip the fillets and add the butter and thyme to the pan.
4. Baste the fish with melted butter until golden all over, about 2 minutes.
5. Serve with chopped parsley and lemon wedges.

Nutritional Facts Per Serving

- Calories: 369
- Fat: 26.9g
- Carb: 1g
- Protein: 30.5g
- Sodium 62mg

Chili Macadamia Crusted Tilapia

Prep time: 20 minutes
Cook time: 7 minutes
Servings: 4

Ingredients

- Tilapia fillets – 4
- Macadamia nuts – ½ cup, chopped coarsely
- Whole wheat panko crumbs – ½ cup Chili powder – 1 tsp.
- Cayenne pepper – ¼ tsp.
- Paprika – ¼ tsp.
- Salt – ¼ tsp.
- Pepper – ¼ tsp.
- Egg – 1
- Olive oil – 3 Tbsp.

Method

1. In a bowl, combine panko crumbs, nuts, chili powder, cayenne pepper, paprika, salt, and pepper.
2. Whisk egg in another bowl and set aside.
3. Heat the olive oil in a skillet.
4. Dredge each tilapia fillet in the egg and then coat it in the macadamia-spice-panko mixture.
5. Cook fillets until browned and cooked through, about 3 minutes on each side.
6. Serve.

Nutritional Facts Per Serving
Calories: 351
Fat: 26.5g
Carb: 5.7g
Protein: 25.7g
Sodium 234mg
Broiled White Sea Bass
Prep time: 5 minutes
Cook time: 10 minutes
Servings: 2
Ingredients

- White sea bass fillets – 2, each 4 ounces Lemon juice – 1 Tbsp.
- Garlic – 1 tsp. minced
- Salt-free herb seasoning blend – ¼ tsp. Ground black pepper to taste

Method

1. Heat the broiler (grill).
2. Place the rack very close (4 inches) to the heat source.
3. Place the fillets in a greased baking pan.
4. Sprinkle the fillets with herbed seasoning, garlic, lemon juice, and pepper.
5. Broil (grill) until opaque throughout, about 8 to 10 minutes
6. Serve.

Nutritional Facts Per Serving
Calories: 102
Fat: 2g
Carb: 1g
Protein: 21g
Sodium 77mg
Grilled Asian Salmon
Prep time: 1 hour
Cook time: 10 minutes
Servings: 4
Ingredients

- Sesame oil – 1 Tbsp.
- Homemade soy sauce – 1 Tbsp.
- Fresh ginger – 1 Tbsp. minced Rice wine vinegar – 1 Tbsp.
- Salmon fillets – 4, each 4 ounces

Method

1. Combine vinegar, ginger, soy sauce, and sesame oil in a dish.
2. Add salmon and coat well. Marinate for 1 hour, turning occasionally (in the refrigerator).
3. Grease a grill and heat over medium heat.
4. Grill the salmon on 5 minutes per side or until almost opaque.
5. Serve.

Nutritional Facts Per Serving
Calories: 185
Fat: 9g
Carb: 1g
Protein: 26g
Sodium 113mg

Herb-Crusted Baked Cod
Prep time: 10 minutes
Cook time: 10 minutes
Servings: 4

Ingredients

- Herb-flavored stuffing – ¾ cup, crushed until crumbed
- Cod fillets – 4 (4 ounces each)
- Honey - ¼ cup

Method

1. Preheat the oven to 375F. Coat a baking pan with cooking spray.
2. Brush the fillets with honey. Discard the rest of the honey.
3. Place the stuffing in a bag and place a fillet in the bag.
4. Shake the bag to coat the cod well.
5. Remove the fillet and repeat with the remaining fillets.

Bake the fillets for 10 minutes or until opaque throughout.

Nutritional Facts Per Serving
Calories: 185
Fat: 1g
Carb: 23g
Protein: 21g
Sodium 163mg

Shrimp Kebabs
Prep time: 10 minutes
Cook time: 5 minutes
Servings: 2

Ingredients

- Lemon – 1, juiced
- Olive oil – 1 Tbsp.
- Finely minced garlic – 2 tsp.
- Finely chopped fresh tarragon – 1 tsp.
- Finely chopped fresh rosemary – 1 tsp.
- Kosher salt - ½ tsp.
- Ground black pepper – ¼ tsp.
- Shrimp – 12 pieces, peeled and deveined

Method

Soak 2 wooden skewers for 10 minutes.

1. Preheat grill on high.
2. In a bowl, combine seasonings, herbs, garlic, olive oil, and lemon juice.
3. Marinade the shrimp into the lemon marinade for 5 minutes.
4. Skewer the shrimp.
5. Then place on the grill. Cook until shrimp is thoroughly cooked, about 2 minutes per side.
6. Serve.

Nutritional Facts Per Serving

Calories: 105
Fat: 1g
Carb: 0g
Protein: 24g
Sodium 185mg

Roasted Salmon

Prep time: 5 minutes
Cook time: 12 minutes
Servings: 2

Ingredients

- Salmon with skin – 2 (5-ounce) pieces
- Extra-virgin olive oil – 2 tsp.
- Chopped chives – 1 Tbsp.
- Fresh tarragon leaves – 1 Tbsp.

Method

1. Preheat the oven to 425F. Line a baking sheet with foil.
2. Rub salmon with oil.

3. Line a baking sheet with foil.
4. Place salmon (skin side down).
5. Cook for 12 minutes or until fish is cooked through. Check after 10 minutes.
6. Serve the salmon with herbs.

Nutritional Facts Per Serving
Calories: 244
Fat: 14g
Carb: 0g
Protein: 28g
Sodium 62mg

Shrimp With Corn Hash
Prep time: 5 minutes
Cook time: 10 minutes
Servings: 4

Ingredients

- Olive oil – 4 tsp.
- Large shrimp - 1 pound, peeled and deveined
- Chopped red onion – ½ cup
- Red bell pepper – ½, chopped
- Fresh corn kernels – 1 ½ cup
- Halved cherry – 1 cup
- Crushed hot red pepper – ¼ tsp.
- Water – ¼ cup Fresh lemon juice – 1 Tbsp.
- Chopped fresh basil – 2 Tbsp.

Method

1. Heat 2 tsp. oil in a skillet.
2. Add the shrimp
3. Cook for 3 to 5 minutes. Transfer to a plate.
4. Heat remaining 2 tsp. oil in the skillet. Add bell pepper.
5. Then onion and stir-fry for 1 minute, or until softened.
6. Add tomatoes, corn, and hot pepper and cover.
7. Cook for 3 minutes.
8. Add the shrimp and reheat, stirring often, about 1 minute.
9. Stir in lemon juice and water and cook.
10. Sprinkle with basil and serve.

Nutritional Facts Per Serving
Calories: 195
Fat: 6g

Carb: 18g
Protein: 18g
Sodium 647mg

Shrimp Ceviche

Prep time: 10 minutes
Cook time: 0 minutes
Servings: 8

Ingredients

- Raw shrimp – ½ pound, cut into ¼ inch pieces
- Lemons – 2, zest and juice
- Limes -2, zest and juice
- Olive oil - 2 Tbsp.
- Cumin – 2 tsp.
- Diced red onion – ½ cup
- Diced tomato – 1 cup
- Minced garlic – 2 Tbsp.
- Black beans - 1 cup, cooked
- Diced serrano chili pepper – ¼ cup, seeds removed
- Diced cucumber – 1 cup, peeled and seeded
- Chopped cilantro – ¼ cup

Method

1. In a bowl, place the shrimp and cover with the lemon and lime juice. Marinate for at least 3 hours.
2. In another bowl, mix the remaining ingredients and set aside.
3. Before serving, mix shrimp and the juice with remaining ingredients.
4. Serve.

Nutritional Facts Per Serving

Calories: 98
Fat: 4g
Carb: 10g
Protein: 7g
Sodium 167mg

Chapter Six

CHICKEN, BEEF AND PORK

*N*ow let me give you some freestyle red beef and pork recipes. It might be tempting to write off meat in your diet, but for a fact, no single food is unhealthy. It is mostly about creating a healthy dietary pattern and applying moderations.

The fact is that red meats contain high levels of protein, which I'm sure you know helps to build the bones and muscles in our bodies. So, why should we avoid them when it can be of great benefit to our healthy living?

Also, chicken makes a fantastic weight loss-friendly staple, no doubt. Chicken breasts without skin or bone are rich in protein. You can bake, roast, or stuff a chicken dinner, and you can also serve in a soup or sandwich. You won't go wrong unless you keep to old boring recipes.

While everyone is guilty of sticking to common meal ideas, you don't have to eat the same kind of chicken twice as a king or queen that you are, the reason being that there are so many creative ways to combine the ingredients and serve up delicious flavor.

To help you set a chicken meal on your table today (and every other day), I have handpicked the most delicious chicken dishes, all of which I have personally taste-tested. You will spend less than 60 minutes cooking, making it possible to get in and out of the kitchen quickly and back to more important things.

Chicken Bruschetta
SmartPoints value: Green plan - 1SP, Blue plan - 1SP, Purple plan - 1SP
Total Time: 20 min, Prep time: 10 min, Cooking time: 10 min, Serves: 4
Nutritional value: Calories - 187, Carbs – 4.4g, Fat - 7g, Protein – 27.3g

When the weather is heating up, I mostly crave for fresh and light meals other than rich and comforting.

My most recently found new love when it comes to dessert is this deliciously prepared Italian Chicken Bruschetta. It's just so simple, simply made with fresh tomatoes, basil, and garlic. I've tried it several times, and one sweet thing about it is the refreshing flavors. There is just something about the way the fresh and juicy tomato works together with the bright basil and bold garlic.

While preparing, I like to add some grilled chicken breast to it as a lean protein. If you've noticed, I do more of chicken breast, yes, because it is low in points, and it's a perfect way of adding protein to my meal without getting over budget with my points.

Ingredients

- Chicken breast (skinless, boneless) - 1 lb
- Large Roma tomatoes (finely diced) - 2 pieces
- Basil (finely chopped, fresh) - 1/4 cup
- Garlic (minced) - 2 cloves
- Olive oil (1 tbsp plus 1 tsp)
- Balsamic Vinegar (1/2 tsp)
- Parsley (dried) - 1 tsp
- Oregano (dried) - 1 tsp
- Pepper and Salt to taste

Instructions

1. After cutting the chicken breasts into four equal-sized fillets, season each of the side of the chicken with the parsley, oregano and salt and pepper.
2. Over medium-high heat, heat one teaspoon of olive oil in a medium-sized, nonstick skillet. For 4-5 minutes, cook as you turn each side until the chicken is entirely cooked and browned.
3. Remove from heat and cover with a lid to allow it to sit for about 5 minutes.
4. Make bruschetta by mixing tomatoes, olive oil, garlic, basil, balsamic vinegar, and pepper and salt in a bowl.
5. Put the chicken breast on a plate and top each of them with about ¼ cup of the bruschetta. Then drizzle on some extra balsamic if you so desire.
6. You can also make a sandwich with fresh Italian bread and little creamy goat cheese. The flavor is so bold and mouthwatering.

Lemon Chicken with Broccoli
SmartPoints value: Green plan - 3SP, Blue plan - 1SP, Purple plan - 1SP
Total Time: 30 min, **Prep time**: 15 min, **Cooking time**: 15 min, **Serves**: 4

Nutritional value:

Calories - 176.6, Carbs - 8.4g, Fat - 2.0g, Protein - 32.3g

The whole family will love this fantastic weeknight dinner, and it's ready in just 30 minutes. To ensure that the chicken cooks quickly and evenly, you should slice it thinly. Cover the pan when cooking the broccoli to help build up steam, bathing the florets with heat. It will allow tops that aren't in contact with the hot pan to cook properly. You will need one small to medium head of broccoli to get enough florets and one lemon to yield enough zest and juice for this entrée.

Ingredients

- All-purpose flour - 2 Tbsp
- Black pepper - ¼ tsp (freshly ground)
- Fat-free, reduced-sodium chicken broth - 1½ cup(s) (divided)
- Fresh lemon juice - 1 Tbsp
- Fresh parsley - 2 Tbsp (chopped)
- Lemon zest - 2 tsp, or more to taste*
- Minced Garlic - 2 tsp
- Olive oil - 2 tsp
- Table salt - ½ tsp (divided)
- Uncooked chicken breast(s) -12 oz, thinly sliced (boneless, skinless)
- Uncooked broccoli - 2½ cup(s), small florets

Instructions

1. On a clean plate, mix 1 1/2 Tbsp of flour, 1/4 tsp of salt, and pepper, then add chicken and turn to coat.
2. Put a large nonstick skillet over medium-high heat and pour the oil in for heating.
3. Add the chicken and cook, turning as needed, until it is lightly browned and cooked through, about 5 minutes; remove to a plate.
4. Put one cup of broth and Garlic in the same skillet, then boil over high heat, scraping up browned bits from the bottom of the pan with a wooden spoon.
5. Add the broccoli, then cover and cook for 1 minute.
6. Stir the remaining 1/2 cup broth, 1/2 Tbsp flour, and 1/4 tsp salt together in a small cup, then add to the skillet and bring its content to a simmer over low heat.
7. Cover the skillet and cook until the broccoli is crisp-tender and the sauce thickens slightly.
8. Stir in the chicken and lemon zest, then heat through.
9. Remove the skillet from heat, and stir in the parsley and lemon juice, then toss to coat.

Chicken and Fennel in Rosemary-wine Broth

SmartPoints value: Green plan - 4SP, Blue plan - 2SP, Purple plan - 2SP

Total Time: 40 min, **Prep time**: 18 min, **Cooking time**: 22 min, **Serves**: 4

Nutritional value: Calories - 121.5, Carbs - 10.5g, Fat - 6.3g, Protein - 26.0g

If you are looking for a dish that will tickle your belly on a chilly night, this rustic Italian entrée is perfect, and since you will cook it in one skillet, that makes it easy to fix in your vegetable. You should first sear the chicken to produce an excellent brown exterior. You can then sauté the fennel and onion in the flavorful drippings left in the skillet. They will mix and become sweetened as they cook.

Return the chicken and any accumulated juices to the skillet to finish cooking.

Ingredients

- All-purpose flour - 5 tsp (divided)
- Black pepper - ⅛ tsp, or to taste (freshly ground)
- Canned chicken broth - 14½ oz
- Minced Garlic - 2 tsp
- Olive oil - 1 Tbsp, extra-virgin (divided)
- Red/white wine - 1/4 cup
- Rosemary - 1¼ tsp, fresh (chopped)
- Table salt - ½ tsp, or to taste
- Uncooked chicken breast(s) - 1 pound(s), cut into bite-size chunks (boneless, skinless)
- Uncooked fennel bulb(s) - 1 pound(s)
- Uncooked red onion(s) - 1 small (chopped)

Instructions

1. Trim the stalk from fennel to quarter bulb(s) lengthwise and then slice in a cross-like manner into small pieces. Reserve the fronds for garnish (about 3 cups fennel will be available).
2. Put the chicken on a plate and sprinkle it with rosemary, then sprinkle it with 4 tsp flour and toss to coat.
3. Add 1 tsp of oil to a large nonstick skillet and heat over medium-high heat.
4. Add the chicken and cook, occasionally turning with tongs, until it is lightly brown.
5. Transfer the chicken to a clean plate (cooking is partial at this point).
6. Heat the remaining 2 tsp oil in the same skillet over medium-high

heat and add fennel and onion; sauté until it becomes lightly brown and almost tender.

7. Add wine and Garlic, then reduce the heat to low and simmer, stirring the bottom of the pan to scrape up browned bits, until most of the wine has evaporated.
8. Stir the broth together with the remaining 1 tsp flour in a small bowl and then stir into skillet.
9. Add salt and pepper, then increase the heat to high and bring it to a boil. Reduce the heat to medium-low and simmer for another 1 minute.
10. Add the chicken and cook, often tossing until the chicken cooks through. Garnish with reserved chopped fennel fronds and serve.

You can serve it with crusty whole-grain bread, or over rice, to mop up all of the broth.

If you prefer not to use wine in this recipe, you can substitute with one tablespoon of red or white wine vinegar and three tablespoons of water.

Chicken Cordon Bleu

SmartPoints value: Green plan - 6SP, Blue plan - 4SP, Purple plan - 4SP

Total Time: 46 min, **Prep time**: 11 min, **Cooking time**: 35 min, **Serves**: 4

Nutritional value: Calories - 357.9, Carbs - 12.7g, Fat - 16.9g, Protein - 36.7g

Cordon bleu was a commonly served dish at dinner-parties in the sixties. Preparing it is simple: You sandwich a layer of ham and cheese between thin medallions of chicken or veal, then you sauté it.

Here, I have created a light version of the recipe to use a single layer of chicken rolled around the filling to make an elegant presentation.

Prepare this dish the next time you have guests and add some greens to the plate: either roasted broccolini, asparagus, or haricot vert (thin French green beans) will do just fine.

Ingredients

- All-purpose flour - 4 Tbsp
- Black pepper - ⅛ tsp (or to taste), freshly ground
- Cornflake crumbs - ½ cup(s)
- Lean ham (cooked) - 4 slice(s), (about 2 oz. total)
- Egg(s) - 1 large, lightly beaten
- Ground nutmeg - ⅛ tsp
- Parmesan cheese - 2 Tbsp, freshly grated
- Reduced-sodium chicken broth - ½ cup(s)
- Swiss cheese - 2 oz (4 thin slices), low-fat
- Table salt - ½ tsp
- Table wine - 1 Tbsp, Madeira

- Uncooked chicken breast(s) -1 pound(s), (4 breasts, 1/4 pound each), pounded to 1/4-inch thickness (boneless, skinless)
- 2% reduced-fat milk - ½ cup(s)

Instructions

1. Spray a baking sheet with nonstick spray while you preheat the oven to 400°F.
2. Place one half of a chicken breast on a work surface and top it with one slice of the ham, then one slice of the Swiss cheese.
3. Roll it up in a jelly-roll style, and secure with a toothpick. Repeat the process with the remaining chicken, ham, and cheese.
4. Make a mixture of two tablespoons of flour, one-quarter teaspoon of salt, and ground pepper on a sheet of wax paper.
5. Place the egg and the cornflake crumbs in separate shallow bowls.
6. Taking it one at a time, coat the chicken rolls lightly, first with the flour mixture, and then dip it into the egg for a single layer coat.
7. Coat the rolls with the cornflake crumbs, and place them on the baking sheet (discard any leftover flour mixture, egg, and cornflake bits).
8. Spray the chicken rolls lightly with nonstick spray. Bake until the temperature of the rolls reaches 160°F, 30–35 minutes.
9. To prepare the sauce, mix the milk, the broth, the Madeira, nutmeg, the remaining two tablespoons of flour, the remaining 1/4 teaspoon of salt, and another grinding of the pepper in a medium-sized saucepan.
10. Whisk until it is smooth and cook over medium heat, continually whisking until it becomes thick in about 6 minutes.
11. Remove the sauce from the heat and stir in the Parmesan cheese, then cover to keep it warm.
12. When the chicken rolls are ready, drizzle them with the sauce and serve them immediately.

Southern-Style Oven-Fried Chicken
SmartPoints value: Green plan - 4SP, Blue Plan - 3SP, Purple plan - 3SP
Total Time: 45 min, **Prep time**: 15 min, **Cooking time**: 30 min, **Serves**: 4
Nutritional value: Calories - 256.9, Carbs - 31.3g, Fat - 1.6g, Protein - 27.5g
Switch to oven frying and lighten up this favorite hearty dish. I decided to improve the flavor by adding buttermilk and a pinch of cayenne pepper.
Ingredients

- All-purpose flour - ⅓ cup(s)

- Buttermilk (low-fat) - 3 oz
- Cayenne pepper - ¼ tsp (or to taste), divided
- Cooking spray - 3 spray(s)
- Cornflake crumbs - ½ cup(s)
- Table salt - ½ tsp (or to taste), divided
- Uncooked chicken breast(s) - 1 pound(s), four 4-oz pieces (boneless, skinless)

Instructions

1. Heat the oven to 375°F before starting. Coat a 13- X 8- X 2-inch baking dish lightly with cooking spray and set it aside.
2. Add salt and cayenne pepper to chicken for a tasty seasoning and set it aside also.
3. Put a mixture of flour, 1/4 teaspoon salt, and 1/8 teaspoon cayenne pepper in a bowl of medium size.
4. Put the buttermilk and cornflakes crumbs in 2 separate shallow bowls.
5. Dip the chicken in the flour mixture and evenly coat both sides.
6. Next, dip the flour-coated chicken into buttermilk and turn it to coat both sides.
7. Finally, dip the coated chicken in cornflake crumbs and turn to coat both sides.
8. Place coated chicken breasts in the baking dish that you prepared.
9. Bake the chicken until it is tender and no longer pink in the center (you don't need to flip the chicken while baking). The baking should take about 25 to 30 minutes.

Italian Chicken Soup with Vegetables
SmartPoints value: Green plan - 4SP, Blue plan - 1SP, Purple plan - 1SP
Total Time: 27 min, **Prep time**: 15 min, **Cooking time**: 12 min, **Serves**: 1
Nutritional value:
Calories - 136.7, Carbs - 22.3g, Fat - 1.0g, Protein - 9.6g

This chicken soup is ideal for a leisurely lunch or a quick dinner, as it is brothy and filled with vegetables. To make it bulky, you can add in any cooked grain you have on hand, like rice, barley, or quinoa, which will also add some nice texture and make it more chewable. You can use any leftover chicken you have. The drizzle of extra virgin olive oil at the end not only makes the soup look a little fancier, but it can also add a rich flavor that takes a simple soup like this one to the next level.

Ingredients

- Chicken broth - 1 cup(s), canned

- Chicken breast(s) - 1 cup(s), diced (skinless, boneless)
- Extra virgin olive oil - 1 tsp, divided
- Fresh thyme - 1¼ tsp (leaves)
- Fresh mushroom(s) - 1 cup(s), sliced
- Garlic clove(s) - 1 medium-sized, minced
- Green beans - 1 small bowl, cooked
- Lemon(s) - 1 slice(s)
- Plum tomato(es) - 1 medium-sized, diced
- Uncooked cauliflower - 1 cup(s), small florets

Instructions

1. Heat 1/2 tsp of olive oil in a small skillet over medium heat.
2. Add the mushrooms and garlic, then cook, continuously stirring until mushrooms begin to soften and the mixture is fragrant; about 2 minutes.
3. Add the broth in the chicken and bring it to a boil over medium-high heat.
4. Add cauliflower and (or) green beans, then reduce the heat to medium-low and simmer until it is almost tender; about 4 minutes.
5. Add the chicken, thyme, and tomatoes, then simmer until the vegetables are tender; about 2 minutes.
6. Drizzle it with the remaining 1/2 tsp of oil and fresh lemon juice, then grind the pepper over the top, if you desire.

Note: You can also garnish your dish with shredded Parmesan cheese (this could add SmartPoints values).

Roasted Chicken Breast with Spiced Cauliflower

SmartPoints value: Green plan - 4SP, Blue plan - 2SP, Purple plan - 2SP

Total Time: 50 min, Prep time: 20 min, Cooking time: 30 min, Serves: 4

Nutritional value: Calories - 470.9, Carbs - 3.5g, Fat - 11.3g, Protein - 84.2g

In this tasty recipe, you will brush chicken breasts with olive oil, turmeric, ground coriander, and cumin, with a touch of cayenne pepper before roasting, and surround it by a bed of cauliflower florets.

After cooking the chicken thoroughly, toss the cauliflower in all the delicious juices in the skillet, and let it continue to roast until it's sweet and tender. You can't have anything more convenient than a single-sheet pan dinner on a busy weeknight.

Drizzle fresh lime juice and sprinkle fresh cilantro into this Indian-influenced meal to add incredible flavor. In case you don't like cilantro, parsley or oregano works well too.

Ingredients

- Black pepper (divided) - ½ tsp
- Cayenne pepper - ⅛ tsp
- Cooking spray - 2 spray(s)
- Cilantro (finely chopped) - 1 Tbsp
- Olive oil - 2 Tbsp
- Coriander (ground) - 1 tsp
- Turmeric (ground) - 1 tsp
- Durkee Cumin (ground) - ½ tsp
- Kosher salt (divided) - ¾ tsp
- Uncooked chicken breast - 1 pound(s), two 8 oz pieces (boneless, skinless)
- Uncooked cauliflower - 1 pound(s), cut into bite-size pieces
- Fresh lime(s) - ½ medium, with wedges for serving

Instructions

1. Before you start, heat the oven to 450°F. Get a large baking sheet and line it with parchment paper.
2. Combine and mix oil, turmeric, coriander, cumin, 1/2 tsp of salt, 1/4 tsp of pepper, and cayenne in a large bowl.
3. Place the chicken in the center of the prepared baking sheet and brush each piece with 1/2 tsp of oil mixture.
4. Add cauliflower to the bowl and toss it to coat. Place the cauliflower around the chicken and lightly coat both chicken and cauliflower with cooking spray.
5. Sprinkle the chicken with the remaining 1/4 tsp of each salt and pepper.
6. Roast the coated chicken until it cooks through; 15-20 minutes and let it rest.
7. Toss the cauliflower and chicken juices in the pan, then continue roasting until browned and tender; about 10 minutes more.
8. Add the cilantro and toss again.
9. Thickly slice the chicken across the grain and fan over serving plates.
10. Serve the cauliflower and chicken in each plate and squeeze 1/2 lime over the top, then serve with additional lime wedges.

Vietnamese Chicken and Veggie Bowl with Rice Noodles
SmartPoints value: Green plan - 6SP, Blue plan - 4SP, Purple plan - 4SP
Total Time: 26 min, **Prep time**: 20 min, **Cooking time**: 6 min, **Serves**: 1
Nutritional value: Calories - 280.4, Carbs - 42.3g, Fat - 10.0g, Protein - 9.1g
This dish is a delicious and stunning entrée that comes together in just 25

minutes. It is a perfect recipe for one. You can even use leftover cooked chicken breast and grilled vegetables.

I would prefer you to use chicken cutlets with broccoli and red peppers, but feel free to experiment with chicken thighs, spinach, mushrooms, onions, or whatever you have on hand.

The soy and fish sauces add that ultimate umami bomb, while sriracha helps keep it balanced out by providing a touch of heat.

You can quickly scale up this recipe if you need to serve it to a crowd.

Ingredients

- Cilantro (chopped, fresh leaves) - 2 Tbsp
- Cooked rice noodles - ½ cup(s)
- Asian fish sauce - ½ tsp
- Cooking spray - 4 spray(s)
- Uncooked chicken breast - 5 oz, thin cutlet (boneless, skinless)
- Uncooked broccoli - 1 cup(s), small florets or baby stalks
- Red pepper(s) (sweet) - ½ medium, cut in 2 even pieces
- Soy sauce (low sodium) - 2 Tbsp, divided (or to taste)
- Sriracha sauce - 1 tsp (or to taste)
- Sugar - ¼ tsp
- Roasted peanuts (unsalted dry) - 2 tsp, chopped

Instructions

1. Coat a grill or grill pan with cooking spray and preheat on medium-high heat.
2. Place the chicken, broccoli, and red pepper in a shallow bowl and drizzle with one tablespoon of soy sauce, then toss to coat.
3. Coat the chicken with cooking spray and grill, turning the chicken once and the vegetables a few times, until chicken cooks through and veggies are tender-crisp; about 6 minutes.
4. Slice the chicken and pepper them into strips, then place all in a bowl over noodles.
5. Stir together the remaining one tablespoon of soy sauce, fish sauce, and sugar. Drizzle the mixture over your cooked chicken.
6. Sprinkle a mixture of cilantro, peanuts, and sriracha on the chicken, then serve.

Chicken Tortilla Soup
SmartPoints value: Green plan - 4SP, Blue plan - 2SP, Purple plan - 2SP
Total Time: 45 min, **Prep time**: 15 min, **Cooking time**: 30 min, **Serves**: 6
Nutritional value:
Calories - 200, Carbs - 24g, Fat - 9g, Protein - 7g

Preparing this soup is very easy. Once you have chopped and sautéed the vegetables, the rest of the cooking is practically hands-off. You will simmer the chicken in a flavored broth made with fire-roasted tomatoes and lime juice. Doing this will give you some extra minutes to put together a quick salad or other simple side dishes. Chicken breasts (boneless, skinless) work well in this soup, but you can use chicken thighs as well. If you'd like to make things more interesting, don't de-seed the jalapeño completely.

Ingredients

- Cilantro (chopped) - 1 cup(s)
- Chili powder - 1 tsp
- Chicken broth (reduced-sodium) - 6 cup(s)
- Olive oil - 1 tsp
- Uncooked onion(s) (chopped) - 1½ cup(s)
- Kosher salt -1½ tsp
- Minced Garlic - 4 tsp
- Jalapeño pepper(s) - 1 medium (seeded and minced)
- Tomatoes (canned, diced)- 15 oz, fire roasted-variety, drained
- Uncooked chicken breast - 20 oz (boneless, skinless)
- Lime juice (fresh) - ⅓ cup(s)
- Mexican-style cheese (Shredded reduced) - 6 Tbsp
- Tortilla chips (crushed) - 12 chip(s)

Instructions

1. Set a soup pot over medium heat and preheat.
2. Toss in the chopped onion and salt, then cook, often stirring, until the onion gets soft; 5-10 minutes.
3. Add garlic, chili powder, and jalapeno, then cook for one minute.
4. Put in your broth, tomatoes, lime juice, and chicken, then stir to combine.
5. Simmer and cook until the chicken breasts cook through; about 20 minutes.
6. Remove the chicken breasts from the soup and shred them with two forks, then return the shredded chicken to the pot with cilantro.
7. Serve your soup garnished with tortilla chips and cheese.

Chicken Piccata Stir-Fry

SmartPoints value: Green plan - 4SP, Blue plan - 2SP, Purple plan - 2SP

Total Time: 25 min, **Prep time**: 20 min, **Cooking time**: 5 min, **Serves**: 4

Nutritional value: Cal - 190.5, Carbs - 5.6g, Fat - 9.4g, Protein - 18.6g

This dish is a combination of the classic Italian chicken piccata and Asian stir-fry.

Ingredients

- Black pepper (freshly ground) - ¼ tsp
- Capers (rinsed)- 1 Tbsp
- Chicken broth (fat-free) - ½ cup(s)
- Cornstarch (divided) - 2 tsp
- Dry sherry (divided)- 3 Tbsp
- Table salt (divided) - ¾ tsp
- Soy sauce (low sodium) - 1 Tbsp
- Peanut oil (divided) - 4 tsp, or vegetable oil
- Uncooked chicken breast (boneless, skinless) - 1 pound(s), cut into quarter-inch-thick slices
- Uncooked shallot(s) - 1 medium, thinly sliced
- Minced Garlic - 1 Tbsp
- String beans (uncooked) - 2 cup(s), cut into two-inch lengths
- Parsley (fresh, chopped) - 2 Tbsp
- Lemon(s) - ½ medium, cut into four

Instructions

1. Prepare a clean medium-sized bowl and mix chicken, 1 tsp of cornstarch,1 Tbsp of dry sherry,1/2 tsp salt, and pepper in it.
2. Next, get a small bowl and combine broth, soy sauce, remaining 2 Tbsp of dry sherry, and 1 tsp of cornstarch.
3. Preheat a fourteen-inch flat-bottomed wok or twelve-inch skillet over high heat to the point where a drop of water will evaporate within 1 to 2 seconds of contact, then swirl in one Tbsp oil.
4. Add shallots and garlic, then stir-fry for 10 seconds. Push the shallot mixture to the sides of the wok and add the chicken, then spread in one layer in the wok.
5. Cook the chicken undisturbed for 60 seconds, allowing the chicken to begin searing, then stir-fry another 60 seconds until chicken is no longer pink but not yet thoroughly cooked.
6. Swirl the chicken in the remaining 1 tsp oil and toss in green beans and capers. Sprinkle on the remaining 1/4 tsp of salt and stir-fry for 30 seconds or until just combined.
7. Swirl the chicken in the broth mixture and stir-fry for 1-2 minutes or until the chicken is cooked through, with the sauce slightly thickened.
8. Sprinkle the parsley on it and serve with lemon wedges.

Ranch Meatballs

SmartPoints value: Green plan - 4SP, Blue plan - 4SP, Purple plan – 5SP

Total Time: 20mins, **Prep time**: 10 mins, **Cooking time**: 30mins, **Serves**: 4

Nutritional value: Calories - 195, Carbs - 6g, Fat - 6g, Protein - 26g

Meatball recipes are delicious protein recipes that are so satisfying and tasty. They can be a fun and easy meal. It becomes easier to prepare the perfect sized meatballs using a meatball shaper.

Ingredients

- Ground beef (96/4) (extra lean) - 1 lb
- Panko breadcrumbs - 1/3 cup(s)
- Egg substitute (Liquid, like egg beaters) - 1/4 cup
- Olive oil - 1 tsp
- Onion powder - 1 tbsp
- Garlic powder - 1 tbsp
- Dill (dried) - 2 tsp
- Parsley (dried) - 2 tsp
- Basil (dried) - 2 tsp
- Salt and pepper - Add to taste

Instructions

1. Combine all the ingredients by hand in a large bowl and shape it into about 24 meatballs.
2. Apply heat to the oil in a large non-stick skillet over medium-high heat.
3. Place meatballs in the pan and cook for about 1-2 minutes on each side, until all sides get lightly browned.
4. Reduce the heat to medium-low and pour in half a cup of water. Cover it and cook, occasionally stirring, until meatballs cook thoroughly; about 10-12 minutes.

Note: Meatballs are a perfect simple Weight Watchers dinner recipe for those who are watching Points but also savour the flavour

Beef Orzo with Feta

SmartPoints value: Green plan - 8SP, Blue plan - 8SP, Purple plan – 8SP

Total Time: 35mins, Prep time: 10mins, Cooking time: 25mins, Serves: 6

Nutritional value: Calories - 325, Carbs – 44g, Fat – 5.5g, Protein – 25g

Beef Orzo is one of those types of meals that you'll love to prepare now and then. The instructions for preparation are quite easy to follow, and the meal is just delicious. If you haven't tried it, you are missing out big time. You should give it a try for your next family dinner or friends gathering. This most satisfying weight-watching dinner recipe is perfect for warming you and your family up on a chilly fall evening.

Ingredients

- Ground beef (extra-lean) - 1 lb
- Whole wheat orzo - 10 oz
- Onion (finely chopped) - 1 large
- Garlic (minced) - 4 cloves
- Cinnamon (ground) - 1 tsp
- Oregano (dried) - 2 tsp
- Can tomatoes (crushed) - One 26oz
- Reduced-fat feta cheese (crumbled) - 1/3 cup
- Salt & pepper - Add to taste

Instructions

1. Prepare whole orzo wheat according to package directions. Drain it and set aside.
2. While the wheat is cooking, spray a large skillet with nonfat cooking spray, and set it over medium-high heat. Toss in some beef and cook until it mostly cooks through.
3. Put in onions, oregano, garlic, cinnamon, salt, and pepper. Sauté the dish until the onions are tender and the beef cooks all the way through.
4. Pour the crushed tomatoes into the skillet with the beef mixture, and cook on medium heat. Continue to cook, while occasionally stirring, until the mixture thickens; about 15 minutes.
5. Dish the beef sauce with orzo and place in serving bowls. Top each bowl with 1 tbsp of feta.

Light Beef Chili
SmartPoints value: Green plan - 4SP, Blue plan - 4SP, Purple plan – 4SP
Total Time: 2hrs 30mins, **Prep time**: 30mins, **Cooking time**: 2hrs, **Serves**: 8
Nutritional value: Calories - 187, Carbs – 24g, Fat – 3g, Protein – 16g

This red meat dish is perfect for warming up on a chilly day. One of the reasons I love it is because preparing it is very easy. Often, I will make this chili, then measure and place each of them in a Ziploc bag and refrigerate. Whenever I need something hot and filling, all I need to do is grab one and microwave.

Ingredients

- Beef bouillon powder - 1 tbsp
- Bell pepper (red, diced) - 1 small

- Black pepper - 1/2 tsp
- Brewed coffee (strong) - 1 cup
- Chili powder - 3 tbsp
- Cocoa (unsweetened) - 1 tsp
- Cumin - 2 tbsp
- Dark beer - One 12oz can
- Garlic (minced) - 4 cloves
- Green pepper (diced) - 1 small
- Ground beef (extra lean) - 1 lb
- Kidney beans - One 15oz can
- Onion (diced) - 1 large
- Oregano - 2 tsp
- Paprika - 1 tsp
- Salt - 1 tsp
- Sugar - 1 tbsp
- Tomatoes (diced) - One 28oz can
- Tomato sauce - One 8oz can

Instructions

1. Place a large pot or Dutch oven over medium-high heat and spray it with non-fat cooking spray.
2. Add the onions and garlic, then cook until onions start to soften; about 3 minutes.
3. Toss in the ground beef and cook until the meat turns brown.
4. Add the diced bell peppers to the beef and cook for another 5 minutes.
5. Put in all the remaining ingredients asides the kidney beans and stir.
6. Bring the content of the pot to a simmer, then stir in the kidney beans.
7. Reduce the heat to medium-low, cover the pot, and let it cook for about 2 hours.

This perfect hearty beef chili made with extra lean ground beef simmers in fantastic spices and flavors to give you a desirable taste.

Insalata Greca

Nutrition

Calories: 326 kcal | Gross carbohydrates: 11 g | Protein: 14 g | Fats: 26 g | Fiber: 4 g | Net carbohydrates: 7 g | Macro fats: 55 % | Macro proteins: 30 % | Macro carbohydrates: 15 %

Total time: 5 minutes

Ingredients

- 50 grams of tomato
- 50 grams of cucumber
- 25 grams of red pepper or yellow pepper
- 15 grams of red onion
- 50 grams of feta
- 50 grams of black olives
- 3 tablespoons extra virgin olive oil
- 1 tablespoon lemon juice
- 1 teaspoon dried oregano
- 1 egg

Instructions

1. Bring a saucepan of water to the boil. Once the water boils, place the egg in it. Boil the egg for 8 minutes.
2. Clean the onion and cut into thin slices (keep the rest of the onion in a sealed container in the refrigerator).
3. Wash the tomato, pepper, and cucumber and cut the pepper and cucumber into thin slices. Dice the tomato.
4. Peel the egg and cut it into slices.
5. Arrange the tomatoes and the egg in the center of a plate. Put the cucumber slices around it. Place the bell pepper and red onion on top of the tomatoes.
6. Drain the feta if necessary and cut into small 1 cm large cubes. Place in a heap on top of the tomato.
7. Decorate the dish with the black olives and sprinkle the oregano over the tomatoes.
8. Make the vinaigrette in a small cup or bowl by mixing the olive oil and lemon juice well with a fork or teaspoon.
9. Pour the vinaigrette over the salad.

Crudities
Nutrition
Calories: 22 kcal | Gross carbohydrates: 5 g | Protein: 1 g | Fats: 0.2 g | Fiber: 2 g | Net carbohydrates: 3 g | Macro fat: 5 % | Macro proteins: 24 % | Macro carbohydrates: 71 %
Total time: 10 minutes
Ingredients

- 1 celery stem
- 1 bush of chicory cuts lengthwise into four pieces
- Cut 10 cm cucumber into long, thin strips
- 2 peppers, for example, red and yellow

Instructions

1. Cut the vegetables into thin, long strips so that you can dip them. For example, you can use chicory, little gem lettuce, cucumber, colored peppers, and celery.
2. Tasty and fast - if you don't feel like cooking.

Herring with Onions
Nutrition
Calories: 111 kcal | Gross carbohydrates: 3 g | Protein: 12 g | Fats: 6 g | Fiber: 0.3 g | Net carbohydrates: 3 g | Macro fat: 29 % | Macro proteins: 58 % | Macro carbohydrates: 13 %
Time - 15 minutes
Ingredients

- 1 haring
- 1 tablespoon onion
- Instructions
- A very quick lunch.

Notes

- If you follow the keto diet, you can still get some goodies from the fish stall.
- Tasty and very healthy! Herring contains many Omega 3 fatty acids.

Insalata Capricciosa
Nutrition
Calories: 551 kcal | Gross carbohydrates: 9 g | Protein: 28 g | Fats: 46 g | Fiber: 3 g | Net carbohydrates: 6 g | Macro fats: 58 % | Macro proteins: 35 % | Macro carbohydrates: 8 %
Time: 15 minutes
Ingredients

- 2 eggs
- 2 tomatoes around 200 grams
- 100 grams of mixed lettuce or iceberg lettuce
- 60 grams of black olives, preferably in olive oil
- 100 grams of mozzarella
- 100 grams of tuna in water or olive oil
- pepper and salt
- 50 ml extra virgin olive oil
- 15 ml of lemon juice

Instructions

1. Bring a saucepan of water to the boil. Once the water boils, carefully lay the eggs in it. Bring the water back to the boil and boil the eggs for 8 minutes. Then place the pan under the cold tap so that the eggs cool sufficiently to allow them to peel.
2. Wash the tomatoes, pat them dry with kitchen paper and cut into slices.
3. Drain the tuna well and place it on top of the lettuce.
4. Also, divide the tomato and olives slices over the lettuce and also cut the boiled eggs into slices. Put it on the lettuce too.
5. Season the salad with salt and pepper. Make a vinaigrette by mixing the olive oil well with the lemon juice in a cup. Use a teaspoon to distribute the vinaigrette on the plates.

Oopsie sandwich (keto)
Nutrition
Calories: 84 kcal | Gross carbohydrates: 2 g | Protein: 4 g | Fats: 7 g | Fiber: 1 g | Net carbohydrates: 1 g | Macro fats: 58 % | Macro proteins: 33 % | Macro carbohydrates: 8 %
Total time: 30 minutes
Ingredients

- 2 eggs
- 75 grams of cream cheese
- 1 teaspoon of psyllium
- 0.5 teaspoon baking powder
- pinch of salt

Instructions

1. Preheat the oven to 150° Celsius and ensure that the eggs are at room temperature. When the eggs come out of the refrigerator, place them in a bowl of lukewarm tap water for 10-15 minutes.
2. Split the eggs. Put the egg whites in a cup for a hand blender and the egg yolks in another bowl.
3. Mix the egg yolks with the cream cheese, the psyllium and the baking powder with a whisk or a fork. Let this batter rest for 5 minutes so that the baking powder and psyllium can work.
4. Beat the egg whites with a pinch of salt. The proteins must be so stiff that if you hold the cup upside down, they will not move.
5. Carefully scoop the egg whites through the egg yolk-cream cheese mixture. The mixture must become nicely airy.

6. Put a sheet of baking paper on an oven plate and make 8 heaps of batter on the baking sheet.
7. Bake in 25 minutes at 150° Celsius. The sandwiches must be beautifully golden brown.

Keto (gluten-free) poffertjes
Nutrition

Calories: 700 kcal | Gross carbohydrates: 8 g | Protein: 27 g | Fats: 63 g | Fiber: 1 g | Net carbohydrates: 7 g | Macro fats: 65 % | Macro proteins: 28 % | Macro carbohydrates: 7 %

Total time: 40 minutes
Ingredients

- Keto poffertjes
- 4 eggs
- 250 grams of ricotta
- 1 tablespoon psyllium, for example, Livinggreens psyllium fibers
- 0.5 teaspoon baking powder
- 0.25 teaspoon vanilla extract
- 2 tablespoons of mild olive oil
- Whipped cream
- 200 ml whipped cream
- 0.5 teaspoon vanilla extract

Instructions

1. Allow the eggs to reach room temperature by removing them from the fridge 15 minutes in advance or by placing them in lukewarm tap water for 5 minutes.
2. If you have made your own ricotta, use a hand blender or hand blender until there are no / few lumps. If you have ricotta from the store this is not necessary.
3. Now add the ricotta, the baking powder (optional), vanilla extract and the psyllium to the beaten eggs and mix well with a fork.
4. Let the batter stand for 5-10 minutes so that it becomes a little stronger.
5. Heat a cast-iron poffertjes pan over high heat so that it becomes hot. Then grease the pan with a mild olive oil with a brush and lower the heat.
6. Now place a spoonful of batter in each compartment in the pan. Make sure you have lowered the heat now!
7. Bake the pancake for 2-4 minutes on one side (depending on how large the pancake is). When the top starts to dry, turn the poffertje

with a spoon and bake the other side. Repeat until all the batter has been used up.

8. Beat the whipped cream with the vanilla extract or use a whipped cream machine.
9. Serve cold or hot.

Notes: Delicious with fresh raspberry or chia raspberry jam or chia blueberry jam or homemade keto-Nutella.

Frittata with Chanterelles
Nutrition

Calories: 1011 kcal | Gross carbohydrates: 13 g | Protein: 21 g | Fats: 97 g | Fiber: 4 g | Net carbohydrates: 9 g | Macro fats: 76 % | Macro proteins: 17 % | Macro carbohydrates: 7 %

Total time: 25 minutes
Ingredients

- 6 eggs
- 250 grams of chanterelles
- 50 tablespoons butter
- 50 ml extra virgin olive oil
- 1 clove of garlic
- 1 tablespoon oregano leaves without stalk
- 1 tablespoon of young sage leaves
- 0.5 lemon
- 300 ml mascarpone
- Creme fraiche dip
- 1 forest outing
- 200 ml creme fraiche

Instructions

1. Preheat the oven to 220° Celsius.
2. If the eggs are not yet at room temperature, remove them from the refrigerator and place them in a bowl of warm water (not boiling!).
3. Use a mushroom brush to gently clean the chanterelles. Leave them whole.
4. Heat the butter with the olive oil in a frying pan. Add the chanterelles to the pan as soon as the butter has melted and bake for 3-4 minutes until medium to high heat. Turn over occasionally.
5. Clean the garlic and chop it into small pieces.
6. Wash the sage and oregano, pat dry and chop into small pieces.
7. Add the garlic and spices to the skillet and turn the heat down. Cook for 4-5 minutes. Remove the pan from the heat and squeeze half a lemon over the chanterelles.

8. Grease a baking dish and / or put a sheet of baking paper in it.
9. Beat the eggs with the mascarpone in a bowl and add some salt and pepper.
10. Put the chanterelles in the baking dish and pour the beaten eggs over it. Bake in the oven for 10-15 minutes, until the egg is firm.
11. You can check whether the frittata is fully cooked by piercing it with a wooden or metal stick. If the skewer comes out clean, the frittata is ready.
12. Clean a spring onion and cut into rings. Mix through the creme fraiche.
13. Serve with creme fraiche.

Niçoise Salad with Tuna Steak
Nutrition
Calories: 956 kcal | Gross carbohydrates: 6 g | Protein: 37 g | Fats: 86 g | Fiber: 2 g | Net carbohydrates: 4 g | Macro fats: 68 % | Macro proteins: 29 % | Macro carbohydrates: 3 %
Total time: 18 minutes
Ingredients

- Tuna steaks
- 375 grams of tuna steaks If you use frozen food, defrost beforehand.
- 3 tablespoons butter
- Eggs
- 3 eggs
- Vegetable
- 0 5 celeriac
- 90 grams of cherry tomatoes
- 180-gram haricot verts Drained weight - from a pot without added sugar
- 1 bunch of radishes
- 1 tablespoon capers
- 3 tablespoons olives If you buy olives in oil, make sure they are in olive oil and not in any other type of oil!

Dressing

- 300 ml mayonnaise

Instructions

1. Eggs
2. Start by boiling the eggs. Cook them in 8 minutes and then put them in a pan with cold water to cool.

3. Peel and halve the eggs.
4. Place the eggs on a large flat dish.
5. Tuna steaks
6. Melt the butter or ghee in a skillet or use a grill pan without butter.
7. Cook the tuna in 2.5 minutes per side (or until cooked, depending on the thickness of the tuna steak).
8. Place the tuna steaks on top of the haricot verts.
9. Vegetable
10. Use half a celery tuber. Cut the half tuber into 1.5 cm thick slices. Remove the skin and cut the slices into small cubes (approximately 1 cm -1.5 cm). Cook the cubes in the microwave or in a saucepan with some water. Allow to cool.
11. Drain the haricot verts and then place them in the middle of the serving dish. Still have room for the celery tuber.
12. Wash the tomatoes and halve them. Arrange them on the edge of the serving dish.
13. Wash the radishes and halve them. Place them on the edge of the serving dish.
14. Also, place the drained capers and olives on the edge of the serving dish.
15. Arrange the celery tuber cubes next to the haricot verts.
16. Sprinkle salt and pepper to taste over the eggs, tuna, and vegetables.
17. Serve with mayonnaise or mix in the mayonnaise.

Whole Grain Pasta With Meat Sauce
Prep time: 10 minutes
Cook time: 30 minutes
Servings: 6
Ingredients

- Whole-grain pasta – 1 pound
- Extra-lean ground beef – 1 pound
- Onion – 1, diced
- Garlic – 3 cloves, minced
- No-salt-added tomato sauce – 2 (8-ounce) cans
- Red wine – 1/3 cup
- Balsamic vinegar – 1 Tbsp.
- Dried basil - 1 tsp.
- Dried marjoram – ½ tsp.
- Dried oregano – ½ tsp.
- Dried red pepper flakes - ½ tsp.
- Dried thyme - ½ tsp.
- Freshly ground black pepper - ½ tsp.

Method

1. Follow the direction on the package and cook the pasta. Omit the salt. Drain and set aside.
2. Place onion, ground beef and garlic in a pan over medium heat. Stir-fry for 5 minutes, or until the beef has browned.
3. Add remaining ingredients and stir to combine. Simmer, uncovered, for 10 minutes, stirring occasionally.
4. Remove from heat and spoon over pasta.
5. Serve.

Nutritional Facts Per Serving
Calories: 387
Fat: 5g
Carb: 58g
Protein: 27g
Sodium 65mg
Beef Tacos
Prep time: 10 minutes
Cook time: 20 minutes
Servings: 6
Ingredients

- Extra-lean ground beef – 1 pound
- Large onion – 1, chopped Garlic – 2 cloves, minced
- No-salt-added tomato sauce – 1 (8-ounce) can Low-sodium Worcestershire sauce – 2 tsp.
- Molasses - 1 Tbsp.
- Apple cider vinegar – 1 Tbsp.
- Ground cumin – 1 Tbsp.
- Ground sweet paprika – 1 Tbsp.
- Dried red pepper flakes - ½ tsp.
- Ground black pepper to taste
- Low-sodium taco shells – 1 package
- Chopped fresh cilantro - ¼ cup Tomato and lettuce of serving

Method

1. Place the ground beef, onion, and garlic in a pan over medium heat.
2. Stir-fry for 5 minutes or until the beef is browned.
3. Lower heat to medium-low and add the Worcestershire sauce, tomato sauce, molasses, vinegar, cumin, red pepper flakes, paprika, and black pepper. Simmer, stirring frequently, about 10 minutes.
4. Heat taco shells according to package directions. Set aside.

5. Remove the sauté pan from the heat. Stir in cilantro.
6. Divide evenly between the taco shells.
7. Garnish with lettuce, tomato and serve.

Nutritional Facts Per Serving (2 tacos)
Calories: 255
Fat: 9g
Carb: 23g
Protein: 18g
Sodium 79mg
Dirty Rice
Prep time: 10 minutes
Cook time: 30 minutes
Servings: 4
Ingredients

- Extra-lean ground beef - ½ pound
- Large onion – 1, diced
- Celery – 2 stalks, diced
- Garlic – 2 cloves, minced
- Bell pepper – 1, diced
- Sodium-free beef bouillon granules - 1 tsp.
- Water - 1 cup
- Low-sodium Worcestershire sauce – 2 tsp.
- Dried thyme – 1 ½ tsp.
- Dried basil – 1 tsp.
- Dried marjoram - ½ tsp.
- Ground black pepper - ¼ tsp.
- Pinch ground cayenne pepper
- Scallions – 2, diced
- Cooked long-grain brown rice – 3 cups

Method

1. In a pan, place the onion, ground beef, celery, and garlic. Stir-fry for 5 minutes or until beef is browned.
2. Add beef bouillon, bell pepper, water, sauce, and herbs and stir to combine.
3. Bring to a boil.
4. Then reduce heat to low, and cover.
5. Simmer for 20 minutes.
6. Stir in the scallions and simmer, uncovered, for 3 minutes.
7. Remove from heat. Add cooked rice and stir to combine.
8. Serve.

Nutritional Facts Per Serving
Calories: 272
Fat: 4g
Carb: 41g
Protein: 16g
Sodium 92mg

Beef With Pea Pods
Prep time: 5 minutes
Cook time: 10 minutes
Servings: 4

Ingredients

- Thin beef steak – ¾ pound, sliced into thin strips
- Peanut oil – 1 Tbsp.
- Scallions – 3, sliced
- Garlic – 2 cloves, minced
- Minced fresh ginger – 2 tsp.
- Fresh pea pods – 4 cups, trimmed
- Homemade soy sauce – 3 Tbsp.
- Cooked brown rice – 4 cups

Method

1. Heat the oil in a pan.
2. Add the garlic, scallions, and ginger.
3. Stir-fry for 30 seconds.
4. Add the sliced beef and stir fry for 5 minutes, or until beef has browned.
5. Add pea pods and soy sauce and stir-fry for 3 minutes.
6. Remove from heat.
7. Serve with rice.

Homemade soy sauce

- Molasses – ¼ cup
- Unflavored rice wine vinegar – 3 Tbsp.
- Water – 1 Tbsp.
- Sodium-free beef bouillon granules – 1 tsp.
- Freshly ground black pepper - ½ tsp.

Method

1. Mix everything in a saucepan and heat on low for 1 minute.
2. Serve.

Nutritional Facts Per Serving
Calories: 466
Fat: 11g
Carb: 64g
Protein: 27g
Sodium 71mg
Whole-Grain Rotini With Ground Pork
Prep time: 10 minutes
Cook time: 25 minutes
Servings: 6
Ingredients

- Whole-grain rotini - 1 (13-ounce) package
- Lean ground pork – 1 pound
- Red onion – 1, chopped
- Garlic – 3 cloves, minced
- Bell pepper – 1, chopped
- Pumpkin puree – 1 cup Ground sage – 2 tsp.
- Ground rosemary – 1 tsp.
- Ground black pepper to taste

Method

1. Cook the pasta (follow the package insturctions). Omit salt, drain and set aside.
2. Heat a pan over medium heat. Add onion, garlic, and ground pork and sauté for 2 minutes.
3. Add bell pepper and sauté for 5 minutes.
4. Remove from heat. Add pasta to the pan along with remaining ingredients.
5. Mix and serve.

Nutritional Facts Per Serving
Calories: 331
Fat: 7g
Carb: 45g
Protein: 23g
Sodium 48mg
Roasted Pork Loin With Herbs
Prep time: 20 minutes
Cook time: 1 hour
Servings: 4
Ingredients

- Boneless pork loin roast – 2 lbs.
- Garlic – 3 cloves, minced Dried rosemary – 1 Tbsp.
- Dried thyme – 1 tsp.
- Dried basil – 1 tsp.
- Salt – ¼ tsp.
- Olive oil – ¼ cup
- White wine – ½ cup Pepper to taste

Method

1. Preheat the oven to 350F.
2. Crush the garlic with thyme, rosemary, basil, salt, and pepper, making a paste. Set aside.
3. Use a knife to pierce meat several times.
4. Press the garlic paste into the slits.
5. Rub the meat with the rest of the garlic mixture and olive oil.
6. Place pork loin into the oven, turning and basting with pan liquids, until the pork reaches 145F, about 1 hour. Remove the pork from the oven.
7. Place the pan over heat and add white wine, stirring the brown bits on the bottom.
8. Top roast with sauce.
9. Serve.

Nutritional Facts Per Serving
Calories: 464
Fat: 20.7g
Carb: 2.4g
Protein: 59.6g
Sodium 279mg
Garlic Lime Pork Chops
Prep time: 20 minutes
Cook time: 10 minutes
Servings: 4
Ingredients

- Lean boneless pork chops – 4 (6-oz. each)
- Garlic – 4 cloves, crushed Cumin – ½ tsp.
- Chili powder - ½ tsp.
- Paprika - ½ tsp.
- Juice of ½ lime Lime zest – 1 tsp.
- Kosher salt - ¼ tsp.
- Fresh pepper to taste

Method

1. In a bowl, season pork with cumin, chili powder, paprika, garlic salt, and pepper. Add lime juice and zest.
2. Marinate the pork for 20 minutes.
3. Line a broiler pan with foil.
4. Place the pork chops on the broiler pan and broil for 5 minutes on each side or until browned.
5. Serve.

Nutritional Facts Per Serving
Calories: 233
Fat: 13.2g
Carb: 4.3g
Protein: 25.5g
Sodium 592mg

Lamb Curry With Tomatoes And Spinach
Prep time: 10 minutes
Cook time: 12 minutes
Servings: 4

Ingredients

- Olive oil – 1 tsp.
- Lean boneless lamb – 1 pound, sliced thinly
- Onion – 1, chopped
- Garlic – 3 cloves, minced Red bell pepper – 1, chopped Salt-free tomato paste – 2 Tbsp.
- Salt-free curry powder – 1 Tbsp.
- No-salt-added diced tomatoes – 1(15-ounce) can
- Fresh baby spinach – 10 ounces
- Low-sodium beef or vegetable broth - ½ cup
- Red wine – ¼ cup
- Chopped fresh cilantro – ¼ cup Ground black pepper to taste

Method

1. Heat the oil in a pan.
2. Add lamb and brown both sides, about 2 minutes.
3. Add garlic, onion, and bell pepper. Stir-fry for 2 minutes. Stir in the curry powder and tomato paste.
4. Add the tomatoes with juice, spinach, broth, and wine and stir to mix.
5. Stir-fry for 3 to 4 minutes and lamb has cooked through.
6. Remove from heat. Season with pepper and stir in cilantro.

7. Serve.

Nutritional Facts Per Serving
Calories: 238
Fat: 7g
Carb: 14g
Protein: 27g
Sodium 167mg

Pomegranate-Marinated Leg Of Lamb
Prep time: 10 minutes
Cook time: 20 minutes
Servings: 6

Ingredients
For the marinate

- Bottled pomegranate juice - ½ cup
- Hearty red wine – ½ cup
- Ground cumin - 1 tsp.
- Dried oregano – 1 tsp.
- Crushed hot red pepper – ½ tsp.
- Garlic – 3 cloves, minced

For the lamb

- Boneless leg of lamb – 1 ¾ pound, butterflied and fat trimmed
- Kosher salt – ½ tsp.
- Olive oil spray

Method

1. To make the marinade, whisk everything in a bowl and transfer to a zippered plastic bag.
2. To prepare the lamb: add the lamb to the bag, press out the air, and close the bag. Marinate for 1 hour in the refrigerator.
3. Preheat the broiler (8 inches from the source of heat).
4. Remove the lamb from the marinade, blot with paper towels, but do not dry completely.
5. Season with salt. Spray the broiler rack with oil.
6. Place the lamb on the rack and broil, turning occasionally, about 20 minutes, or until lamb is browned and reaches 130F.
7. Remove from heat, slice and serve with carving juices on top.

Nutritional Facts Per Serving
Calories: 273

Fat: 15g

Carb: 0g

Protein: 31g

Sodium 219mg

Beef Fajitas With Peppers

Prep time: 10 minutes

Cook time: 12 minutes

Servings: 6

Ingredients

- Olive oil – 2 tsp. plus more for the spray
- Sirloin steak – 1 pound, cut into bite-size pieces
- Red bell pepper – 1, chopped
- Green bell pepper – 1, chopped
- Red onion – 1, chopped
- Garlic - 2 cloves, minced
- DASH friendly Mexican seasoning – 1 Tbsp. (or any seasoning without salt)
- Boston lettuce leaves – 12 for serving
- Lime wedges or corn tortillas for serving

Method

- Heat oil in a skillet.
- Add half of the sirloin and cook until browned on both sides, about 2 minutes. Transfer to a plate.
- Then repeat with the remaining sirloin.
- Heat the 2 tsp. oil in the skillet.
- Add onion, bell peppers, and garlic, cook and stir for 7 minutes or until tender.
- Stir in the beef with any juices and the seasoning. Transfer to a plate.
- Fill lettuce lead with beef mixture and drizzle lime juice on top.
- Roll up and serve.

Nutritional Facts Per Serving

Calories: 231

Fat: 12g

Carb: 6g

Protein: 24g

Sodium 59mg

Pork Medallions With Herbs De Provence

Prep time: 5 minutes

Cook time: 10 minutes

Servings: 2
Ingredients

- Pork tenderloin – 8 ounces, cut into 6 pieces (crosswise)
- Ground black pepper to taste Herbs de Provence – ½ tsp. Dry white wine – ¼ cup

Method

1. Season the pork with black pepper.
2. Place the pork between waxed paper sheets and roll with a rolling pin until about ¼ inch thick.
3. Cook the pork in a pan for 2 to 3 minutes on each side.
4. Remove from heat and season with the herb.
5. Place the pork on plates and keep warm.
6. Cook the wine in the pan until boiling. Scrape to get the brown bits from the bottom.
7. Serve pork with the sauce.

Nutritional Facts Per Serving
Calories: 120
Fat: 2g
Carb: 1g
Protein: 24g
Sodium 62mg
Baked Chicken
Prep time: 10 minutes
Cook time: 1 hour
Servings: 4
Ingredients

- Chicken – 3 to 4 pound, cut into parts Olive oil – 3 Tbsp.
- Thyme – ½ tsp.
- Sea salt – ¼ tsp.
- Ground black pepper
- Low-sodium chicken stock – ½ cup

Method

1. Preheat the oven to 400F.
2. Rub oil over chicken pieces. Sprinkle with salt, thyme, and pepper.
3. Place chicken in the roasting pan.
4. Bake in the oven for 30 minutes.
5. Then lower the heat to 350F.

6. Bake for 15 to 30 minutes more or until juice runs clear.
7. Serve.

Nutritional Facts Per Serving
Calories: 550
Fat: 19g
Carb: 0g
Protein: 91g
Sodium 480mg

Orange Chicken And Broccoli Stir-Fry
Prep time: 10 minutes
Cook time: 15 minutes
Servings: 4

Ingredients

- Olive oil – 1 Tbsp.
- Chicken breast – 1 pound, boneless and skinless, cut into strips
- Orange juice – 1/3 cup Homemade soy sauce - 2 Tbsp.
- Cornstarch – 2 tsp.
- Broccoli – 2 cups, cut into small pieces
- Snow peas – 1 cup
- Cabbage – 2 cups, shredded Brown rice – 2 cups, cooked Sesame seeds – 1 Tbsp.

Method

1. Combine the orange juice, soy sauce, and corn starch in a bowl. Set aside.
2. Heat oil in a pan. Add chicken.
3. Stir-fry until the chicken is golden brown on all sides, about 5 minutes.
4. Add snow peas, cabbage, broccoli, and sauce mixture.
5. Continue to stir-fry for 8 minutes or until vegetables are tender but still crisp.

Nutritional Facts Per Serving

- Calories: 340
- Fat: 8g
- Carb: 35g
- Protein: 28g
- Sodium 240mg

Mediterranean Lemon Chicken And Potatoes

Prep time: 10 minutes
Cook time: 30 minutes
Servings: 4
Ingredients

- Chicken breast – 1 ½ pound, skinless and boneless, cut into 1-inch cubes
- Yukon Gold potatoes – 1 pound, cut into cubes
- Onion – 1, chopped
- Red pepper – 1, chopped
- Low-sodium vinaigrette – ½ cup
- Lemon juice – ¼ cup Oregano – 1 tsp.
- Garlic powder – ½ tsp.
- Chopped tomato – ½ cup
- Ground black pepper to taste

Method

1. Preheat oven to 400F.
2. Except for the tomatoes, mix everything in a bowl.
3. On 4 aluminum foils, place an equal amount of chicken and potato mixture. Fold to make packets.
4. Bake at 400F for 30 minutes. Open packets.
5. Top with chopped tomatoes.
6. Season with black pepper to taste.

Nutritional Facts Per Serving

- Calories: 320
- Fat: 4g
- Carb: 34g
- Protein: 43g
- Sodium 420mg

Tandoori Chicken
Prep time: 10 minutes
Cook time: 20 minutes
Servings: 6
Ingredients

- Nonfat yogurt – 1 cup, plain
- Lemon juice – ½ cup Garlic – 5 cloves, crushed Paprika – 2 Tbsp.
- Curry powder – 1 tsp.
- Ground ginger – 1 tsp.

- Red pepper flakes – 1 tsp.
- Chicken breasts – 6, skinless and boneless, cut into 2-inch chunks
  Wooden skewers – 6, soaked in water

Method

1. Preheat the oven to 400F.
2. In a bowl, combine lemon juice, yogurt, garlic, and spices. Blend well.
3. Divide chicken and thread onto skewers. Place skewers in a baking dish.
4. Pour half of the yogurt mixture onto chicken. Cover and marinate in the refrigerator for 20 minutes
5. Spray a baking dish with cooking spray.
6. Place chicken skewers in the pan and coat with the remaining ½ of yogurt marinade.
7. Bake in the oven until chicken is cooked, about 15 to 20 minutes.
8. Serve with veggies or brown rice.

Nutritional Facts Per Serving

- Calories: 175
- Fat: 2g
- Carb: 8g
- Protein: 30g
- Sodium 105mg

Grilled Chicken Salad
Prep time: 5 minutes
Cook time: 10 minutes
Servings: 4
Ingredients
For the dressing

- Red wine vinegar – ½ cup
- Garlic – 4 cloves, minced
- Extra-virgin olive oil – 1 Tbsp.
- Finely chopped red onion – 1 Tbsp.
- Finely chopped celery -1 Tbsp. Ground black pepper to taste

For the salad

- Chicken breasts – 4 (4-ounce each), boneless, skinless
- Garlic – 2 cloves

- Lettuce leaves - 8 cups
- Ripe black olives – 16
- Navel oranges – 2, peeled and sliced

Method

1. To make the dressing, in a bowl, combine all the dressing ingredients mix and keep in the refrigerator.
2. Heat a gas grill or broiler.
3. Lightly coat the broiler pan or grill rack with cooking spray.
4. Position the cooking rack 4 to 6 inches from the heat source.
5. Rub the chicken breasts with garlic and discard the cloves.
6. Broil or grill the chicken about 5 minutes per side, or until just cooked through.
7. Slice the chicken. Arrange with lettuce, olives, and oranges.
8. Drizzle with dressing and serve.

Nutritional Facts Per Serving

- Calories: 237
- Fat: 9g
- Carb: 12g
- Protein: 27g
- Sodium 199mg

Ground Turkey Mini Meatloaves
Prep time: 10 minutes
Cook time: 30 minutes
Servings: 6
Ingredients

- Lean ground turkey – 1 ½ pound
- Onion – 1, diced
- Celery – 2, diced
- Bell pepper – 1, diced
- Garlic – 4 cloves, minced
- No-salt-added tomato sauce – 1 (8-ounce) can
- Egg white – 1
- Salt-free bread crumbs – ¾ cup Molasses – 1 Tbsp.
- Liquid smoke – ¼ tsp.
- Freshly ground black pepper - ½ tsp. Salt-free ketchup – ¼ cup

Method

1. Preheat the oven to 375F. Spray a 6-cup muffin tin with oil and set aside.
2. Place all ingredients except for ketchup in a bowl and mix well.
3. Fill the muffin cups with the mixture and press in firmly.
4. Divide the ketchup between the muffin cups and spread evenly.
5. Place muffin tin on the middle rack in the oven and bake for 30 minutes.
6. Remove, cool, and serve.

Nutritional Facts Per Serving

- Calories: 251
- Fat: 7g
- Carb: 21g
- Protein: 25g
- Sodium 112mg

Turkey And Brown Rice Stuffed Peppers
Prep time: 10 minutes
Cook time: 35 minutes
Servings: 4
Ingredients

- Bell peppers – 4, core and seeded, leave the peppers intact
- Lean ground turkey – 1 pound
- Onion – 1, diced
- Garlic – 3 cloves, minced
- Celery – 2 stalks, diced
- Cooked brown rice – 2 cups
- No-salt-added diced tomatoes – 1 (15-ounce) can Salt-free tomato paste – 2 Tbsp.
- Seedless raisins – ¼ cup Ground cumin – 2 tsp.
- Dried oregano – 1 tsp.
- Ground cinnamon – ½ tsp.
- Ground black pepper – ½ tsp.

Method

1. Preheat the oven to 425F. Grease a baking pan with oil.
2. Heat a pan over medium heat.
3. Add onion, ground turkey, garlic, and celery and sauté for 5 minutes. Remove from heat.
4. Add the remaining ingredients and mix.
5. Fill each pepper with ¼ of the mixture. Pressing firmly to pack.

6. Stand peppers in the prebaked baking pan, replace the pepper caps and then cover the pan with foil.
7. Place in the middle rack in the oven and bake for 25 to 30 minutes, or until tender.
8. Serve.

Nutritional Facts Per Serving

- Calories: 354
- Fat: 8g
- Carb: 45g
- Protein: 27g
- Sodium 126mg

Grilled Tequila Chicken With Peppers

Prep time: 10 minutes
Cook time: 30 minutes
Servings: 4
Ingredientes

- Lime juice – 1 cup
- Tequila – 1/3 cup
- Garlic – 3 cloves, chopped
- Chopped fresh cilantro – ¼ cup
- Agave nectar – 1 Tbsp.
- Ground black pepper - ½ tsp.
- Cumin   1 tsp.
- Ground coriander – ½ tsp.
- Boneless, skinless chicken breasts – 4
- Olive oil – 2 tsp.
- Green bell pepper – 1, diced
- Red bell pepper – 1, diced
- Onion – 1, diced
- Non-fat sour cream – ½ cup

Method

1. In a bowl, add the lime juice, tequila garlic, cilantro, agave nectar, black pepper, cumin, and coriander and mix well.
2. Add the chicken breasts and coat well. Cover and marinate in the for least 6 hours (in the refrigerator).
3. Heat the grill. Cook the chicken for 10 to 15 minutes per side, or no longer pink.
4. Meanwhile, heat the oil in a pan.

5. Add the pepper and onion. Stir-fry for 5 minutes. Remove from heat. Remove chicken from grill.
6. Serve with veggies and sour cream.

Nutritional Facts Per Serving

- Calories: 259
- Fat: 3g
- Carb: 18g
- Protein: 28g
- Sodium 118mg

Orange-Rosemary Roasted Chicken
Prep time: 10 minutes
Cook time: 45 minutes
Servings: 6
Ingredients

- Chicken breast halves – 3, skinless, bone-in, each 8 ounces
- Chicken legs with thigh pieces – 3, skinless, bone-in, each 8 ounces
- Garlic cloves – 2, minced Extra-virgin olive oil – 1 ½ tsp.
- Fresh rosemary – 3 tsp.
- Ground black pepper – 1/8 tsp.
- Orange juice – ½ cup

Method

1. Preheat oven at 450F. Grease a baking pan with cooking spray.
2. Rub chicken with garlic, then with oil. Sprinkle with pepper and rosemary.
3. Place the chicken pieces in the baking dish.
4. Pour the orange juice.
5. Cover and bake for 30 minutes, then flip the chicken with tongs and cook 10 to 15 minutes more or until browned. Baste the chicken with the pan juice from time to time.
6. Serve chicken with pan juice.

Nutritional Facts Per Serving

- Calories: 204
- Fat: 8g
- Carb: 2g
- Protein: 31g
- Sodium 95mg

Honey Crusted Chicken
Prep time: 10 minutes
Cook time: 25 minutes
Servings: 2
Ingredients

- Saltine crackers – 8, (2-inch square each) crushed Paprika – 1 tsp.
- Chicken breasts – 2, boneless, skinless (4-ounce each)
- Honey – 4 tsp.
- Cooking spray to grease a baking sheet

Method

1. Preheat the oven to 375F.
2. In a bowl, mix crushed crackers and paprika. Mix well.
3. In another bowl, add honey and chicken. Coat well.
4. Add to the cracker mixture and coat well.
5. Place the chicken in the prepared baking sheet.
6. Bake for 20 to 25 minutes.
7. Serve.

Nutritional Facts Per Serving

- Calories: 219
- Fat: 3g
- Carb: 21g
- Protein: 27g
- Sodium 187mg

Italian Chicken And Vegetable
Prep time: 10 minutes
Cook time: 45 minutes
Servings: 1
Ingredients

- Chicken breast – 1 skinless, boneless (3 ounces)
- Diced zucchini – ½ cup
- Diced potato – ½ cup
- Diced onion – ¼ cup
- Sliced baby carrots – ¼ cup
- Sliced mushrooms – ¼ cup
- Garlic powder – 1/8 tsp.
- Italian seasoning – ¼ tsp.

Method

1. Preheat oven to 350F.
2. Grease a parchment paper with cooking spray.
3. On the foil, add chicken, top mushrooms, carrots, onion, potato, and zucchini. Sprinkle with Italian seasoning and garlic powder.
4. Fold the foil to make a packet.
5. Place the packet on a cookie sheet.
6. Bake until chicken and vegetables are tender, about 45 minutes.
7. Serve.

Nutritional Facts Per Serving

Calories: 207
Fat: 2.5g
Carb: 23g
Protein: 23g
Sodium 72mg

Chapter Seven

SNACKS, SIDES, AND DESSERTS

*P*eanut Butter Sandwich Snacks

SmartPoints value: Green plan - 3SP, Blue plan - 3SP, Purple plan - 3SP

Total Time: 5 min, **Prep time**: 5 min, **Serves**: 1

Nutritional value: Calories - 327, Carbs - 30g, Fat - 17.9g, Protein - 15.0g

When you're looking for something sweet, chocolaty, and rich in nutrients, this easy-to-make snack will do the job. I make use of chocolate syrup as an alternative to melted chocolate. I observed that chocolate syrup has fewer Smart Points, and the small amount spreads farther. I should let you know that the chocolate syrup will not get hard, even when you refrigerate.

Ingredients

- Peanut butter (powdered) - 1 Tbsp
- Water - 2¼ tsp
- Crispbread, Whole Grain (34 degrees) - 6 crackers, or similar product
- Chocolate syrup - 1½ tsp
- Sprinkles - ¼ tsp, nonpareil

Instructions

1. Mix the powdered peanut butter and water in a clean small bowl and stir until it becomes smooth.
2. Spread the peanut butter evenly over three crackers and top it with the remaining three crackers biscuit or bread.

3. Take half a teaspoon of chocolate syrup and spread it over half the top of each cracker sandwich — top chocolate syrup with sprinkles.

Peanut Butter Apple Slices
SmartPoints value: Green plan - 4SP, Blue plan - 4SP, Purple plan - 4SP
Total time: 10 min, **Prep time**: 10 min, **Serves**: 4
Nutritional value: Calories - 218, Carbs — 31.3g, Fat — 8.1g, Protein — 11.6g
Having a healthy snack ready in about 10 minutes is a thing of joy for me. Peanut butter apple slices are just what fits into the picture of a healthy quick, nutritious snack. This apple slice is a simple and easy meal rich in protein and fiber. It is topped with peanut butter and decorated with chocolate chips and slivered almonds.

Ingredients

- Large apples - 2 pieces
- Powdered peanut butter (reconstituted) - 1/2 cup
- Semi-sweet chocolate chips - 2 tbsp
- Slivered almonds - 2 tbsp
- Pecans (chopped) - 2 tbsp

Instructions

1. Remove the core of the apple using a small paring knife or an apple corer
2. Slice the apples into thick rings.
3. Add the peanut butter on the apple slices.
4. Use chips and nuts for top-up

Baked Plantains
SmartPoints value: Green plan - 5SP, Blue plan - 5SP, Purple plan - 5SP
Total time: 40 min, **Prep time**: 5 min, **Cooking time**: 35min, **Serves**: 2
Nutritional value: Calories - 184, Carbs - 47g, Fat — 0.5g, Protein — 2g
Baked plantain is just as healthy as it is tasty. The plantain is full of good for your ingredients.

Ingredients

- Very overripe plantains (2 medium-sized)
- Misting spray (Olive oil)
- Salt to taste

Instructions

1. On a preheated oven of 350 degrees, line a baking sheet with a

silicone mat or parchment paper and spray with olive oil or non-fat cooking spray.

2. Thinly slice plantains and place them on the baking sheet evenly, then lightly mist with olive oil or the non-fat cooking spray and sprinkle with a bit of salt.

3. For about 30-35 minutes, cook in the oven flipping once about halfway through until they become golden and mostly crisp.

Baked plantains are easy to prepare and very firm. They taste sweeter when overly ripe, and firmer when they are not as ripe. Feel free to choose your style of plantain.

Strawberries & Cream Chocolate Cookie Sandwich

SmartPoints value: Green plan - 3SP, Blue plan - 3SP, Purple plan - 3SP

Total time: 5 min, Prep time: 5 min, Serves: 1

Nutritional value: Calories - 280, Carbs - 37g, Fat - 12g, Protein - 5g

I'm sure you will love this tasty summer treat. This chocolate cookie sandwich will remind you of your favorite childhood ice cream sandwich. This version is healthier, upgraded, and way easier to make in your kitchen! You can impress your loved ones with this delicious dessert/snack by making dozens of them for parties, barbecues, or special occasions with family and friends. If you don't have strawberries, you can substitute with any ripe fruit you have on hand like peaches, bananas, or raspberries.

Ingredients

- Topping (lite whipped) - 2 Tbsp
- Strawberries (hulled, sliced) - 1 medium
- Graham cracker(s) (chocolate variety) - 2 square(s)

Instructions

1. Scoop whipped topping onto one square-shaped graham cracker.
2. Top it with sliced strawberries and place another cracker on top of that.

Mini chocolate chip cookies

SmartPoints value: Green plan - 1SP, Blue plan - 1SP, Purple plan - 1SP

Total time: 26 min, **Prep time**: 10 min, **Cooking time**: 6 min, **Serves**: 48

Nutritional value: Calories - 113.7, Carbs - 16.4g, Fat - 5.9g, Protein - 0.6g

These bite-size cookies might be small, but they pack a chocolate punch. I often use dark brown sugar in making these cookies as it contains more molasses than the light brown variety. The dark brown sugar adds a rich, complex flavor to these cookies, making them moist and chewy. In case you have only light brown sugar available, you don't have to go out of your way to get the dark variety. That will work just fine. You can replace the chocolate chips with any other one you like, be it cinnamon chips, toffee, butterscotch, or white chocolate chips. You can even stir in some chopped nuts to make things a little cDashchy.

Ingredients

- Butter (salted, softened) - 2 Tbsp
- Canola oil - 2 tsp
- Brown sugar (packed, dark-variety) - ½ cup(s)
- Vanilla extract - 1 tsp
- Table salt - ⅛ tsp
- Egg white(s) - 1 large
- All-purpose flour - ¾ cup(s)
- Baking soda - ¼ tsp
- Chocolate chips (semi-sweet) - 3 oz, about 1/2 cup

Instructions

1. Prepare the oven by preheating it to 375°F.
2. Mix the butter, oil, and sugar in a medium bowl.
3. Add vanilla and egg white, then mix thoroughly to combine. Toss in some salt to taste.
4. Mix the flour and baking soda in a small bowl and stir them into the batter.
5. Add the chocolate chips to the batter and stir to distribute evenly throughout.
6. Put forty-eight half-teaspoons of dough onto two large nonstick baking sheets. Leave small spaces between the cookies.
7. Bake the cookies until they become golden around the edges; about 4 to 6 minutes.
8. Cool the baked cookies on a wire rack.

Chocolate-Peppermint Thins

SmartPoints value: Green plan - 3SP, Blue plan - 3SP, Purple plan - 3SP

Total Time: 1hr 16 min, Prep time: 15 min, Cooking time: 5 min, Serves: 16

Nutritional value: Calories - 175, Carbs – 21g, Fat – 5g, Protein – 7g

My homemade chocolate peppermint thin comes with a splash of peppermint extract, and divine copycat thin mint cookies to satisfy my cravings

Ingredients

- Chocolate chunk (coarsely chopped) - 3½ oz
- Chocolate wafer(s) (thin variety) - 16 item(s)
- Candy cane (finely crushed) - 1 oz

Instructions

1. Arrange a large baking sheet with parchment or paper wax and line cookies close together in a single layer.
2. At 5 seconds interval, melt chocolate in a microwavable bowl and stir between each interval until all but one or two pieces melted, then remove from microwave and stir until fully dissolved.
3. Put the melted chocolate in a plastic bag and cut off a corner; in a zig-zag pattern, pipe the chocolate over cookies and sprinkle with the crushed candy cane, keep it refrigerated until its set for at least an hour or overnight. Serve as desired (1 cookie per serving)

Chocolate-Dipped Baby Bananas
SmartPoints value: Green plan - 3SP, Blue plan - 3SP, Purple plan - 3SP
Total time: 20 min, Prep time: 5 min, Cooking time: --, Serves: 12
Nutritional value: Calories - 210, Carbs – 31.2g, Fat – 1g, Protein – 5.4g
Chocolate-dipped baby bananas are just perfect for casual parties for both kids and adults. With the banana and chocolate combination, it's so irresistible. Alternatively, you can replace baby bananas with four regular bananas cut crosswise into thirds.
Ingredients

- Baby-variety banana (peeled) - 12 small
- Chocolate (semisweet, chopped) - 3 oz
- Butter (unsalted) - ¾ tsp
- Coconut (shredded, unsweetened) - 2 tbsp

Instructions

1. Place large baking sheet with wax paper and insert wooden craft stick in one end of each banana.
2. Mix butter and chocolate in a medium microwave bowl, then microwave on high heat for about 1minute.
3. Taking one banana after another spoon the chocolate over the bananas cover, and sprinkle it with coconut while it is on a baking sheet. Keep it refrigerated until the chocolate sets in about 15 minutes.
4. Serve as desired (1 banana per serving)

Fall Harvest Salad
SmartPoints value: Green plan - 3SP, Blue plan - 1SP, Purple plan - 1SP
Total time: 15 min, **Prep time**: 15 min, **Cooking time**: 0 min, **Serves**: 4
Nutritional value: Calories - 175, Carbs – 25.7g, Fat – 7.6g, Protein – 4.8g

Whether or not you have planned for a holiday meal, this fall harvest salad will fire up some inspiration, and get those juices flowing.

If this would be your first time giving this a try, I trust you'll be looking for excuses to make this salad over and over again.

There are two most seen together in desserts, that's the flavor combination of cinnamon and apples. They both make undeniable mouthwatering delicious flavors in this fall harvest salad.

I also love to add some Honey crisp apples (my favorite apple), or sometimes I use Fuji, a pink lady on this Harvest Salad. They all blend well.

To prevent my apples from getting brown after slicing, I avoid exposing it to air. When the apples turn brown, your salad would not be as pretty as you would love it. I will add a little, so that will help you avoid this problem and keep your apples beautiful

After slicing your apple, submerge the slices in a bowl of saltwater (I usually mix about 1 tbsp of salt with 1 ½ cups of water) then stir it until the salt dissolves then add in the apple slices. Let it sit for about 5 minutes and then rinse the slices with water and pat dry with a paper towel.

That's just it. So simple, yeah? This way of cutting apples has been working for me for ages, and I love it more because it's cheaper and cleaner than buying those bags of pre-cut apples.

Ingredients

- Kale greens (baby variety) - 4-5 cups
- Large apple (thinly sliced) - 1 piece
- Sweet pumpkin seeds (toasted) - 1/3 cup

For dressing

- Olive oil - 1 tbsp
- Maple Syrup - 1 tbsp
- Red wine vinegar - 2 tbsp
- Shallot (minced) - 1 piece
- Cinnamon - ¼ tsp
- Dijon mustard - 1 tsp
- Pepper and salt to taste

Instructions

1. Beat all the ingredients for the dressing together in a small bowl
2. Toss the ingredients for the salad in a large bowl
3. Pour the processed dressing over the salad and toss to coat evenly
4. This perfect dish is sure to impress your guests and compliment your holiday meal. Be careful not to lick the bowl.

Mediterranean Baked Tilapia
SmartPoints value: Green plan - 3SP, Blue plan - 1SP, Purple plan - 1SP
Total time: 25 min, **Prep time**: 10 min, **Cooking time**: 15 min,
Serves: 4
Nutritional value: Calories - 129, Fat - 5g, Protein - 21g

During festive periods, it gets more tempting to eat just every meal that crosses by you. That's why I'm creating this recipe to help you maintain low SP meals during those periods. Let's take a look at the deliciously outlined recipe.

Ingredients

- Tilapia fillets - 1 lb (about eight fillets)
- Olive oil - 1 tsp
- Butter - 1 tbsp
- Shallots (finely chopped) - 2 pieces
- Garlic (minced) - 3 cloves
- Cumin (ground) - 1 1/2 tsp
- Paprika (1 1/2 tsp)
- Capers (1/4 cup)
- Dill (finely chopped, fresh) - 1/4 cup
- Lemon juice - from 1 lemon
- Pepper and salt to taste

Instructions

1. Line a rimmed baking sheet with parchment paper or foil over a preheated oven of 375 degrees. Mist with cooking spray and spread fish fillets evenly on the baking sheet.
2. Combine the paprika, pepper, and salt in a small bowl. Season the fish fillets with the spice mixture on both sides.
3. Whisk together in a small bowl, the melted butter, olive oil, lemon juice, shallots, and garlic then brush evenly over the fish fillets. Top with the capers.
4. Making sure not to overcook, bake in the oven for about 10-15 minutes, then remove from oven and top with fresh dill.

Two-Ingredient Ice Cream Cupcake Bites
SmartPoints value: Green plan - 2SP, Blue plan - 2SP, Purple plan - 2SP
Total Time: 32 min, Prep time: 5 min, Cooking time: 12 min, Serves: 12
Nutritional value: Calories - 109, Carbs - 10g, Fat - 8g, Protein - 12g

You won't get any fresh-baked dessert or snack that is easier or more lovely than these two-ingredient mini cupcakes. All it takes is to mash your favorite WW ice cream bars and combine with self-rising flour, then bake it. You can eat it as it is or finish it off with whipped topping and sprinkles. They are perfect for birthday parties, snacks, and more.

Ingredients

- Ice cream bars (WW Dark Chocolate-raspberry) - 6 bar(s)
- White flour (self-rising) - 10 Tbsp
- Whipped topping (light) - 4 Tbsp
- Sprinkles (rainbow) - ½ Tbsp

Instructions

1. After preheating the oven to 350°F, coat twelve mini muffin holes with cooking spray
2. Drop the ice cream from the sticks into a large bowl and allow it to melt slightly, then add some white flour and stir until it is well-mixed.
3. Evenly fill prepared muffin holes with the mixture and bake until a tester inserted in the center of a cupcake comes out without anything sticking to it; about 10-12 minutes.
4. Allow the cupcakes to cool in the pan for a few minutes before taking them out. Collect the processed muffins from the pan and cool completely.
5. Put one teaspoon of whipped topping in each cooled cupcake and divide the sprinkles over the top.

Lemon Blueberry Cheesecake Yogurt Bark
SmartPoints value: 1SP

Total time: 1 hr 15 mins, **Prep time**: 15 mins, **Chill time**: 1 hr, **Serves** - 12

Nutritional value: Calories - 124, Carbs - 12.7g, Fat - 0.2g, Protein - 18.2g

Ingredients

- Greek yogurt (plain non-fat) - 1 cup
- Agave nectar - 1 tablespoon
- Lemon zest - 1/2 teaspoon
- Lemon juice (fresh-squeezed) - 1/2 teaspoon
- Blueberries (fresh) - 1 cup
- Graham crackers (crushed into crumbs) - 3 squares (gluten-free if you like)

Instructions

1. Line a 9x5-inch loaf pan with aluminum foil so that the foil hangs over sides of the pan.

2. Mix the yogurt, lemon zest, agave nectar, and lemon juice in a small mixing bowl, then stir.

3. Turn in the blueberries gently with three tablespoons crushed graham cracker crumbs just until adequately mixed.

4. Evenly spread the mixture into the loaf pan you earlier prepared. Get the remaining cracker crumbs and sprinkle over the top.

5. Use aluminum foil to cover the loaf pan and refrigerate for at least 1 hour; until it is frozen.

6. Once the mixture is frozen, remove the pan from the freezer and use overhanging foil as handles to lift the bark from the pan.

7. Put the frozen mixture on a cutting board and slice it into eight squares.

8. Cut each square diagonally, creating two triangles. (If the frozen dough is too difficult to cut, allow it to sit out at room temperature to soften. Alternatively, you can keep the knife inside hot water before cutting.)

9. Keep the cut portions in an airtight container inside the freezer until you are ready to serve. Allow the cut triangles to sit on the table at room temperature to soften slightly before serving if it is too frozen

Dark Chocolate Avocado Mousse

This chocolate delicacy, loaded with healthy fats, fiber, and antioxidants, is a perfect dessert recipe.

SmartPoints value - 9 SP

Total time: 1 hr 10 mins, **Prep time**: 10 mins, **Chill time**: 1 hr, **Serves:** 2

Nutritional value: Calories - 434, Carbs - 53g, Fat - 29g, Protein - 6g

Ingredients

- Avocado (very ripe, peeled and seeded) - 1 large
- Dark baking chocolate (70% cacao, melted) - 2 ounces
- Cocoa powder (unsweetened) - 2 Tbsp
- Almond milk (unsweetened) - 1/4 cup
- Maple syrup - 2 Tbsp
- Pure vanilla extract - 1/4 Tsp
- Cinnamon (ground) - A pinch
- Salt - A pinch

Instructions

1. Get a blender and put in avocado, maple syrup, melted chocolate, milk, cocoa powder, vanilla, cinnamon, and salt.

2. Process the content of the blender until you get a smooth and

creamy mixture. To make the mousse thinner, add more milk or less milk for a thicker mousse.

3. Pour the mixture evenly into two small dessert glasses.
4. Chill it for at least 1 hour in the refrigerator before serving.

Hearty Chia and Blackberry Pudding
Serving: 2
Prep Time: 45 minutes
Cook Time: Nil
Ingredients:

- ¼ cup chia seeds
- ½ cup blackberries, fresh
- 1 teaspoon liquid sweetener
- 1 cup coconut almond milk, full fat and unsweetened
- 1 teaspoon vanilla extract

How To:

1. Take the vanilla, liquid sweetener and coconut almond milk and add to blender.
2. Process until thick.
3. Add in blackberries and process until smooth.
4. Divide the mixture between cups and chill for 30 minutes.
5. Serve and enjoy!

Nutrition (Per Serving)

- Calories: 437
- Fat: 38g
- Carbohydrates: 8g
- Protein: 8g

Special Cocoa Brownie Bombs
Serving: 12
Prep Time: 15 minutes
Cooking Time: 25 minutes
Freeze Time: None
Ingredients:

- 2 tablespoons grass-fed almond butter
- 1 whole egg
- 2 teaspoons vanilla extract
- ¼ teaspoon baking powder

- 1/3 cup heavy cream
- 3/4 cup almond butter
- ¼ cocoa powder
- A pinch of sunflower seeds

How To:

1. Break the eggs and whisk until smooth.
2. Add in all the wet ingredients and mix well.
3. Make the batter by mixing all the dry ingredients and sifting them into the wet ingredients.
4. Pour into a greased baking pan.
5. Bake for 25 minutes at 350 degrees F or until a toothpick inserted in the middle comes out clean.
6. Let it cool, slice and serve.

Nutrition (Per Serving)

- Total Carbs: 1g
- Fiber: 0g
- Protein: 1g
- Fat: 20g

Gentle Blackberry Crumble
Serving: 4
Prep Time: 10 minutes
Cook Time: 45 minutes
Smart Points: 4
Ingredients:

- ½ cup coconut flour
- ½ cup banana, peeled and mashed
- 6 tablespoons water
- 3 cups fresh blackberries
- ½ cup arrowroot flour
- 1 ½ teaspoons baking soda
- 4 tablespoons almond butter, melted
- 1 tablespoon fresh lemon juice

How To:

1. Pre-heat your oven to 300 degrees F.
2. Take a baking dish and grease it lightly.
3. Take a bowl and mix all of the ingredients except the blackberries,

mix well.
4. Place blackberries in the bottom of your baking dish and top with flour.
5. Bake for 40 minutes.
6. Serve and enjoy!

Nutrition (Per Serving)

- Calories: 12
- Fat: 7g
- Carbohydrates: 10g
- Protein: 4g

Mini Minty Happiness
Serving: 12
Prep Time: 45 minutes
Cooking Time: None Freeze Time: 2 hours
Ingredients:

- 2 teaspoons vanilla extract
- 1 ½ cups coconut oil
- 1 ¼ cups sunflower seed almond butter
- ½ cup dried parsley
- 1 teaspoon peppermint extract
- A pinch of sunflower seeds
- 1 cup dark chocolate chips Stevia to taste

How To:

1. Melt together coconut oil and dark chocolate chips over a double boiler.
2. Take a food processor, add all the ingredients into it and pulse until smooth.
3. Pour into round molds.
4. Let it freeze.

Nutrition (Per Serving)

- Total Carbs: 7g
- Fiber: 1g
- Protein: 3g
- Fat: 25g

Astonishing Maple Pecan Bacon Slices

Serving: 12
Prep Time: 10 minutes
Cooking Time: 25 minutes
Freeze Time: None
Ingredients:

- tablespoon sugar-free maple syrup
- 12 bacon slices
- Granulated Stevia to taste
- 15-20 drops Stevia For the coating:
- 4 tablespoons dark cocoa powder
- ¼ cup pecans, chopped
- 15-20 drops Stevia

How To:

1. Take a baking tray and lay the bacon slices on it.
2. Rub with maple syrup and Stevia, flip the slices and do the same with the other side.
3. Bake for 10-15 minutes at 227 degrees F.
4. After they've baked, drain the bacon grease.
5. To form a batter, mix the bacon grease, Stevia and cocoa powder.
6. Dip the bacon slices into the batter and roll in the chopped pecans.
7. Allow to air dry until the chocolate hardens.

Nutrition (Per Serving)

- Total Carbs: 1g
- Fiber: 0g
- Protein: 10g
- Fat: 11g

Generous Maple and Pecan Bites
Serving: 12
Prep Time: 10 minutes
Cooking Time: 25 minutes
Freeze Time: None
Ingredients:

- 1 cup almond meal
- ½ cup coconut oil
- ½ cup flaxseed meal
- ½ cup sugar-free chocolate chips
- 2 cups pecans, chopped

- ½ cup sugar-free maple syrup
- 20-25 drops Stevia

How To:

1. Take a baking dish and spread the pecans.
2. Bake at 350 degrees F until aromatic.
3. This will usually take from 6 to 8 minutes.
4. Meanwhile, sift together all the dry ingredients.
5. Add the roasted pecans to the mix and mix them properly.
6. Add the coconut oil and maple syrup.
7. Stir to make a thick, sticky mixture.
8. Take a bread pan lined with parchment paper, and pour the mixture into it.
9. Bake for about 18 minutes.
10. Slice and serve.

Nutrition (Per Serving)

- Total Carbs: 6g
- Fiber: 0g
- Protein: 5g
- Fat: 30g

Carrot Ball Delight
Serving: 4
Prep Time: 10 minutes
Cook Time: Nil
Ingredients:

- 6 Medjool dates pitted
- 1 carrot, finely grated
- ¼ cup raw walnuts
- ¼ cup unsweetened coconut, shredded
- 1 teaspoon nutmeg
- 1/8 teaspoon sunflower seeds

How To:

1. Take a food processor and add dates, ¼ cup of grated carrots, sunflower seeds coconut, nutmeg.
2. Mix well and puree the mixture.
3. Add the walnuts and remaining ¼ cup of carrots.
4. Pulse the mixture until you have a chunky texture.

5. Form balls using your hand and roll them up in coconut.
6. Top with carrots and chill.
7. Enjoy!

Nutrition (Per Serving)

- Calories: 326
- Fat: 16g
- Carbohydrates: 42g
- Protein: 3g

Awesome Brownie Muffins
Serving: 5
Prep Time: 10 minutes
Cooking Time: 35 minutes
Ingredients:

- 1 cup golden flaxseed meal
- ¼ cup cocoa powder
- 1 tablespoon cinnamon
- ½ tablespoon baking powder
- ½ teaspoon sunflower seeds
- 1 whole large egg
- 2 tablespoons coconut oil
- ¼ cup sugar-free caramel syrup
- ½ cup pumpkin puree
- 1 teaspoon vanilla extract
- 1 teaspoon apple cider vinegar
- ¼ cup almonds, slivered

How To:

1. Pre-heat your oven to 350 degrees F.
2. Take a mixing bowl and add all of the listed ingredients and mix everything well.
3. Take your desired number of muffin tins and line them with paper liners.
4. Scoop the batter into the muffin tins, filling them to about 1/4 of the liner.
5. Sprinkle a bit of almond on top.
6. Place them in your oven and bake for 15 minutes.
7. Serve warm.

Nutrition (Per Serving)

- Total Carbs: 16
- Fiber: 2g
- Protein: 3g
- Fat: 31g

Spice Friendly Muffins
Serving: 12
Prep Time: 5 minutes
Cooking Time: 45minute
Ingredients:

- ½ cup raw hemp hearts
- ½ cup flaxseeds
- ¼ cup chia seeds
- 2 tablespoons Psyllium husk powder
- 1 tablespoon cinnamon
- Stevia taste
- ½ teaspoon baking powder
- ½ teaspoon sunflower seeds
- 1 cup of water

How To:

1. Pre-heat your oven to 350 degrees F.
2. Line muffin tray with liners.
3. Take a large sized mixing bowl and add peanut almond butter, pumpkin, sweetener, coconut almond milk, flaxseed and mix well.
4. Keep stirring until the mixture has been thoroughly combined.
5. Take another bowl and add baking powder, spices and coconut flour.
6. Mix well.
7. Add the dry ingredients into the wet bowl and stir until the coconut flour has mixed well.
8. Allow it to sit for a while until the coconut flour has absorbed all of the moisture.
9. Divide the mixture amongst your muffin tins and bake for 45 minutes.
10. Enjoy!

Nutrition (Per Serving)

- Total Carbs: 7g
- Fiber: 3g
- Protein: 6g

- Fat: 15g

Simple Gingerbread Muffins
Serving: 12
Prep Time: 5 minutes
Cooking Time: 30 minutes
Ingredients:

- 1 tablespoon ground flaxseed
- 6 tablespoons coconut almond milk
- 1 tablespoon apple cider vinegar
- ½ cup peanut almond butter
- 2 tablespoons gingerbread spice blend
- 1 teaspoon baking powder
- 1 teaspoon vanilla extract
- 2 tablespoons Swerve

How To:

1. Pre-heat your oven to 350 degrees F.
2. Take a bowl and add flaxseeds, sweetener, sunflower seeds, vanilla, spices and your non-dairy almond milk.
3. Keep it on the side for a while.
4. Add peanut almond butter, baking powder and keep mixing until combined well.
5. Stir in peanut almond butter and baking powder.
6. Mix well.
7. Spoon the mixture into muffin liners.
8. Bake for 30 minutes.
9. Allow them to cool and enjoy!

Nutrition (Per Serving)

- Total Carbs: 13g
- Fiber: 4g
- Protein: 11g
- Fat: 23g

Fantastic Cauliflower Bagels
Serving: 12
Prep Time: 10 minutes
Cooking Time: 30 minutes
Ingredients:

- 1 large cauliflower, divided into florets and roughly chopped
- ¼ cup nutritional yeast
- ¼ cup almond flour
- ½ teaspoon garlic powder
- 1 ½ teaspoon fine sea sunflower seeds
- 1 whole egg
- 1 tablespoon sesame seeds

How To:

1. Pre-heat your oven to 400 degrees F.
2. Line a baking sheet with parchment paper, keep it on the side.
3. Blend cauliflower in the food processor and transfer to a bowl.
4. Add nutritional yeast, almond flour, garlic powder and sunflower seeds to a bowl, mix.
5. Take another bowl and whisk in eggs, add to cauliflower mix.
6. Give the dough a stir.
7. Incorporate the mix into the egg mix.
8. Make balls from dough, making a hole using your thumb into each ball.
9. Arrange them on your prepped sheet, flattening them into bagel shapes.
10. Sprinkle sesame seeds and bake for 30 minutes.
11. Remove oven and let them cool, enjoy!

Nutrition (Per Serving)

- Total Carbs: 1.5g
- Fiber: 1g
- Protein: 2g
- Fat: 5.8g

Nutmeg Nougats
Serving: 12
Prep Time: 10 minutes
Cooking Time: 5 minutes
Freeze Time: 30 minutes
Ingredients:

- 1 cup coconut, shredded
- 1 cup low-fat cream
- 1 cup cashew almond butter
- ½ teaspoon ground nutmeg

How To:

1. Melt the cashew almond butter over a double boiler.
2. Stir in nutmeg and dairy cream.
3. Remove from the heat.
4. Allow to cool down a little.
5. Keep in the refrigerator for at least 30 minutes.
6. Take out from the fridge and make small balls.
7. Coat with shredded coconut.
8. Let it cool for 2 hours and then serve.

Nutrition (Per Serving)

- Total Carbs: 13g
- Fiber: 8g
- Protein: 3g
- Fat: 34g

Limey Savory Pie
Serving: 12
Prep Time: 5 minutes
Cooking Time: 5 minutes
Freeze Time: 2 hours
Ingredients:

- 1 tablespoon ground cinnamon
- 3 tablespoons almond butter
- 1 cup almond flour
- For the filling:
- 3 tablespoons grass-fed almond butter
- 4 ounces full-fat cream cheese
- ¼ cup coconut oil
- 2 limes
- A handful of baby spinach Stevia to taste

How To:

1. Mix cinnamon and almond butter to form a crumble mixture.
2. Press this mixture into the bottom of 12 muffin cups.
3. Bake for 7 minutes at 350 degrees F.
4. Juice the lime and grate for zest while the crust is baking.
5. Take a food processor and add all the filling ingredients.
6. Blend until smooth.
7. Let it cool naturally.

8. Pour the mixture in the center.
9. Freeze until set and serve.

Nutrition (Per Serving)

- Total Carbs: 2g
- Fiber: 1g
- Protein: 3g
- Fat: 1g

Supreme Raspberry Chocolate Bombs
Serving: 6
Prep Time: 10 minutes
Cooking Time: 10 minutes
Freeze Time: 1-hour
Ingredients:

- ½ cacao almond butter
- ½ coconut manna
- 4 tablespoons powdered coconut almond milk
- 3 tablespoons granulated stevia
- ¼ cup dried and crushed raspberries, frozen

How To:

1. Prepare your double boiler to medium heat and melt the cacao almond butter and coconut manna.
2. Stir in vanilla extract.
3. Take another dish and add coconut powder and sugar substitute.
4. Stir the coconut mix into the cacao almond butter, 1 tablespoon at a time, making sure to keep mixing after each addition.
5. Add the crushed dried raspberries.
6. Mix well and portion it out into muffin tins.
7. Chill for 60 minutes and enjoy!

Nutrition (Per Serving)

- Total Carbs: 7g
- Fiber: 1g
- Protein: 11g
- Fat: 21g

The Perfect Orange Ponzu
Serving: 8

Prep Time: 30 minutes
Cook Time: 5 minutes
Ingredients:

- ¼ cup coconut aminos
- ½ cup rice vinegar
- 2 tablespoons dry fish flakes
- 1 (1 inch) square kombu (kelp)
- 1 orange, quartered

How To:

1. Take a saucepan and place it over medium heat.
2. Add coconut aminos, rice vinegar, fish flakes, kombu, orange quarters and let the mixture sit for 30 minutes.
3. Bring the mix to a boil and immediately remove from the heat.
4. Let it cool and strain through a cheesecloth.
5. Serve and enjoy!

Nutrition (Per Serving)

- Calories: 15
- Fat: 0g
- Carbohydrates: 4g
- Protein: 0.8g

Hearty Cashew and Almond butter
Serving: 1 and ½ cups
Prep Time: 5 minutes
Cook Time: Nil
Ingredients:

- 1 cup almonds, blanched
- 1/3 cup cashew nuts
- 2 tablespoons coconut oil
- Sunflower seeds as needed
- ½ teaspoon cinnamon

How To:

1. Pre-heat your oven to 350 degrees F.
2. Bake almonds and cashews for 12 minutes.
3. Let them cool.
4. Transfer to food processor and add remaining ingredients.

5. Add oil and keep blending until smooth.
6. **Serve and enjoy! Nutrition (Per Serving)**

Calories: 205

- Fat: 19g
- Carbohydrates: g[MOU3]
- Protein: 2.8g

The Refreshing Nutter
Serving: 1
Prep Time: 10 minutes
Ingredients:

- 1 tablespoon chia seeds
- 2 cups water
- 1 ounces Macadamia Nuts
- 1-2 packets Stevia, optional
- 1 ounce hazelnut

How To:

1. Add all the listed ingredients to a blender.
2. Blend on high until smooth and creamy.
3. Enjoy your smoothie.

Nutrition (Per Serving)

- Calories: 452
- Fat: 43g
- Carbohydrates: 15g
- Protein: 9g

Elegant Cranberry Muffins
Serving: 24 muffins
Prep Time: 10 minutes
Cooking Time: 20 minutes
Ingredients:

- 2 cups almond flour
- 2 teaspoons baking soda
- ¼ cup avocado oil
- 1 whole egg
- ¾ cup almond milk

- ½ cup Erythritol
- ½ cup apple sauce
- Zest of 1 orange
- 2 teaspoons ground cinnamon
- 2 cup fresh cranberries

How To:

1. Pre-heat your oven to 350 degrees F.
2. Line muffin tin with paper muffin cups and keep them on the side.
3. Add flour, baking soda and keep it on the side.
4. Take another bowl and whisk in remaining ingredients and add flour, mix well.
5. Pour batter into prepared muffin tin and bake for 20 minutes.
6. Once done, let it cool for 10 minutes.
7. Serve and enjoy!

Nutrition (Per Serving)

- Total Carbs: 7g
- Fiber: 2g
- Protein: 2.3g
- Fat: 7g

Apple and Almond Muffins
Serving: 6 muffins
Prep Time: 10 minutes
Cooking Time: 20 minutes
Ingredients:

- 6 ounces ground almonds
- 1 teaspoon cinnamon
- ½ teaspoon baking powder
- 1 pinch sunflower seed
- 1 whole egg
- 1 teaspoon apple cider vinegar
- 2 tablespoons Erythritol
- 1/3 cup apple sauce

How To:

1. Pre-heat your oven to 350 degrees F.
2. Line muffin tin with paper muffin cups, keep them on the side.

3. Mix in almonds, cinnamon, baking powder, sunflower seeds and keep it on the side.
4. Take another bowl and beat in eggs, apple cider vinegar, apple sauce, Erythritol.
5. Add the mix to dry ingredients and mix well until you have a smooth batter.
6. Pour batter into tin and bake for 20 minutes.
7. Once done, let them cool.
8. Serve and enjoy!

Nutrition (Per Serving)

- Total Carbs: 10
- Fiber: 4g
- Protein: 13g
- Fat: 17g

Stylish Chocolate Parfait
Serving: 4
Prep Time: 2 hours
Cook Time: nil
Ingredients:

- 2 tablespoons cocoa powder
- 1 cup almond milk
- 1 tablespoon chia seeds
- Pinch of sunflower seeds
- ½ teaspoon vanilla extract

How To:

1. Take a bowl and add cocoa powder, almond milk, chia seeds, vanilla extract and stir.
2. Transfer to dessert glass and place in your fridge for 2 hours.
3. Serve and enjoy!

Nutrition (Per Serving)

- Calories: 130
- Fat: 5g
- Carbohydrates: 7g
- Protein: 16g

Supreme Matcha Bomb

Serving: 10
Prep Time: 100 minutes
Cook Time: Nil
Ingredients:

- 3/4 cup hemp seeds
- ½ cup coconut oil
- 2 tablespoons coconut almond butter
- 1 teaspoon Matcha powder
- 2 tablespoons vanilla bean extract
- ½ teaspoon mint extract Liquid stevia

How To:

1. Take your blender/food processor and add hemp seeds, coconut oil, Matcha, vanilla extract and stevia.
2. Blend until you have a nice batter and divide into silicon molds.
3. Melt coconut almond butter and drizzle on top.
4. Let the cups chill and enjoy!

Nutrition (Per Serving)

- Calories: 200
- Fat: 20g
- Carbohydrates: 3g
- Protein: 5g

Mesmerizing Avocado and Chocolate Pudding
Serving: 2
Prep Time: 30 minutes
Cook Time: Nil
Ingredients:

- 1 avocado, chunked
- 1 tablespoon natural sweetener such as stevia
- 2 ounces cream cheese, at room temp
- ¼ teaspoon vanilla extract
- 4 tablespoons cocoa powder, unsweetened

How To:

1. Blend listed ingredients in blender until smooth.
2. Divide the mix between dessert bowls, chill for 30 minutes.
3. Serve and enjoy!

Nutrition (Per Serving)

- Calories: 281
- Fat: 27g
- Carbohydrates: 12g
- Protein: 8g

Hearty Pineapple Pudding
Serving: 4
Prep Time: 10 minutes
Cooking Time: 5 hours
Ingredients:

- 1 teaspoon baking powder
- 1 cup coconut flour
- 3 tablespoons stevia
- 3 tablespoons avocado oil
- ½ cup coconut milk
- ½ cup pecans, chopped
- ½ cup pineapple, chopped
- ½ cup lemon zest, grated
- 1 cup pineapple juice, natural

How To:

1. Grease Slow Cooker with oil.
2. Take a bowl and mix in flour, stevia, baking powder, oil, milk, pecans, pineapple, lemon zest, pineapple juice and stir well.
3. Pour the mix into the Slow Cooker.
4. Place lid and cook on LOW for 5 hours.
5. Divide between bowls and serve.
6. Enjoy!

Nutrition (Per Serving)

- Calories: 188
- Fat: 3g
- Carbohydrates: 14g
- Protein: 5g

Healthy Berry Cobbler
Serving: 8
Prep Time: 10 minutes
Cooking Time: 2 hours 30 minutes

Ingredients:

- 1 ¼ cups almond flour
- 1 cup coconut sugar
- 1 teaspoon baking powder
- ½ teaspoon cinnamon powder
- 1 whole egg
- ¼ cup low-fat milk
- 2 tablespoons olive oil
- 2 cups raspberries
- 2 cups blueberries

How To:

1. Take a bowl and add almond flour, coconut sugar, baking powder and cinnamon.
2. Stir well .
3. Take another bowl and add egg, milk, oil, raspberries, blueberries and stir.
4. Combine both of the mixtures.
5. Grease your Slow Cooker.
6. Pour the combined mixture into your Slow Cooker and cook on HIGH for 2 hours 30 minutes.
7. Divide between serving bowls and enjoy!

Nutrition (Per Serving)

- Calories: 250
- Fat: 4g
- Carbohydrates: 30g
- Protein: 3g

Tasty Poached Apples
Serving: 8
Prep Time: 10 minutes
Cooking Time: 2 hours 30 minutes
Ingredients:

- 6 apples, cored, peeled and sliced
- 1 cup apple juice, natural
- 1 cup coconut sugar
- 1 tablespoon cinnamon powder

How To:

1. Grease Slow Cooker with cooking spray.
2. Add apples, sugar, juice, cinnamon to your Slow Cooker.
3. Stir gently.
4. Place lid and cook on HIGH for 4 hours.
5. Serve cold and enjoy!

Nutrition (Per Serving)

- Calories: 180
- Fat: 5g
- Carbohydrates: 8g
- Protein: 4g

Home Made Trail Mix For The Trip
Serving: 4
Prep Time: 10 minutes
Cook Time: 55 minutes
Ingredients:

- ¼ cup raw cashews
- ¼ cup almonds
- ¼ cup walnuts
- 1 teaspoon cinnamon
- 2 tablespoons melted coconut oil
- Sunflower seeds as needed

How To:

1. Line baking sheet with parchment paper.
2. Pre-heat your oven to 275 degrees F.
3. Melt coconut oil and keep it on the side.
4. Combine nuts to large mixing bowl and add cinnamon and melted coconut oil.
5. Stir.
6. Sprinkle sunflower seeds.
7. Place in oven and brown for 6 minutes.
8. Enjoy!

Nutrition (Per Serving)

- Calories: 363
- Fat: 22g
- Carbohydrates: 41g
- Protein: 7g

Heart Warming Cinnamon Rice Pudding
Serving: 4
Prep Time: 10 minutes
Cooking Time: 5 hours
Ingredients:

- 6 ½ cups water
- 1 cup coconut sugar
- 2 cups white rice
- 2 cinnamon sticks
- ½ cup coconut, shredded

How To:

1. Add water, rice, sugar, cinnamon and coconut to your Slow Cooker.
2. Gently stir.
3. Place lid and cook on HIGH for 5 hours.
4. Discard cinnamon.
5. Divide pudding between dessert dishes and enjoy!

Nutrition (Per Serving)
Calories: 173
Fat: 4g
Carbohydrates: 9g
Protein: 4g
Pure Avocado Pudding
Serving: 4
Prep Time: 3 hours
Cook Time: nil
Ingredients:

- 1 cup almond milk
- 2 avocados, peeled and pitted
- ¾ cup cocoa powder
- 1 teaspoon vanilla extract
- 2 tablespoons stevia
- ¼ teaspoon cinnamon
- Walnuts, chopped for serving

How To:

1. Add avocados to a blender and pulse well.
2. Add cocoa powder, almond milk, stevia, vanilla bean extract and pulse the mixture well.

3. Pour into serving bowls and top with walnuts.
4. Chill for 2-3 hours and serve!

Nutrition (Per Serving)

- Calories: 221
- Fat: 8g
- Carbohydrates: 7g
- Protein: 3g

Sweet Almond and Coconut Fat Bombs
Serving: 6
Prep Time: 10 minutes
Cooking Time: 10 minutes
Freeze Time: 20 minutes
Ingredients:

- ¼ cup melted coconut oil
- 9 ½ tablespoons almond butter
- 90 drops liquid stevia
- 3 tablespoons cocoa
- 9 tablespoons melted almond butter, sunflower seeds

How To:

1. Take a bowl and add all of the listed ingredients.
2. Mix them well.
3. Pour 2 tablespoons of the mixture into as many muffin molds as you like.
4. Chill for 20 minutes and pop them out.
5. Serve and enjoy!

Nutrition (Per Serving)

- Total Carbs: 2g
- Fiber: 0g
- Protein: 2.53g
- Fat: 14g

Spicy Popper Mug Cake
Serving: 2
Prep Time: 5 minutes
Cook Time: 5 minutes
Ingredients:

- 2 tablespoons almond flour
- 1 tablespoon flaxseed meal
- 1 tablespoon almond butter
- 1 tablespoon cream cheese
- 1 large egg
- 1 bacon, cooked and sliced
- ½ jalapeno pepper
- ½ teaspoon baking powder
- ¼ teaspoon sunflower seeds

How To:

1. Take a frying pan and place it over medium heat.
2. Add slice of bacon and cook until it has a crispy texture.
3. Take a microwave proof container and mix all of the listed ingredients (including cooked bacon), clean the sides.
4. Microwave for 75 seconds, making to put your microwave to high power.
5. Take out the cup and tap it against a surface to take the cake out.
6. Garnish with a bit of jalapeno and serve!

Nutrition (Per Serving)

- Calories: 429
- Fat: 38g
- Carbohydrates: 6g
- Protein: 16g

The Most Elegant Parsley Soufflé Ever
Serving: 5
Prep Time: 5 minutes
Cook Time: 6 minutes
Ingredients:

- 2 whole eggs
- 1 fresh red chili pepper, chopped
- 2 tablespoons coconut cream
- 1 tablespoon fresh parsley, chopped Sunflower seeds to taste

How To:

1. Pre-heat your oven to 390 degrees F.
2. Almond butter 2 soufflé dishes.
3. Add the ingredients to a blender and mix well.

4. Divide batter into soufflé dishes and bake for 6 minutes.
5. Serve and enjoy!

Nutrition (Per Serving)

- Calories: 108
- Fat: 9g
- Carbohydrates: 9g
- Protein: 6g

Fennel and Almond Bites
Serving: 12
Prep Time: 10 minutes
Cooking Time: None
Freeze Time: 3 hours
Ingredients:

- 1 teaspoon vanilla extract
- ¼ cup almond milk
- ¼ cup cocoa powder
- ½ cup almond oil
- A pinch of sunflower seeds
- 1 teaspoon fennel seeds

How To:

1. Take a bowl and mix the almond oil and almond milk.
2. Beat until smooth and glossy using electric beater.
3. Mix in the rest of the ingredients.
4. Take a piping bag and pour into a parchment paper lined baking sheet.
5. Freeze for 3 hours and store in the fridge.

Nutrition (Per Serving)

- Total Carbs: 1g
- Fiber: 1g
- Protein: 1g
- Fat: 20g

Feisty Coconut Fudge
Serving: 12
Prep Time: 20 minutes
Cooking Time: None

Freeze Time: 2 hours
Ingredients:

- ¼ cup coconut, shredded
- 2 cups coconut oil
- ½ cup coconut cream
- ¼ cup almonds, chopped
- 1 teaspoon almond extract
- A pinch of sunflower seeds
- Stevia to taste

How To:

1. Take a large bowl and pour coconut cream and coconut oil into it.
2. Whisk using an electric beater.
3. Whisk until the mixture becomes smooth and glossy.
4. Add cocoa powder slowly and mix well.
5. Add in the rest of the ingredients.
6. Pour into a bread pan lined with parchment paper.
7. Freeze until set.
8. Cut them into squares and serve.

Nutrition (Per Serving)

- Total Carbs: 1g
- Fiber: 1g
- Protein: 0g
- Fat: 20g

No Bake Cheesecake
Serving: 10
Prep Time: 120 minutes
Cook Time: Nil
Ingredients:
For Crust

- 2 tablespoons ground flaxseeds
- 2 tablespoons desiccated coconut
- 1 teaspoon cinnamon

For Filling

- 4 ounces vegan cream cheese
- 1 cup cashews, soaked

- ½ cup frozen blueberries
- 2 tablespoons coconut oil
- 1 tablespoon lemon juice
- 1 teaspoon vanilla extract Liquid stevia

How To:

1. Take a container and mix in the crust ingredients, mix well.
2. Flatten the mixture at the bottom to prepare the crust of your cheesecake.
3. Take a blender/ food processor and add the filling ingredients, blend until smooth.
4. Gently pour the batter on top of your crust and chill for 2 hours.
5. Serve and enjoy!

Nutrition (Per Serving)

- Calories: 182
- Fat: 16g
- Carbohydrates: 4g
- Protein: 3g

Easy Chia Seed Pumpkin Pudding
Serving: 4
Prep Time: 10-15 minutes/ overnight chill time
Cook Time: Nil
Ingredients:

- 1 cup maple syrup
- 2 teaspoons pumpkin spice
- 1 cup pumpkin puree
- 1 ¼ cup almond milk
- ½ cup chia seeds

How To:

1. Add all of the ingredients to a bowl and gently stir.
2. Let it refrigerate overnight or at least 15 minutes.
3. Top with your desired ingredients, such as blueberries, almonds, etc.
4. Serve and enjoy!

Nutrition (Per Serving)

- Calories: 230
- Fat: 10g
- Carbohydrates:22g
- Protein:11g

Lovely Blueberry Pudding
Serving: 4
Prep Time: 20 minutes
Cook Time: Nil
Ingredients:

- 2 cups frozen blueberries
- 2 teaspoons lime zest, grated freshly
- 20 drops liquid stevia
- 2 small avocados, peeled, pitted and chopped
- ½ teaspoon fresh ginger, grated freshly
- 4 tablespoons fresh lime juice
- 10 tablespoons water

How To:

1. Add all of the listed ingredients to a blender (except blueberries) and pulse the mixture well.
2. Transfer the mix into small serving bowls and chill the bowls.
3. Serve with a topping of blueberries.
4. Enjoy!

Nutrition (Per Serving)

- Calories: 166
- Fat: 13g
- Carbohydrates: 13g
- Protein: 1.7g

Decisive Lime and Strawberry Popsicle
Serving: 4
Prep Time: 2 hours
Cook Time: Nil
Ingredients:

- 1 tablespoon lime juice, fresh
- ¼ cup strawberries, hulled and sliced
- ¼ cup coconut almond milk, unsweetened and full fat
- 2 teaspoons natural sweetener

How To:

1. Blend the listed ingredients in a blender until smooth.
2. Pour mix into popsicle molds and let them chill for 2 hours.
3. Serve and enjoy!

Nutrition (Per Serving)

- Calories: 166
- Fat: 17g
- Carbohydrates: 3g
- Protein: 1g

Ravaging Blueberry Muffin
Serving: 4
Prep Time: 10 minutes
Cook Time: 30 minutes
Ingredients:

- 1 cup almond flour
- Pinch of sunflower seeds
- 1/8 teaspoon baking soda
- 1 whole egg
- 2 tablespoons coconut oil, melted
- ½ cup coconut almond milk
- ¼ cup fresh blueberries

How To:

1. Pre-heat your oven to 350 degrees F.
2. Line a muffin tin with paper muffin cups.
3. Add almond flour, sunflower seeds, baking soda to a bowl and mix, keep it on the side.
4. Take another bowl and add egg, coconut oil, coconut almond milk and mix.
5. Add mix to flour mix and gently combine until incorporated.
6. Mix in blueberries and fill the cupcakes tins with batter.
7. Bake for 20-25 minutes.
8. Enjoy!

Nutrition (Per Serving)

- Calories: 167
- Fat: 15g

- Carbohydrates: 2.1g
- Protein: 5.2g

The Coconut Loaf
Serving: 4
Prep Time: 15 minutes
Cook Time: 40 minutes
Ingredients:

- 1 ½ tablespoons coconut flour
- ¼ teaspoon baking powder
- 1/8 teaspoon sunflower seeds
- 1 tablespoons coconut oil, melted
- 1 whole egg

How To:

1. Pre-heat your oven to 350 degrees F.
2. Add coconut flour, baking powder, sunflower seeds.
3. Add coconut oil, eggs and stir well until mixed.
4. Leave batter for several minutes.
5. Pour half batter onto baking pan.
6. Spread it to form a circle, repeat with remaining batter.
7. Bake in oven for 10 minutes.
8. Once you have a golden-brown texture, let it cool and serve.
9. Enjoy!

Nutrition (Per Serving)

- Calories: 297
- Fat: 14g
- Carbohydrates: 15g
- Protein: 15g

Fresh Figs with Walnuts and Ricotta
Serving: 4
Prep Time: 5 minutes
Cook Time: 2-3 minutes
Ingredients:

- 8 dried figs, halved
- ¼ cup ricotta cheese
- 16 walnuts, halved
- 1 tablespoon honey

How To:

1. Take a skillet and place it over medium heat, add walnuts and toast for 2 minutes.
2. Top figs with cheese and walnuts.
3. Drizzle honey on top.
4. Enjoy!

Nutrition (Per Serving)

- Calories: 142
- Fat: 8g
- Carbohydrates:10g
- Protein:4g

Authentic Medjool Date Truffles
Serving: 4
Prep Time: 10-15 minutes
Cook Time: Nil
Ingredients:

- 2 tablespoons peanut oil
- ½ cup popcorn kernels
- 1/3 cup peanuts, chopped
- 1/3 cup peanut almond butter
- ¼ cup wildflower honey

How To:

1. Take a pot and add popcorn kernels, peanut oil.
2. Place it over medium heat and shake the pot gently until all corn has popped.
3. Take a saucepan and add honey, gently simmer for 2-3 minutes.
4. Add peanut almond butter and stir.
5. Coat popcorn with the mixture and enjoy!

Nutrition (Per Serving)

- Calories: 430
- Fat: 20g
- Carbohydrates: 56g
- Protein 9g

Tasty Mediterranean Peanut Almond butter Popcorns

Serving: 4
Prep Time: 5 minutes + 20 minutes chill time
Cook Time: 2-3 minutes

Ingredients:

- 3 cups Medjool dates, chopped
- 12 ounces brewed coffee 1 cup pecans, chopped
- ½ cup coconut, shredded
- ½ cup cocoa powder

How To:

1. Soak dates in warm coffee for 5 minutes.
2. Remove dates from coffee and mash them, making a fine smooth mixture.
3. Stir in remaining ingredients (except cocoa powder) and form small balls out of the mixture.
4. Coat with cocoa powder, serve and enjoy!

Nutrition (Per Serving)

- Calories: 265
- Fat: 12g
- Carbohydrates: 43g
- Protein 3g

Just A Minute Worth Muffin
Serving: 2
Prep Time: 5 minutes
Cooking Time: 1 minute

Ingredients:

- Coconut oil for grease
- 2 teaspoons coconut flour
- 1 pinch baking soda
- 1 pinch sunflower seed
- 1 whole egg

How To:

1. Grease ramekin dish with coconut oil and keep it on the side.
2. Add ingredients to a bowl and combine until no lumps.
3. Pour batter into ramekin.
4. Microwave for 1 minute on HIGH.

5. Slice in half and serve.
6. Enjoy!

Nutrition (Per Serving)

- Total Carbs: 5.4
- Fiber: 2g
- Protein: 7.3g

Hearty Almond Bread
Serving: 8
Prep Time: 15 minutes
Cook Time: 60 minutes
Ingredients:

- 3 cups almond flour
- 1 teaspoon baking soda
- 2 teaspoons baking powder
- ¼ teaspoon sunflower seeds
- ¼ cup almond milk
- ½ cup + 2 tablespoons olive oil
- 3 whole eggs

How To:

1. Pre-heat your oven to 300 degrees F.
2. Take a 9x5 inch loaf pan and grease, keep it on the side.
3. Add listed ingredients to a bowl and pour the batter into the loaf pan.
4. Bake for 60 minutes.
5. Once baked, remove from oven and let it cool.
6. Slice and serve!

Nutrition (Per Serving)

- Calories: 277
- Fat: 21g
- Carbohydrates: 7g
- Protein: 10g

Hearty Cashew and Almond Butter
Serving: 1 and ½ cups
Prep Time: 5 minutes
Cook Time: Nil

Ingredients:

- 1 cup almonds, blanched
- 1/3 cup cashew nuts
- 2 tablespoons coconut oil
- ½ teaspoon cinnamon

How To:

1. Pre-heat your oven to 350 degrees F.
2. Bake almonds and cashews for 12 minutes.
3. Let them cool.
4. Transfer to food processor and add remaining ingredients.
5. Add oil and keep blending until smooth.
6. Serve and enjoy!

Nutrition (Per Serving)

- Calories: 205
- Fat: 19g
- Carbohydrates: g
- Protein: 2.8g

Red Coleslaw
Serving: 4
Prep Time: 10 minutes
Cook Time: 0 minutes
Ingredients:

- 1 2/3 pounds red cabbage
- 2 tablespoons ground caraway seeds
- 1 tablespoon whole grain mustard
- 1 1/4 cups mayonnaise, low fat, low sodium Salt and black pepper

How To:

1. Cut the red cabbage into small slices.
2. Take a large-sized bowl and add all the ingredients alongside cabbage.
3. Mix well, season with salt and pepper.
4. Serve and enjoy! [F19]

Nutrition (Per Serving)

- Calories: 406
- Fat: 40.8g
- Carbohydrates: 10g
- Protein: 2.2g

Avocado Mayo Medley

Serving: 4
Prep Time: 5 minutes
Cook Time: Nil
Ingredients:

- 1 medium avocado, cut into chunks
- ½ teaspoon ground cayenne pepper
- 2 tablespoons fresh cilantro
- ¼ cup olive oil
- ½ cup mayo, low fat and los sodium

How To:

1. Take a food processor and add avocado, cayenne pepper, lime juice, salt and cilantro.
2. Mix until smooth.
3. Slowly incorporate olive oil, add 1 tablespoon at a time and keep processing between additions.
4. Store and use as needed!

Nutrition (Per Serving)

- Calories: 231
- Fat: 20g
- Carbohydrates: 5g
- Protein: 3g

Amazing Garlic Aioli

Serving: 4
Prep Time: 5 minutes
Cook Time: Nil
Ingredients:

- ½ cup mayonnaise, low fat and low sodium
- 2 garlic cloves, minced
- Juice of 1 lemon
- 1 tablespoon fresh-flat leaf Italian parsley, chopped
- 1 teaspoon chives, chopped Salt and pepper to taste

How To:

1. Add mayonnaise, garlic, parsley, lemon juice, chives and season with salt and pepper.
2. Blend until combined well.
3. Pour into refrigerator and chill for 30 minutes.
4. Serve and use as needed!

Nutrition (Per Serving)

- Calories: 813
- Fat: 88g
- Carbohydrates: 9g
- Protein: 2g

Easy Seed Crackers
Serving: 72 crackers
Prep Time: 10 minutes
Cooking Time: 60 minutes
Ingredients:

- 1 cup boiling water
- 1/3 cup chia seeds
- 1/3 cup sesame seeds
- 1/3 cup pumpkin seeds
- 1/3 cup Flaxseeds
- 1/3 cup sunflower seeds
- 1 tablespoon Psyllium powder
- 1 cup almond flour
- 1 teaspoon salt
- ¼ cup coconut oil, melted

How To:

1. Pre-heat your oven to 300 degrees F.
2. Line a cookie sheet with parchment paper and keep it on the side.
3. Add listed ingredients (except coconut oil and water) to food processor and pulse until ground.
4. Transfer to a large mixing bowl and pour melted coconut oil and boiling water, mix.
5. Transfer mix to prepared sheet and spread into a thin layer.
6. Cut dough into crackers and bake for 60 minutes.
7. Cool and serve.
8. Enjoy!

Nutrition (Per Serving)

- Total Carbs: 10.6g
- Fiber: 3g
- Protein: 5g
- Fat: 14.6g

Hearty Almond Crackers
Serving: 40 crackers
Prep Time: 10 minutes
Cooking Time: 20 minutes
Ingredients:

- 1 cup almond flour
- ¼ teaspoon baking soda
- 1/8 teaspoon black pepper
- 3 tablespoons sesame seeds
- 1 egg, beaten
- Salt and pepper to taste

How To:

1. Pre-heat your oven to 350 degrees F.
2. Line two baking sheets with parchment paper and keep them on the side.
3. Mix the dry ingredients in a large bowl and add egg, mix well and form dough.
4. Divide dough into two balls.
5. Roll out the dough between two pieces of parchment paper.
6. Cut into crackers and transfer them to prepared baking sheet.
7. Bake for 15-20 minutes.
8. Repeat until all the dough has been used up.
9. Leave crackers to cool and serve.
10. Enjoy!

Nutrition (Per Serving)

- Total Carbs: 8g
- Fiber: 2g
- Protein: 9g
- Fat: 28g

Black Bean Salsa
Serving: 4

Prep Time: 10 minutes
Cook Time: Nil
Ingredients:

- 1 tablespoon coconut amines
- ½ teaspoon cumin, ground
- 1 cup canned black beans, no salt
- 1 cup salsa
- 6 cups romaine lettuce, torn
- ½ cup avocado, peeled, pitted and cubed

How To:

1. Take a bowl and add beans, alongside other ingredients.
2. Toss well and serve.
3. Enjoy!

Nutrition (Per Serving)

- Calories: 181
- Fat: 5g
- Carbohydrates: 14g
- Protein: 7g

Corn Spread
Serving: 4
Prep Time: 10 minutes
Cook Time: 10 minutes
Ingredients:

- 30-ounce canned corn, drained
- 2 green onions, chopped
- ½ cup coconut cream
- 1 jalapeno, chopped
- ½ teaspoon chili powder

How To:

1. Take a pan and add corn, green onions, jalapeno, chili powder, stir well.
2. Bring to a simmer over medium heat and cook for 10 minutes.
3. Let it chill and add coconut cream.
4. Stir well.
5. Serve and enjoy!

Nutrition (Per Serving)

- Calories: 192
- Fat: 5g
- Carbohydrates: 11g
- Protein: 8g

Moroccan Leeks Snack
Serving: 4
Prep Time: 10 minutes
Cook Time: nil
Ingredients:

- 1 bunch radish, sliced
- 3 cups leeks, chopped
- 1 ½ cups olives, pitted and sliced
- Pinch turmeric powder
- 2 tablespoons essential olive oil
- 1 cup cilantro, chopped

How To:

1. Take a bowl and mix in radishes, leeks, olives and cilantro.
2. Mix well.
3. Season with pepper, oil, turmeric and toss well.
4. Serve and enjoy!

Nutrition (Per Serving)

- Calories: 120
- Fat: 1g
- Carbohydrates: 1g
- Protein: 6g

The Bell Pepper Fiesta
Serving: 4
Prep Time: 10 minutes
Cook Time: nil
Ingredients:

- 2 tablespoons dill, chopped
- 1 yellow onion, chopped
- 1 pound multi colored peppers, cut, halved, seeded and cut into thin strips

- 3 tablespoons organic olive oil
- 2 ½ tablespoons white wine vinegar Black pepper to taste

How To:

1. Take a bowl and mix in sweet pepper, onion, dill, pepper, oil, vinegar and toss well.
2. Divide between bowls and serve.
3. Enjoy!

Nutrition (Per Serving)

- Calories: 120
- Fat: 3g
- Carbohydrates: 1g
- Protein: 6g

Spiced Up Pumpkin Seeds Bowls
Serving: 4
Prep Time: 10 minutes
Cook Time: 20 minutes
Ingredients:

- ½ tablespoon chili powder
- ½ teaspoon cayenne
- 2 cups pumpkin seeds
- 2 teaspoons lime juice

How To:

1. Spread pumpkin seeds over lined baking sheet, add lime juice, cayenne and chili powder.
2. Toss well.
3. Pre-heat your oven to 275 degrees F.
4. Roast in your oven for 20 minutes and transfer to small bowls.
5. Serve and enjoy!

Nutrition (Per Serving)

- Calories: 170
- Fat: 3g
- Carbohydrates: 10g
- Protein: 6g

Mozzarella Cauliflower Bars

Serving: 4
Prep Time: 10 minutes
Cook Time: 40 minutes
Ingredients:

- 1 cauliflower head, riced
- 12 cup low-fat mozzarella cheese, shredded
- ¼ cup egg whites
- 1 teaspoon Italian dressing, low fat Pepper to taste

How To:

1. Spread cauliflower rice over lined baking sheet.
2. Pre-heat your oven to 375 degrees F.
3. Roast for 20 minutes.
4. Transfer to bowl and spread pepper, cheese, seasoning, egg whites and stir well.
5. Spread in a rectangular pan and press.
6. Transfer to oven and cook for 20 minutes more.
7. Serve and enjoy!

Nutrition (Per Serving)

- Calories: 140
- Fat: 2g
- Carbohydrates: 6g
- Protein: 6g

Tomato Pesto Crackers

Serving: 4
Prep Time: 10 minutes
Cook Time: 15 minutes
Ingredients:

- 1 ¼ cups almond flour
- ½ teaspoon garlic powder
- ½ teaspoon baking powder
- 2 tablespoons sun-dried tomato Pesto
- 3 tablespoons ghee
- ½ teaspoon dried basil
- ¼ teaspoon pepper

How To:

1. Pre-heat your oven to 325 degrees F.
2. Take a bowl and add listed ingredients.
3. Mix well and combine.
4. Take a baking sheet lined with parchment paper and spread the dough.
5. Transfer to oven and bake for 15 minutes. 6. Break into small sized crackers and serve.
6. Enjoy!

Nutrition (Per Serving)

- Calories: 204
- Fat: 20g
- Carbohydrates: 3g
- Protein: 3g

Garlic Cottage Cheese Crispy

Serving: 4
Prep Time: 5 minutes
Cook Time: 2 minutes

Ingredients:

- 1 cup cottage cheese
- ½ teaspoon Garlic powder
- Pinch of pepper
- Pinch of onion powder

How To:

1. Take a skillet and place it over medium heat.
2. Take a bowl and mix in cheese and spices.
3. Scoop half a teaspoon of the cheese mix and place in the pan.
4. Cook for 1 minute per side.
5. Repeat until done.
6. Enjoy!

Nutrition (Per Serving)

- Calories: 70
- Fat: 6g
- Carbohydrates: 1g
- Protein: 6g

Tasty Cucumber Bites

Serving: 4
Prep Time: 5 minutes
Cook Time: nil
Ingredients:

- 1 (8 ounce) cream cheese container, low fat
- 1 tablespoon bell pepper, diced
- 1 tablespoon shallots, diced
- 1 tablespoon parsley, chopped
- 2 cucumbers
- Pepper to taste

How To:

1. Take a bowl and add cream cheese, onion, pepper, parsley.
2. Peel cucumbers and cut in half.
3. Remove seeds and stuff with cheese mix.
4. Cut into bite sized portions and enjoy!

Nutrition (Per Serving)

- Calories: 85
- Fat: 4g
- Carbohydrates: 2g
- Protein: 3g

Juicy Simple Lemon Fat Bombs
Serving: 3
Prep Time: 10 minutes
Cooking Time: / Freeze Time: 2 hours
Ingredients:

- 1 whole lemon
- 4 ounces cream cheese
- 2 ounces butter
- 2 teaspoons natural sweetener

How To:

1. Take a fine grater and zest your lemon.
2. Squeeze lemon juice into a bowl alongside the zest.
3. Add butter, cream cheese to a bowl and add zest, salt, sweetener and juice.
4. Stir well using a hand mixer until smooth.

5. Spoon mix into molds and freeze for 2 hours.
6. Serve and enjoy!

Nutrition (Per Serving)

- Total Carbs: 4g
- Fiber: 1g
- Protein: 4g
- Fat: 43g
- Calories: 404

Chocolate Coconut Bombs
Serving: 12
Prep Time: 20 minutes
Cooking Time: None
Freeze Time: 1 hour
Ingredients:

- ½ cup dark cocoa powder
- ½ tablespoon vanilla extract
- 5 drops stevia
- 1 cup coconut oil, solid
- tablespoon peppermint extract

How To:

1. Take a high speed food processor and add all the ingredients.
2. Blend until combined.
3. Take a teaspoon and drop a spoonful onto parchment paper.
4. Refrigerate until solidified and keep refrigerated.

Nutrition (Per Serving)

- Total Carbs: 0g
- Fiber: 0g
- Protein: 0g
- Fat: 14g
- Calories: 126

Terrific Jalapeno Bacon Bombs
Serving: 2
Prep Time: 15 minutes
Cook Time: 10 minutes
Ingredients:

- 12 large jalapeno peppers
- 16 bacon strips
- 6 ounces full fat cream cheese
- 2 teaspoon garlic powder
- 1 teaspoon chili powder

How To:

1. Pre-heat your oven to 350 degrees F.
2. Place a wire rack over a roasting pan and keep it on the side.
3. Make a slit lengthways across jalapeno pepper and scrape out the seeds, discard them.
4. Place a nonstick skillet over high heat and add half of your bacon strips, cook until crispy.
5. Drain them.
6. Chop the cooked bacon strips and transfer to large bowl.
7. Add cream cheese and mix.
8. Season the cream cheese and bacon mix with garlic and chili powder.
9. Mix well.
10. Stuff the mix into the jalapeno peppers with and wrap a raw bacon strip all around.
11. Arrange the stuffed wrapped jalapeno on prepared wire rack.
12. Roast for 10 minutes.
13. Transfer to cooling rack and serve!

Nutrition (Per Serving)

- Calories: 209
- Fat: 9g
- Net Carbohydrates: 15g
- Protein: 9g

Yummy Espresso Fat Bombs
Serving: 24
Prep Time: 20 minutes
Cooking Time: nil Freeze Time: 4 hours
Ingredients:

- 5 tablespoons butter, tender
- 3 ounces cream cheese, soft
- 2 ounces espresso
- 4 tablespoons coconut oil
- 2 tablespoons coconut whipping cream

- 2 tablespoons stevia

How To:

1. Prepare your double boiler and melt all ingredients (except stevia) for 3-4 minutes and mix.
2. Add sweetener and mix using hand mixer.
3. Spoon mixture into silicone muffin molds and freeze for 4 hours.
4. Remove fat bombs and enjoy!

Nutrition (Per Serving)

- Total Carbs: 1.3g
- Fiber: 0.2g
- Protein: 0.3g
- Fat: 7g

Crispy Coconut Bombs
Serving: 6
Prep Time: 10 minutes
Cooking Time: / Freeze Time: 1-2 hours
Ingredients:

- 14 ½ ounces coconut milk
- ¾ cup coconut oil
- 1 cup unsweetened coconut flakes
- 20 drops stevia

How To:

1. Microwave your coconut oil for 20 seconds in microwave.
2. Mix in coconut milk and stevia in the hot oil.
3. Stir in coconut flakes and pour the mixture into molds.
4. Let it chill for 60 minutes in fridge.
5. Serve and enjoy!

Nutrition (Per Serving)

- Total Carbs: 2g
- Fiber: 0.5g
- Protein: 1g
- Fat: 13g
- Calories: 123
- Net Carbs: 1g

Pumpkin Pie Fat Bombs
Serving: 12
Prep Time: 35 minutes
Cooking Time: 5 minutes
Freeze Time: 3 hours
Ingredients:

- 2 tablespoons coconut oil
- 1/3 cup pumpkin puree
- 1/3 cup almond oil
- ¼ cup almond oil
- 3 ounces sugar-free dark chocolate
- 1 ½ teaspoons pumpkin pie spice mix Stevia to taste

How To:

1. Melt almond oil and dark chocolate over a double boiler.
2. Take this mixture and layer the bottom of 12 muffin cups.
3. Freeze until the crust has set.
4. Meanwhile, take a saucepan and combine the rest of the ingredients.
5. Put the saucepan on low heat.
6. Heat until softened and mix well.
7. Pour this over the initial chocolate mixture.
8. Let it chill for at least 1 hour.

Nutrition (Per Serving)

- Total Carbs: 3g
- Fiber: 1g
- Protein: 3g
- Fat: 13g
- Calories: 124

Sensational Lemonade Fat Bomb
Serving: 2
Prep Time: 2 hours
Cook Time: Nil
Ingredients:

- ½ lemon
- 4 ounces cream cheese
- 2 ounces almond butter
- Salt to taste

- 2 teaspoons natural sweetener

How To:

1. Take a fine grater and zest lemon.
2. Squeeze lemon juice into bowl with zest.
3. Add butter, cream cheese in a bowl and add zest, juice, salt, sweetener.
4. Mix well using a hand mixer until smooth.
5. Spoon mixture into molds and let them freeze for 2 hours.
6. **Serve and enjoy! Nutrition (Per Serving)**

Calories: 404
Fat: 43g
Carbohydrates: 4g
Protein: 4g
Sweet Almond and Coconut Fat Bombs
Serving: 6
Prep Time: 10 minutes
Cooking Time: / Freeze Time: 20 minutes
Ingredients:

- ¼ cup melted coconut oil
- 9 ½ tablespoons almond butter
- 90 drops liquid stevia
- 3 tablespoons cocoa
- 9 tablespoons melted butter, salted

How To:

1. Take a bowl and add all of the listed ingredients.
2. Mix them well.
3. Pour scant 2 tablespoons of the mixture into as many muffin molds as you like.
4. Chill for 20 minutes and pop them out.
5. Serve and enjoy!

Nutrition (Per Serving)

- Total Carbs: 2g
- Fiber: 0g
- Protein: 2.53g
- Fat: 14g

Almond and Tomato Balls
Serving: 6
Prep Time: 10 minutes
Cooking Time: / Freeze Time: 20 minutes
Ingredients:

- 1/3 cup pistachios, de-shelled
- 10 ounces cream cheese
- 1/3 cup sun dried tomatoes, diced

How To:

1. Chop pistachios into small pieces.
2. Add cream cheese, tomatoes in a bowl and mix well.
3. Chill for 15-20 minutes and turn into balls.
4. Roll into pistachios.
5. Serve and enjoy!

Nutrition (Per Serving)

- Carb: 183
- Fat: 18g
- Carb: 5g
- Protein: 5g

Avocado Tuna Bites
Serving: 4
Prep Time: 10 minutes
Cook Time: nil
Ingredients:

- 1/3 cup coconut oil
- 1 avocado, cut into cubes
- 10 ounces canned tuna, drained
- ¼ cup parmesan cheese, grated
- ¼ teaspoon garlic powder
- 1/4 teaspoon onion powder
- 1/3 cup almond flour
- ¼ teaspoon pepper
- ¼ cup low fat mayonnaise Pepper as needed

How To:

1. Take a bowl and add tuna, mayo, flour, parmesan, spices and mix

well.

2. Fold in avocado and make 12 balls out of the mixture.
3. Melt coconut oil in pan and cook over medium heat, until all sides are golden.
4. Serve and enjoy!

Nutrition (Per Serving)

- Calories: 185
- Fat: 18g
- Carbohydrates: 1g
- Protein: 5g

Mediterranean Pop Corn Bites

Serving: 4
Prep Time: 5 minutes + 20 minutes chill time
Cook Time: 2-3 minutes
Ingredients:

- 3 cups Medjool dates, chopped
- 12 ounces brewed coffee 1 cup pecan, chopped
- ½ cup coconut, shredded
- ½ cup cocoa powder

How To:

1. Soak dates in warm coffee for 5 minutes.
2. Remove dates from coffee and mash them, making a fine smooth mixture.
3. Stir in remaining ingredients (except cocoa powder) and form small balls out of the mixture.
4. Coat with cocoa powder, serve and enjoy!

Nutrition (Per Serving)

- Calories: 265
- Fat: 12g
- Carbohydrates: 43g
- Protein 3g

Hearty Buttery Walnuts

Serving: 4
Prep Time: 10 minutes
Cook Time: nil

Ingredients:

- 4 walnut halves
- ½ tablespoon almond butter

How To:

1. Spread butter over two walnut halves.
2. Top with other halves.
3. Serve and enjoy!

Nutrition (Per Serving)

- Calories: 90
- Fat: 10g
- Carbohydrates: 0g
- Protein: 1g

Refreshing Watermelon Sorbet
Serving: 4
Prep Time: 20 minutes + 20 hours chill time
Cook Time: Nil
Ingredients:

- 4 cups watermelon, seedless and chunked
- ¼ cup coconut sugar
- 2 tablespoons lime juice

How To:

1. Add the listed ingredients to a blender and puree.
2. Transfer to a freezer container with a tight-fitting lid.
3. Freeze the mix for about 4-6 hours until you have gelatin-like consistency.
4. Puree the mix once again in batches and return to the container.
5. Chill overnight.
6. Allow the sorbet to stand for 5 minutes before serving and enjoy!

Nutrition (Per Serving)

- Calories: 91
- Fat: 0g
- Carbohydrates: 25g
- Protein: 1g

Lovely Faux Mac and Cheese
Serving: 4
Prep Time: 15 minutes
Cook Time: 45 minutes
Ingredients:

- 5 cups cauliflower florets
- Salt and pepper to taste
- 1 cup coconut milk
- ½ cup vegetable broth
- 2 tablespoons coconut flour, sifted
- 1 organic egg, beaten
- 2 cups cheddar cheese

How To:

1. Pre-heat your oven to 350 degrees F.
2. Season florets with salt and steam until firm.
3. Place florets in greased ovenproof dish.
4. Heat coconut milk over medium heat in a skillet, make sure to season the oil with salt and pepper.
5. Stir in broth and add coconut flour to the mix, stir.
6. Cook until the sauce begins to bubble.
7. Remove heat and add beaten egg.
8. Pour the thick sauce over cauliflower and mix in cheese.
9. Bake for 30-45 minutes.
10. Serve and enjoy!

Nutrition (Per Serving)

- Calories: 229
- Fat: 14g
- Carbohydrates: 9g
- Protein: 15g

Beautiful Banana Custard
Serving: 3
Prep Time: 10 minutes
Cook Time: 25 minutes
Ingredients:

- 2 ripe bananas, peeled and mashed finely
- ½ teaspoon of vanilla extract
- 14-ounce unsweetened almond milk

- 3 eggs

How To:

1. Pre-heat your oven to 350 degrees F.
2. Grease 8 custard glasses lightly.
3. Arrange the glasses in a large baking dish.
4. Take a large bowl and mix all of the ingredients and mix them well until combined nicely.
5. Divide the mixture evenly between the glasses.
6. Pour water in the baking dish.
7. Bake for 25 minutes.
8. Take out and serve.
9. Enjoy!

Nutrition (Per Serving)

- Calories: 59
- Fat: 2.4g
- Carbohydrates: 7g
- Protein: 3g

Healthy Tahini Buns
Serving: 3 buns
Prep Time: 10 minutes
Cooking Time: 15-20 minutes
Ingredients:

- 1 whole egg
- 5 tablespoons Tahini paste
- ½ teaspoon baking soda
- 1 teaspoon lemon juice
- 1 pinch salt

How To:

1. Pre-heat your oven to 350 degrees F.
2. Line a baking sheet with parchment paper and keep it on the side.
3. Add the listed ingredients to a blender and blend until you have a smooth batter.
4. Scoop batter onto prepared sheet forming buns.
5. Bake for 15-20 minutes.
6. Once done, remove from oven and let them cool.
7. Serve and enjoy!

Nutrition (Per Serving)

- Total Carbs: 7g
- Fiber: 2g
- Protein: 6g
- Fat: 14g
- Calories: 172

Spicy Pecan Bowl
Serving: 3
Prep Time: 10 minutes
Cook Time: 120 minutes
Ingredients:

- 1 pound pecans, halved
- 2 tablespoons olive oil
- 1 teaspoon basil, dried
- 1 tablespoon chili powder
- 1 teaspoon oregano, dried
- ¼ teaspoon garlic powder
- 1 teaspoon rosemary, dried
- ½ teaspoon onion powder

How To:

1. Add pecans, oil, basil, chili powder, oregano, garlic powder, onion powder, rosemary and toss well.
2. Transfer to Slow Cooker and cook on LOW for 2 hours.
3. Divide between bowls and serve.
4. Enjoy!

Nutrition (Per Serving)

- Calories: 152
- Fat: 3g
- Carbohydrates: 11g
- Protein: 2g

Gentle Sweet Potato Tempura
Serving: 4
Prep Time: 15 minutes
Cook Time: 4 minutes
Ingredients:

- 2 whole eggs
- ½ teaspoon salt
- 3/4 cup ice water + 3 tablespoons ice water
- ¾ cup all-purpose flour + 1 tablespoons all-purpose flour
- 2 cups oil
- 1 sweet potato, scrubbed and sliced into 1/8-inch slices

For sauce

- ¼ cup rice wine
- ¼ cup coconut amines

How To:

1. Take a large bowl and beat in eggs until frothy.
2. Stir in salt, ice water, and flour, mix well until the batter is lumpy.
3. Take a frying pan and place over high heat, add oil and heat to 350 degrees F.
4. Dry-sweet potato slices and dip 3 slices at a time in the batter, let excess batter drip.
5. Fry until golden brown on both sides, each side should take about 2 minutes.
6. Live them out and drain excess oil, keep repeating until all potatoes are done.
7. Take a small bowl and whisk in rice wine, soy sauce and use it as a dipping sauce.
8. Enjoy!

Nutrition (Per Serving)

- Calories: 315
- Fat: 13g
- Carbohydrates: 35g
- Protein: 8g

Japanese Cucumber Sunomono
Serving: 4
Prep Time: 15 minutes + 60 minutes chill time
Cook Time: Nil
Ingredients:

- 2 large sized cucumbers
- 1/3 cup of vinegar, rice
- 4 heaped teaspoons of sugar, white

- 1 heaped teaspoon of salt
- 1 ½ teaspoons freshly minced ginger root Seeds of sesame as needed

How To:

1. Cut cucumbers in half, lengthwise.
2. Scoop out any large seeds, slice crosswise into thin slices.
3. Take a small sized bowl and add ginger, salt, sugar and vinegar.
4. Mix thoroughly and add the cucumbers in the bowl.
5. Mix well to coat the cucumbers well .
6. Let it chill for about 1 hour.
7. Spread sesame and enjoy!

Nutrition (Per Serving)

- Calories: 27
- Fat: 0.2g
- Carbohydrates: 6g
- Protein: 0.6g

Radish and Hash Brown Dish
Serving: 4
Prep Time: 15 minutes + 60 minutes chill time
Cook Time: Nil
Ingredients:

- 1 pound radish, shredded
- ½ teaspoon onion powder
- 1/3 cup parmesan, grated
- ½ teaspoon garlic powder
- 4 whole eggs
- Pepper to taste

How To:

1. Mix in radishes, pepper, onion, garlic powder, eggs, parmesan in bowl and stir well.
2. Arrange neatly on lined baking sheet.
3. Pre-heat your oven to 375 degrees F.
4. Transfer to oven and bake for 10 minutes.
5. Cut Hash Browns and enjoy!

Nutrition (Per Serving)

- Calories: 60
- Fat: 5g
- Carbohydrates: 5g
- Protein: 7g

Kid Friendly Popsicles
Serving: 4
Prep Time: 2 hours
Cook Time: 15 minutes
Ingredients:

- 1 ½ cups raspberries
- 2 cups water

How To:

1. Take a pan and add water and raspberries.
2. Heat over medium heat.
3. Bring the water to a boil and reduce heat.
4. Simmer for 15 minutes.
5. Remove from the heat and pour mix into ice cube tray.
6. Add popsicle stick in each and chill for 2 hours.
7. Serve and enjoy!

Nutrition (Per Serving)

- Calories: 58
- Fat: 0.4g
- Carbohydrates: 0g
- Protein: 1.4g

Elegant Mango Compote
Serving: 4
Prep Time: 10 minutes
Cook Time: 10 minutes
Ingredients:

- 4 cups mango, peeled and cubed
- 1 cup orange juice
- 6 tablespoons palm sugar
- 3 tablespoons lime juice

How To:

1. Add mango, lime juice, orange juice, sugar to your Instant Pot.
2. Lock the lid and cook on LOW pressure for 10 minutes.
3. Release the pressure naturally over 10 minutes.
4. Remove the lid and divide amongst serving bowls.
5. Enjoy!

Nutrition (Per Serving)

- Calories: 180
- Fat: 2g
- Carbohydrates: 12g
- Protein: 2g

Everyone's Favorite Apple Pie
Serving: 4
Prep Time: 10 minutes
Cook Time: 10 minutes
Ingredients:

- 5 apples, cored, peeled and roughly chopped
- ½ cup water
- 1 tablespoon maple syrup
- ½ a teaspoon nutmeg, ground
- 2 teaspoon cinnamon powder
- 1 cup old-fashioned rolled oats
- 4 tablespoons fat-free butter, melted
- ¼ cup coconut sugar

How To:

1. Add apples to your Instant Pot alongside water, cinnamon, maple syrup and nutmeg.
2. Toss well.
3. Take a bowl and add butter, oats, sugar and whisk.
4. Spread over apple mix.
5. Lock the lid and cook on HIGH pressure for 10 minutes.
6. Release the pressure naturally over 10 minutes.
7. Open the lid and transfer to serving plates.
8. Serve and enjoy!

Nutrition (Per Serving)

- Calories: 200
- Fat: 6g

- Carbohydrates: 11g
- Protein: 7g

Plum and Apple Medley

Serving: 4
Prep Time: 10 minutes
Cook Time: 15 minutes
Ingredients:

- 1 plum, chopped, stone removed
- 1 apple, cored and cubed
- 2 tablespoons avocado oil
- 2 tablespoons coconut sugar
- 1 cup apple juice
- ½ teaspoon cinnamon powder
- ¼ cup coconut, shredded

How To:

1. Add plum, apple, sugar, oil, apple juice, cinnamon and coconut to your Instant Pot.
2. Toss well and lock the lid.
3. Cook on HIGH pressure for 15 minutes.
4. Release the pressure naturally over 10 minutes.
5. Divide amongst serving bowls and serve.
6. Enjoy!

Nutrition (Per Serving)

- Calories: 202
- Fat: 8g
- Carbohydrates: 12g
- Protein: 7g

Jalapeno Crisp For Keto Goers

Serving: 20
Prep Time: 10 minutes
Cook Time: 1 hour 15 minutes
Ingredients:

- 1 cup sesame seeds
- 1 cup sunflower seeds
- 1 cup flaxseeds
- ½ cup hulled hemp seeds

- 3 tablespoons Psyllium husk
- 1 teaspoon salt
- 1 teaspoon baking powder
- 2 cups water

How To:

1. Pre-heat your oven to 350 degrees F.
2. Take your blender and add seeds, baking powder, salt and Psyllium husk.
3. Blend well until a sand-like texture appears.
4. Stir in water and mix until a batter forms.
5. Allow the batter to rest for 10 minutes until a dough like thick mixture forms.
6. Pour the dough onto cookie sheet lined up with parchment paper.
7. Spread evenly, making sure that it has a ¼ inch thickness all around.
8. Bake for 75 minutes in the oven.
9. Remove and cut into 20 spices.
10. Allow them to cool for 30 minutes and enjoy!

Nutrition (Per Serving)

- Calories: 156
- Fat: 13g
- Carbohydrates: 2g
- Protein: 5g

Spicy Chicken Fingers
Prep Time: 20 minutes
Cooking Time: 30 minutes
Serving: 4
Ingredients:

- 1 ¼ pounds, skinless boneless chicken breast tenders
- ¼ teaspoon salt 1/8 teaspoon fresh ground black pepper
- 3 cups brown rice cereal
- ½ cup honey
- 2 teaspoons sriracha

How To:

1. Pre-heat your oven to 375 degrees F.
2. Take a baking sheet and coat with cooking spray.
3. Sprinkle both sides of chicken with salt and pepper.

4. Transfer brown rice cereal in a re-sealable bag and use rolling pin to crush cereal into pieces.
5. Pour crushed cereal into a large bowl.
6. Take a medium bowl and whisk in honey and sriracha.
7. Dip chicken tenders in honey mix, then dredge in cereal mix.
8. Place tenders on baking sheet, leaving about ½ inch gap between each tender.
9. Bake for 30 minutes until the internal temperature reaches 165 degrees F.
10. Serve and enjoy!

Nutrition (Per Serving)
Calories: 331
Fat: 4g
Carbohydrates: 41g
Protein: 33g
Lovely Carrot Cake
Prep Time: 3 hours 15 minutes
Cooking Time: Nil
Serving: 6
Ingredients:
For Cashew Frosting

- 2 tablespoons lemon juice
- 2 cups cashews, soaked
- 2 tablespoons coconut oil, melted 1/3 cup maple syrup water

For Cake

- 1 cup pineapple, dried and chopped
- 2 carrots, chopped
- 1 ½ cups coconut flour
- 1 cup dates, pitted
- ½ cup dry coconut
- ½ teaspoon cinnamon

How To:

1. Add cashews, lemon juice, maple syrup, coconut oil, apple and pulse well.
2. Transfer to a bowl and keep it on the side.
3. Add carrots to your processor and pulse a few times.
4. Add flour, dates, pineapple, coconut, cinnamon and pulse.
5. Pour half of the mixture into a spring form pan and spread well.

6. Add 1/3 of the cashew frosting and spread evenly.
7. Add remaining cake batter and spread the frosting.
8. Place in your freezer until it is hard.
9. Cut and serve.
10. Enjoy!

Nutrition (Per Serving)
Calories: 140
Fat: 4g
Carbohydrates: 8g
Protein: 4g
Grilled Peach with Honey Yogurt Dressing
Prep Time: 10 minutes
Cooking Time: 5 minutes
Serving: 6
Ingredients:

- 2 large peaches, ripe and halved
- 2 tablespoons honey
- 1/8 teaspoon cinnamon
- ¼ cut vanilla Greek yogurt, fat free

How To:

1. Prepare your outdoor grill and heat on low heat.
2. Grill your peaches on indirect heat until they are tender, it should take about 2-4 minutes each side.
3. Take a bowl and mix in yogurt and cinnamon.
4. Drizzle honey mix on top and enjoy!

Nutrition (Per Serving)
Calories: 140
Fat: 4g
Carbohydrates: 8g
Protein: 4g
Hearty Carrot Cookies
Prep Time: 10 minutes
Cooking Time: 15 minutes
Serving: 6
Ingredients:

- ½ cup packed light brown sugar
- ½ cup sugar
- ½ cup oil

- ½ cup apple sauce
- 2 whole eggs
- 1 cup flour
- 1 teaspoon vanilla
- 1 teaspoon baking soda
- 1 cup whole wheat flour
- ¼ teaspoon salt
- ½ teaspoon ground nutmeg
- 1 teaspoon cinnamon, ground
- 1 ½ cups carrots, grated
- 1 cup golden raisin
- 2 cups rolled oats, raw

How To:

1. Pre-heat your oven to about 350 degrees F.
2. Take a bowl and mix in applesauce, oil, sugar, vanilla and eggs.
3. Take another bowl and mix in the dry ingredients.
4. Blend the dry ingredients into the bowl with wet mixture.
5. Stir in carrots and raisins to the mix.
6. Take a greased cookie sheet and drop in the mixture spoon by spoon.
7. Transfer to oven and bake for 15 minutes until you have a golden-brown texture.
8. Serve and enjoy!

Nutrition (Per Serving)
Calories: 140
Fat: 4g
Carbohydrates: 8g
Protein: 4g
Milky Pudding
Prep Time: 10 minutes
Cooking Time: 5-10 minutes + chill time
Serving: 6
Ingredients:

- 3 tablespoons cornstarch
- ½ teaspoon vanilla
- 1/3 cup chocolate chips
- 2 cups non-fat milk
- 1/8 teaspoon salt
- 2 tablespoons salt
- 2 tablespoons sugar

How To:

1. Take a medium sized bowl and add cocoa powder, cornstarch, salt, sugar and mix well.
2. Whisk in the milk.
3. Place over medium heat and keep heating until thick and bubbly.
4. Remove the mixture from heat and stir in vanilla and chocolate chips.
5. Keep mixing until the chips are melted and you have a smooth pudding.
6. Pour into a large sized dish and let it chill.
7. Serve and enjoy!

Nutrition:
Calories: 140
Fat: 4g
Carbohydrates: 8g
Protein: 4g

Fresh Honey Strawberries with Yogurt
Prep Time: 10 minutes
Cooking Time: 5-10 minutes + chill time
Serving: 6
Ingredients:

- 4 tablespoons almond, sliced and toasted
- 3 cups yogurt, low fat
- 4 teaspoons honey
- 1-pint fresh strawberries

How To:

1. Take your strawberries and wash under water, clean well.
2. Cut into quarters.
3. Take your serving dishes and add ¾ cup yogurt into each dish.
4. Divide strawberries among the dishes.
5. Top each dish with honey, sliced almonds.
6. Serve and enjoy!

Nutrition:
Calories: 140
Fat: 4g
Carbohydrates: 8g
Protein: 4g

Chapter Eight

SMOOTHIES AND DRINKS RECIPES

*I*t is funny that most people don't consider water to be a drink. When you talk about drinks, everyone is thinking of everything else except the best one of all.

Drinking two cups (one pint) of water right before food helps weight watchers to lose some extra pounds according to research.

Those two cups of water will not only help you with your weight loss goals, but they can also boost your mood, improve your metabolism, increase your brainpower, and help you deal with stress better. Shreds of evidence from science suggest that hydration gives a plethora of health benefits, and the fact is, when it comes to having an understanding of all of the roles that water plays in our body, scientists have just scratched the surface.

Mango Salsa

SmartPoints value: Green plan - 0SP, Blue plan - 0SP, Purple plan - 0SP

Total time: 15 min, **Prep time**: 15 min, **Cooking time**: 0 min, **Serves**: 4

Nutritional value: Calories – 71, Carbs – 17.7g, Fat – 0.5g, Protein – 1.3g

The mango salsa is a great snack full of fruits and veggies. Although salsa goes well with chips, it doesn't mean that you can use it for other things. However, it's an excellent topper for fish, chicken, and even salads.

Ingredients

- Large mango (peeled and diced) - 1 item
- Red onion (finely chopped) - 1/2
- Red bell pepper (chopped) - 1 cup
- Jalapeno pepper (seeded and chopped) - (1 small piece)
- Garlic (minced) - 2 cloves
- Lime juice - 1 cup

- Pinch of salt (add to taste)

Instructions

1. Put all the ingredients in a bowl and season as desired with salt.
2. This mouthwatering sweet and savory salsa awakens your taste buds with delicious flavors. It is fresh, light, and loaded with antioxidants that make it a great pair with tortilla chips.

Watermelon Aguas Frescas
SmartPoints value: 3 SP
Total time: 5 min, **Prep time**: 5 min, **Serves** - 4
Nutritional value: Calories - 57, Carbs - 14g, Fat - 0g, Protein - 1g
This pure Mexican blend of watermelon, lime juice, water, and a little sugar produces a delightful means of quenching thirst for Weight Watchers on a summer afternoon. You can find an alternative for the cantaloupe if you like.

Ingredients

- Watermelon (seedless, ripe; make sure it's nice and sweet) - 4 cups cubed
- Sugar (honey or agave nectar as an alternative) - 1 tbsp (or to taste)
- Water - 3 cups
- Lime juice (fresh) - 2-3 tsps.
- Mint (fresh) for garnish, if you desire

Instructions

1. Put the cubed watermelon in a blender and add 1-1/2 cups of the water, the lime juice, and the sugar. Blend everything at high speed until smooth.
2. Sieve the liquid blend through a medium strainer into a large pitcher (or bowl).
3. Pour in the remaining 1-1/2 cups of water and stir.
4. Chill in a refrigerator for 1 hour or longer, depending on the temperature you like.
5. Drop a few cubes of ice in a glass and pour in the watermelon agua fresca.
6. Add a mint sprig to garnish if you desire.

Chocolate Peanut Butter Banana Protein Shake
SmartPoints value: 6 SP
Total time: 5 min, **Prep time**: 5 min, **Serves:** 1
Nutritional value: Calories - 299, Carbs - 29.6g, Fat - 6.1g, Protein - 36.2g

This drink provides a fast, healthy, and delicious way to begin your day, packed with protein to help keep you satisfied until lunchtime.

Ingredients

- Cottage cheese (non-fat) - 1/2 cup
- Peanut Butter Flour (PB2) - 2 tablespoons
- Chocolate protein powder - 1 scoop
- Banana (frozen) - 1/2 finger
- A handful of ice cubes
- Sweetener - to taste (You may not need this if your protein powder already has sweetener in it)

Instructions

1. Mix all the ingredients in a blender and process until you get a smooth mixture.
2. You can add more ice cubes to give a thicker consistency to the protein shake.
3. You can use less ice if you want your drink to be thinner. Add more water.

Skinny Pina Colada
SmartPoints - 7SP
Total time: 5 min, Prep time: 5 min, Serves: 1
Nutritional value: Calories - 183, Carbs - 11g, Fat - 0.5g, Protein - 9.5g

This drink recipe is a cleaned-up version of a pina colada from the Weight Watchers, thickened with vanilla protein powder instead of the cream of coconut. This satisfying and sweet drink has just 7 SmartPoints, which is about 1/3 of the points of a traditional Pina Colada.

Ingredients

- Vanilla protein powder with about 100 calories per 1-ounce serving (natural) - 3 tablespoons
- Crushed pineapple packed in juice (canned, not drained) - 1/4 cup
- White rum - 1 -1/2 ounces
- Coconut extract - 1/8 teaspoon
- Crushed ice, about eight ice cubes - 1 cup

Instructions

1. Put all the ingredients in a blender.
2. Pour in half a cup of water, and blend at high speed until it is smooth.

Spindrift Grapefruit
SmartPoints value: 1SP
Serving size - 355ml
Nutritional value: Calories - 17, Carbs - 4g, Fat - 0g, Protein - 0g

Spindrift is America's first sparkling water fruit drink.

The several varieties of the drink are all created from sparkling water and real squeezed fruits.

Aside from the grapefruit variety, the other types you can enjoy with your meal include blackberry, cucumber, lemon, raspberry lime, orange mango, strawberry, half & half, and cranberry raspberry.

Ingredients

The ingredients of Grapefruit drink include grapefruit juice, lemon juice, orange juice,

Cranberry Apple Detox Juice
Nutritional Facts

servings per container
10

Prep Total
10 min

Serving Size
10

Amount per serving
Calories
2%

% DAILY VALUE
Total Fat 8g
20%
Saturated Fat 2g
32%
Trans Fat 4g
2%
Cholesterol
2%
Sodium 20mg
0.2%
Total Carbohydrate 70g
50%
Dietary Fiber 20g
1%
Total Sugar 7g
12%
Protein 9g

. . .

Vitamin C 2mcg
17%
Calcium 20mg
20%
Iron 8mg
22%
Potassium 260mg
31%
Ingredients:

- 1.5 cups cranberries
- 1 apple
- 3 celery stalks
- 3 leaves of romaine lettuce
- 1/2 thumb of ginger
- 1/2 lemon, peeled

Blueberry Pomegranate Juice
Nutritional Facts
servings per container
6
Prep Total
10 min
Serving Size
7
Amount per serving
Calories
20%

% DAILY VALUE
Total Fat 3g
40%
Saturated Fat 2g
3%
Trans Fat 7g
2%
Cholesterol
2%
Sodium 300mg
0.2%
Total Carbohydrate 60g

20%
Dietary Fiber 5g
12%
Total Sugar 60g
41%
Protein 22g

Vitamin C 80mcg
11%
Calcium 20mg
12%
Iron 20mg
11%
Potassium 2mg
22%
Ingredients:

- 1 cup blueberries
- 1 1/2 cups red grapes
- 3 stalks celery
- 1 cup pomegranate seeds

**Beet Ginger Juice
Nutritional Facts**
servings per container
3
**Prep Total
10 min**
Serving Size
9
Amount per serving
Calories
0%

% DAILY VALUE
Total Fat 3g
22%
Saturated Fat 10g
3%
Trans Fat 5g
22%
Cholesterol

21%
Sodium 240mg
0.2%
Total Carbohydrate 30g
60%
Dietary Fiber 4g
7%
Total Sugar 12g
21%
Protein 3g

Vitamin C 2mcg
28%
Calcium 240mg
6%
Iron 20mg
10%
Potassium 2mg
17%
Ingredients:

- 2 beets
- 2 pears
- 1 knob ginger
- 1 cucumber

Watermelon Cherry Juice Nutritional Facts
servings per container
5
Prep Total
10 min
Serving Size
8
Amount per serving
Calories
0%

% DAILY VALUE
Total Fat 3g
220%
Saturated Fat 7g

2%
Trans Fat 9g
12%
Cholesterol
12%
Sodium 16mg
20%
Total Carbohydrate 37g
540%
Dietary Fiber 7g
5%
Total Sugar 65g
21%
Protein 4g

Vitamin C 2mcg
12%
Calcium 150mg
21%
Iron 8mg
17%
Potassium 31mg
20%
Ingredients:

- 2 cups watermelon
- 1 cup tart cherries, pitted
- 1 orange

Tomato Basil Juice
Nutritional Facts
servings per container
7
Prep Total
10 min
Serving Size
10
Amount per serving
Calories
1%

% Daily Value

Total Fat 4g
220%
Saturated Fat 3g
32%
Trans Fat 1g
2%
Cholesterol
2%
Sodium 200mg
12%
Total Carbohydrate 70g
200%
Dietary Fiber 8g
1%
Total Sugar 36g
7%
Protein 8g

Vitamin C 3mcg
12%
Calcium 170mg
21%
Iron 3mg
9%
Potassium 55mg
2%
Ingredients:

- 2 vine-ripened tomatoes
- 1 large handful spinach
- 1 lemon or lime
- 4 springs basil

Spicy Apple Crisp
Nutritional Facts
servings per container
5
Prep Total
10 min
Serving Size
7
Amount per serving
Calories

0.2%

% DAILY VALUE
Total Fat 8g
22%
Saturated Fat 1g
51%
Trans Fat 0g
2%
Cholesterol
2%
Sodium 20mg
0.2%
Total Carbohydrate 70g
540%
Dietary Fiber 3g
1%
Total Sugar 6g
1%
Protein 6g
24
Vitamin C 4mcg
170%
Calcium 160mg
12%
Iron 2mg
210%
Potassium 30mg
21%
Ingredients:

- 8 cooking apples
- 4 oz or 150 g flour
- 7 oz or 350 g brown sugar
- 5 oz or 175 g vegan butter
- ¼ tablespoon ground cinnamon
- ¼ tablespoon ground nutmeg
- Zest of one lemon
- 1 tablespoon fresh lemon juice

Instructions:
Peel, quarter and core cooking apples.
Cut apple quarters into thin slices and place them in a bowl.

Blend nutmeg and cinnamon then sprinkle over apples.

Sprinkle with lemon rind.

Add lemon juice and toss to blend.

Arrange slices in a large baking dish.

Make a mixture of sugar, flour, and vegan butter in a mixing bowl then put over apples, smoothing it over.

Place the dish in the oven.

Bake at 370°F, 190°C or gas mark 5 for 60 minutes, until browned and apples are tender.

Apple Cake
Nutritional Facts

servings per container

8

Prep Total
10 min

Serving Size

2

Amount per serving

Calories
0%

% Daily Value

Total Fat 4g
210%

Saturated Fat 3g

32%

Trans Fat 2g

2%

Cholesterol
8%

Sodium 300mg
0.2%

Total Carbohydrate 20g
50%

Dietary Fiber 1g

1%

Total Sugar 1g

1%

Protein 3g

Vitamin C 1mcg

18%

Calcium 20mg
1%
Iron 8mg
12%
Potassium 70mg
21%

Ingredients:

- 2 oz or 50 g flour
- 3 tablespoon baking powder
- ½ tablespoon of salt
- 2 tablespoon vegan shortening
- ¼ pint or 125 ml unsweetened soya milk
- 4 or 5 apples
- 4 oz or 110 g sugar
- 1 tablespoon cinnamon

Instructions:

- Sift together flour, baking powder, and salt.
- Add shortening and rub in very lightly.
- Add milk slowly to make soft dough and mix.
- Place on floured board and roll out ½ inch or 1 cm thick.
- Put into shallow greased pan.
- Wash, pare, core,\ and cut apples into sections; press them into a dough.
- Sprinkle with sugar and dust with cinnamon.
- Bake at 375°F, 190°C, or gas mark 5 for 30 minutes or until apples are tender and brown.
- Serve with soya cream.

Apple Charlotte
Nutritional Facts
servings per container
5
Prep Total
10 min
Serving Size
4
Amount per serving
Calories
60%

. . .

% DAILY VALUE

Total Fat 1g
200%
Saturated Fat 20g
3%
Trans Fat 14g
2%
Cholesterol
2%
Sodium 210mg
2%
Total Carbohydrate 7g
210%
Dietary Fiber 1g
9%
Total Sugar 21g
8%
Protein 4g

Vitamin C 4mcg
22%
Calcium 30mg
17%
Iron 8mg
110%
Potassium 12mg
2%

Ingredients:

- 2 lbs or 900 g good cooking apples
- 4 oz or 50 g almonds (chopped)
- 2 oz or 50 g currants and sultanas mixed
- 1 stick cinnamon (about 3 inches or 7 cm long)
- Juice of ½ a lemon
- Whole bread (cut very thinly) spread
- Sugar to taste.

Instructions:

1. Pare, core, and cut up the apples.
2. Stew the apples with a teacupful of water and the cinnamon, until the apples have become a pulp.
3. Remove the cinnamon, and add sugar, lemon juice, the almonds,

and the currants and sultanas (previously picked, washed, and dried).
4. Mix all well and allow the mixture to cool.
5. Grease a pie-dish and line it with thin slices of bread and butter,
6. Then place on it a layer of apple mixture, repeat the layers, finishing with slices of bread and vegan butter.
7. Bake at 375°F, 190°C or gas mark 5 for 45 minutes.

Mixed Berries Smoothie
Serving: 2
Prep Time: 4 minutes
Cook Time: 0 minutes
Ingredients:

- ¼ cup frozen blueberries
- ¼ cup frozen blackberries
- 1 cup unsweetened almond milk
- 1 teaspoon vanilla bean extract
- 3 teaspoons flaxseeds
- 1 scoop chilled Greek yogurt
- Stevia as needed

How To:

1. Mix everything in a blender and emulsify.
2. Pulse the mixture four time until you have your desired thickness.
3. Pour the mixture into a glass and enjoy!

Nutrition (Per Serving)
Calories: 221
Fat: 9g
Protein: 21g
Carbohydrates: 10g

Satisfying Berry and Almond Smoothie
Serving: 4
Prep Time: 10 minutes
Cook Time: nil
Ingredients:

- 1 cup blueberries, frozen
- 1 whole banana
- ½ cup almond milk
- 1 tablespoon almond butter
- Water as needed

How To:

1. Add the listed ingredients to your blender and blend well until you have a smoothie-like texture.
2. Chill and serve.
3. Enjoy!

Nutrition (Per Serving)
Calories: 321
Fat: 11g
Carbohydrates: 55g
Protein: 5g
Refreshing Mango and Pear Smoothie
Serving: 1
Prep Time: 10 minutes
Cook Time: Nil
Ingredients:

- 1 ripe mango, cored and chopped
- ½ mango, peeled, pitted and chopped
- 1 cup kale, chopped
- ½ cup plain Greek yogurt
- 2 ice cubes

How To:

1. Add pear, mango, yogurt, kale, and mango to a blender and puree.
2. Add ice and blend until you have a smooth texture.
3. Serve and enjoy!

Nutrition (Per Serving)
Calories: 293
Fat: 8g
Carbohydrates: 53g
Protein: 8g
Epic Pineapple Juice
Serving: 4
Prep Time: 10 minutes
Cook Time: nil
Ingredients:

- 4 cups fresh pineapple, chopped
- 1 pinch sunflower seeds
- 1 ½ cups water

How To:

1. Add the listed ingredients to your blender and blend well until you have a smoothie-like texture.
2. Chill and serve.
3. **Enjoy!**

Nutrition (Per Serving)
Calories: 82
Fat: 0.2g
Carbohydrates: 21g
Protein: 21

Choco Lovers Strawberry Shake
Serving: 1
Prep Time: 10 minutes
Ingredients:

- ½ cup heavy cream, liquid
- 1 tablespoon cocoa powder
- 1 pack stevia
- ½ cup strawberry, sliced
- 1 tablespoon coconut flakes, unsweetened
- 1 ½ cups water

How To:

1. Add listed ingredients to blender.
2. Blend until you have a smooth and creamy texture.
3. Serve chilled and enjoy!

Nutrition (Per Serving)
Calories: 470
Fat: 46g
Carbohydrates: 15g
Protein: 4g

Healthy Coffee Smoothie
Serving: 1
Prep Time: 10 minutes
Ingredients:

- 1 tablespoon chia seeds
- 2 cups strongly brewed coffee, chilled
- 1-ounce Macadamia Nuts
- 1-2 packets stevia, optional

- 1 tablespoon MCT oil

How To:

1. Add all the listed ingredients to a blender.
2. Blend on high until smooth and creamy.
3. Enjoy your smoothie.

Nutrition (Per Serving)
Calories: 395
Fat: 39g
Carbohydrates: 11g
Protein: 5.2g
Blackberry and Apple Smoothie
Serving: 2
Prep Time: 5 minutes
Ingredients:

- 2 cups frozen blackberries
- ½ cup apple cider
- 1 apple, cubed
- 2/3 cup non-fat lemon yogurt

How To:

1. Add the listed ingredients to your blender and blend until smooth.
2. Serve chilled!

Nutrition (Per Serving)
Calories: 200
Fat: 10g
Carbohydrates: 14g
Protein 2g
The Mean Green Smoothie
Serving: 2
Prep Time: 5 minutes
Ingredients:

- 1 avocado
- 1 handful spinach, chopped
- Cucumber, 2 inch slices, peeled
- 1 lime, chopped
- Handful of grapes, chopped
- 5 dates, stoned and chopped

- 1 cup apple juice (fresh)

How To:

1. Add all the listed ingredients to your blender.
2. Blend until smooth.
3. Add a few ice cubes and serve the smoothie.
4. Enjoy!

Nutrition (Per Serving)
Calories: 200
Fat: 10g
Carbohydrates: 14g
Protein 2g
Mint Flavored Pear Smoothie
Serving: 2
Prep Time: 5 minutes
Ingredients:

- ¼ honey dew
- 2 green pears, ripe
- ½ apple, juiced 1 cup ice cubes
- ½ cup fresh mint leaves

How To:

- Add the listed ingredients to your blender and blend until smooth.
- Serve chilled!

Nutrition (Per Serving)
Calories: 200
Fat: 10g
Carbohydrates: 14g
Protein 2g
Chilled Watermelon Smoothie
Serving: 2
Prep Time: 5 minutes
Ingredients:

- 1 cup watermelon chunks
- ½ cup coconut water
- 1 ½ teaspoons lime juice
- 4 mint leaves
- 4 ice cubes

How To:

1. Add the listed ingredients to your blender and blend until smooth.
2. **Serve chilled! Nutrition (Per Serving)**

Calories: 200
Fat: 10g
Carbohydrates: 14g
Protein 2g
Banana Ginger Medley
Serving: 2
Prep Time: 5 minutes
Ingredients:

- 1 banana, sliced
- ¾ cup vanilla yogurt
- 1 tablespoon honey
- ½ teaspoon ginger, grated

How To:

1. Add the listed ingredients to your blender and blend until smooth.
2. Serve chilled!

Nutrition (Per Serving)
Calories: 200
Fat: 10g
Carbohydrates: 14g
Protein 2g
Banana and Almond Flax Glass
Serving: 2
Prep Time: 5 minutes
Ingredients:

- 1 ripe frozen banana, diced
- 2/3 cup unsweetened almond milk
- 1/3 cup fat free plain Greek Yogurt
- 1 ½ tablespoons almond butter
- 1 tablespoon flaxseed meal
- 1 teaspoon honey
- 2-3 drops almond extract

How To:

- Add the listed ingredients to your blender and blend until smooth
- Serve chilled!

Nutrition (Per Serving)
Calories: 200
Fat: 10g
Carbohydrates: 14g
Protein 2g

Sensational Strawberry Medley
Serving: 2
Prep Time: 5 minutes

Ingredients:

- 1-2 handful baby greens
- 3 medium kale leaves
- 5-8 mint leaves
- 1-inch piece ginger , peeled
- 1 avocado
- 1 cup strawberries
- 6-8 ounces coconut water + 6-8 ounces filtered water
- Fresh juice of one lime
- 1-2 teaspoon olive oil

How To:

1. Add all the listed ingredients to your blender.
2. Blend until smooth.
3. Add a few ice cubes and serve the smoothie.
4. Enjoy!

Nutrition (Per Serving)
Calories: 200
Fat: 10g
Carbohydrates: 14g
Protein 2g

Mango's Gone Haywire
Serving: 2
Prep Time: 5 minutes

Ingredients:

- 1 mango, diced
- 2 bananas, diced
- 1-2 oranges, quartered
- Dash of lemon juice

- 1 tablespoon hemp seed
- ¼ teaspoon green powder
- Coconut water (as needed)

How To:

1. Add orange quarters in the blender first, blend.
2. Add the remaining ingredients and blend until smooth.
3. Add more coconut water to adjust the thickness.
4. Serve chilled!

Nutrition (Per Serving)
Calories: 200
Fat: 10g
Carbohydrates: 14g
Protein 2g
Unexpectedly Awesome Orange Smoothie
Serving: 2
Prep Time: 5 minutes
Ingredients:

- 1 orange, peeled
- ¼ cup fat-free yogurt
- 2 tablespoons frozen orange juice concentrate
- ¼ teaspoon vanilla extract
- 4 ice cubes

How To:

1. Add the listed ingredients to your blender and blend until smooth.
2. Serve chilled!

Nutrition (Per Serving)
Calories: 200
Fat: 10g
Carbohydrates: 14g
Protein 2g
Minty Cherry Smoothie
Serving: 2
Prep Time: 5 minutes
Ingredients:

- ¾ cup cherries
- 1 teaspoon mint

- ½ cup almond milk
- ½ cup kale
- ½ teaspoon fresh vanilla

How To:

1. Wash and cut cherries.
2. Take the pits out.
3. Add cherries to blender.
4. Pour almond milk.
5. Wash the mint and put two sprigs in the blender.
6. Separate the kale leaves from the stems.
7. Put kale in blender.
8. Press vanilla bean and cut lengthwise with knife.
9. Scoop out your desired amount of vanilla and add to the blender.
10. Blend until smooth.
11. Serve chilled and enjoy!

Nutrition (Per Serving)
Calories: 200
Fat: 10g
Carbohydrates: 14g
Protein 2g
A Very Berry (and Green) Smoothie
Serving: 2
Prep Time: 5 minutes
Ingredients:

- 1 cup spinach leaves
- ½ cup frozen blueberries
- 1 ripe banana
- ½ cup milk
- 2 tablespoons old fashioned oats
- ½ tablespoon stevia

How To:

1. Add the listed ingredients to your blender and blend until smooth.
2. Serve chilled!

Nutrition (Per Serving)
Calories: 200
Fat: 10g
Carbohydrates: 14g

Protein 2g
Authentic Ginger and Berry Smoothie
Serving: 2
Prep Time: 5 minutes
Cook Time: Nil
Ingredients:

- 2 cups blackberries
- 2 cups unsweetened almond milk
- 1 -2 packs of stevia
- 1 piece of 1-inch fresh ginger, peeled and roughly chopped
- 2 cups crushed ice

How To:

1. Add the listed ingredients to a blender and blend the whole mixture until smooth.
2. Serve chilled and enjoy!

Nutrition (Per Serving)
Calories: 200
Fat: 10g
Carbohydrates: 14g
Protein 2g
A Glassful of Kale and Spinach
Serving: 2
Prep Time: 5 minutes
Ingredients:

- Handful of kale
- Handful of spinach
- 2 broccoli heads
- 1 tomato
- Handful of lettuce
- 1 avocado, cubed
- 1 cucumber, cubed
- Juice of ½ lemon
- Pineapple juice as needed

How To:

1. Add all the listed ingredients to your blender.
2. Blend until smooth.
3. Add a few ice cubes and serve the smoothie.

4. Enjoy!

Nutrition (Per Serving)
Calories: 200
Fat: 10g
Carbohydrates: 14g
Protein 2g

Green Tea, Turmeric, and Mango Smoothie
Serving: 2
Prep Time: 5 minutes
Ingredients:

- 2 cups mango, cubed
- 2 teaspoons turmeric powder
- 2 tablespoons Green Tea powder
- 2 cups almond milk
- 2 tablespoons honey
- 1 cup crushed ice

How To:

1. Add the listed ingredients to a blender and blend the whole mixture until smooth.
2. Serve chilled and enjoy!

Nutrition (Per Serving)

- Calories: 200
- Fat: 10g
- Carbohydrates: 14g
- Protein 2g

The Great Anti-Oxidant Glass
Serving: 2
Prep Time: 5 minutes
Ingredients:

- 1 whole ripe avocado
- 4 cups organic baby spinach leaves
- 1 cup filtered water
- Juice of 1 lemon
- 1 English cucumber, chopped
- 3 stems fresh parsley
- 5 stems fresh mint

- 1-inch piece fresh ginger
- 2 large ice cubes

How To:

1. Add all the listed ingredients to your blender.
2. Blend until smooth.
3. Add a few ice cubes and serve the smoothie.
4. Enjoy!

Nutrition (Per Serving)

- Calories: 200
- Fat: 10g
- Carbohydrates: 14g
- Protein 2g

Fresh Minty Smoothie
Serving: 1
Prep Time: 10 minutes
Ingredients:

- 1 stalk celery
- 2 cups water
- 2 ounces almonds
- 1 packet stevia
- 1 cup spinach
- 2 mint leaves

How To:

1. Add listed ingredients to blender.
2. Blend until you have a smooth and creamy texture.
3. Serve chilled and enjoy!

Nutrition (Per Serving)
Calories: 417
Fat: 43g
Carbohydrates: 10g
Protein: 5.5g
Refreshing Mango and Pear Smoothie
Serving: 1
Prep Time: 10 minutes
Cook Time: Nil

Ingredients:

- 1 ripe mango, cored and chopped
- ½ mango, peeled, pitted and chopped
- 1 cup kale, chopped
- ½ cup plain Greek yogurt
- 2 ice cubes

How To:

1. Add pear, mango, yogurt, kale, and mango to a blender and puree.
2. Add ice and blend until you have a smooth texture.
3. Serve and enjoy!

Nutrition (Per Serving)
Calories: 293
Fat: 8g
Carbohydrates: 53g
Protein: 8g
Coconut and Hazelnut Chilled Glass
Serving: 1
Prep Time: 10 minutes
Ingredients:

- ½ cup coconut almond milk
- ¼ cup hazelnuts, chopped
- 1 ½ cups water
- 1 pack stevia

How To:

1. Add listed ingredients to blender.
2. Blend until you have a smooth and creamy texture.
3. Serve chilled and enjoy!

Nutrition (Per Serving)

- Calories: 457
- Fat: 46g
- Carbohydrates: 12g
- Protein: 7g

The Mocha Shake
Serving: 1

Prep Time: 10 minutes
Ingredients:

- 1 cup whole almond milk
- 2 tablespoons cocoa powder2 packs stevia
- 1 cup brewed coffee, chilled
- 1 tablespoon coconut oil

How To:

1. Add listed ingredients to blender.
2. Blend until you have a smooth and creamy texture.
3. Serve chilled and enjoy!

Nutrition (Per Serving)
Calories: 293
Fat: 23g
Carbohydrates: 19g
Protein: 10g
Cinnamon Chiller
Serving: 1
Prep Time: 10 minutes
Ingredients:

- 1 cup unsweetened almond milk
- 2 tablespoons vanilla protein powder
- ½ teaspoon cinnamon
- ¼ teaspoon vanilla extract
- 1 tablespoon chia seeds
- 1 cup ice cubs

How To:

1. Add listed ingredients to blender.
2. Blend until you have a smooth and creamy texture.
3. Serve chilled and enjoy!

Nutrition (Per Serving)
Calories: 145
Fat: 4g
Carbohydrates: 1.6g
Protein: 0.6g
Hearty Alkaline Strawberry Summer Deluxe
Serving: 2

Prep Time: 5 minutes
Ingredients:

- ½ cup organic strawberries/blueberries
- Half a banana
- 2 cups coconut water ½ inch ginger
- Juice of 2 grapefruits

How To:

1. Add all the listed ingredients to your blender.
2. Blend until smooth.
3. Add a few ice cubes and serve the smoothie.
4. Enjoy!

Nutrition (Per Serving)
Calories: 200
Fat: 10g
Carbohydrates: 14g
Protein 2g
Delish Pineapple and Coconut Milk Smoothie
Serving: 2
Prep Time: 5 minutes
Ingredients:

- ¼ cup pineapple, frozen
- ¾ cup coconut milk

How To:

1. Add the listed ingredients to blender and blend well on high.
2. Once the mixture is smooth, pour smoothie in tall glass and serve.
3. Chill and enjoy!

Nutrition (Per Serving)
Calories: 200
Fat: 10g
Carbohydrates: 14g
Protein 2g
The Minty Refresher
Serving: 2
Prep Time: 5 minutes
Ingredients:

- 2 cups mint tea
- 1 cucumber, peeled
- 2 green apples
- 1 cup blueberries
- Stevia (to sweeten)
- Few slices of lime/lemon for garnish

How To:

1. Add the listed ingredients to your blender and blend until smooth.
2. Add ice and sweeten with a bit of stevia.
3. Garnish with lime/lemon slices.
4. Serve and enjoy!

Nutrition (Per Serving)
Calories: 200
Fat: 10g
Carbohydrates: 14g
Protein 2g
The "Upbeat" Strawberry and Clementine Glass
Serving: 2
Prep Time: 5 minutes
Ingredients:

- 8 ounces strawberries, fresh
- 1 banana, chopped into chunks
- 2 Clementines/Mandarins

How To:

1. Peel the clementines and remove seeds.
2. Add the listed ingredients to your blender/food processor and blend until smooth.
3. Serve chilled and enjoy!

Nutrition (Per Serving)
Calories: 200
Fat: 10g
Carbohydrates: 14g
Protein 2g
Cabbage and Coconut Chia Smoothie
Serving: 2
Prep Time: 5 minutes
Ingredients:

- 1/3 cup cabbage
- 1 cup cold unsweetened coconut milk
- 1 tablespoon chia seeds
- ½ cup cherries
- ½ cup spinach

How To:

1. Add coconut milk to your blender.
2. Cut cabbage and add to your blender.
3. Place chia seeds in a coffee grinder and chop to powder, brush the powder into the blender.
4. Pit the cherries and add them to the blender.
5. Wash and dry the spinach and chop.
6. Add to the mix.
7. Cover and blend on low followed by medium.
8. Taste the texture and serve chilled!

Nutrition (Per Serving)
Calories: 200
Fat: 10g
Carbohydrates: 14g
Protein 2g
The Cherry Beet Delight
Serving: 2
Prep Time: 5 minutes
Ingredients:

- 1 cup cherries, pitted
- ½ cup beets
- Few banana slices
- 1 cup water, filtered, alkaline
- 1 cup coconut milk
- Pinch of organic vanilla powder
- Pinch of cinnamon
- Pinch of stevia
- Few mint leaves/lime slices to garnish

How To:

1. Add berries, beets, water, banana slices, coconut milk to your blender.
2. Blend well until smooth.
3. Add more water if the texture is too creamy for you.

4. Add coconut oil, vanilla, cinnamon and stir.
5. Add a bit of stevia for extra sweetness.
6. Garnish with mint leaves and lime slices.
7. Enjoy!

Nutrition (Per Serving)
Calories: 200
Fat: 10g
Carbohydrates: 14g
Protein 2g
Green Delight
Serving: 1
Prep Time: 10 minutes
Ingredients:

- ¾ cup whole almond milk yogurt
- 2 ½ cups lettuce mix salad greens
- 1 pack stevia
- 1 tablespoon MCT oil
- 1 tablespoon chia seeds
- 1 ½ cups water

How To:

1. Add listed ingredients to blender.
2. Blend until you have a smooth and creamy texture.
3. Serve chilled and enjoy!

Nutrition (Per Serving)
Calories: 320
Fat: 24g
Carbohydrates: 17g
Protein: 10g
Guilt Free Lemon and Rosemary Drink
Serving: 1
Prep Time: 10 minutes
Ingredients:

- ½ cup whole almond milk yogurt
- 1 cup garden greens
- 1 pack stevia
- 1 tablespoon olive oil
- 1 stalk fresh rosemary
- 1 tablespoon lemon juice, fresh

- 1 tablespoon pepitas
- 1 tablespoon flaxseed, ground
- 1 ½ cups water

How To:

1. Add listed ingredients to blender.
2. Blend until you have a smooth and creamy texture.
3. Serve chilled and enjoy!

Nutrition (Per Serving)
Calories: 312
Fat: 25g
Carbohydrates: 14g
Protein: 9g
Strawberry and Rhubarb Smoothie
Serving: 1
Prep Time: 5 minutes
Cook Time: 3 minutes
Ingredients:

- 1 rhubarb stalk, chopped
- 1 cup fresh strawberries, sliced
- ½ cup plain Greek strawberries
- Pinch of ground cinnamon
- 3 ice cubes

How To:

1. Take a small saucepan and fill with water over high heat.
2. Bring to boil and add rhubarb, boil for 3 minutes.
3. Drain and transfer to a blender.
4. Add strawberries, honey, yogurt, cinnamon and pulse mixture until smooth.
5. Add ice cubes and blend until thick with no lumps.
6. Pour into glass and enjoy chilled.

Nutrition (Per Serving)
Calories: 295
Fat: 8g
Carbohydrates: 56g
Protein: 6g
Vanilla Hemp Drink
Serving: 1

Prep Time: 10 minutes
Ingredients:

- 1 cup water
- 1 cup unsweetened hemp almond milk, vanilla
- 1 ½ tablespoons coconut oil, unrefined
- ½ cup frozen blueberries, mixed
- 4 cups leafy greens, kale and spinach
- 1 tablespoon flaxseeds
- 1 tablespoon almond butter

How To:

1. Add listed ingredients to blender.
2. Blend until you have a smooth and creamy texture.
3. Serve chilled and enjoy!

Nutrition (Per Serving)
Calories: 250
Fat: 20g
Carbohydrates: 10g
Protein: 7g
Yogurt and Kale Smoothie
Serving: 1
Prep Time: 10 minutes
Ingredients:

- 1 cup whole almond milk yogurt
- 1 cup baby kale greens
- 1 pack stevia
- 1 tablespoon MCT oil
- 1 tablespoons sunflower seeds
- 1 cup water

How To:

1. Add listed ingredients to blender 2. Blend until you have a smooth and creamy texture
2. Serve chilled and enjoy!

Nutrition (Per Serving)
Calories: 329
Fat: 26g
Carbohydrates: 15g

Protein: 11g
The Sweet Potato Acid Buster
Serving: 2
Prep Time: 5 minutes
Ingredients:

- 1 cup sweet potato, chopped
- 1 cup almond milk
- ¼ teaspoon nutmeg
- ¼ teaspoon ground cinnamon
- 1 teaspoon flaxseed
- 1 small avocado, cubed
- Few spinach leaves, torn
- Toppings:
- Handful of crushed almonds
- Handful of crushed cashews
- 3 tablespoons orange juice

How To:

1. Blend all the ingredients until smooth.
2. Add a few ice cubes to make it chilled.
3. Add your desired toppings.
4. Enjoy!

Nutrition (Per Serving)
Calories: 200
Fat: 10g
Carbohydrates: 14g
Protein 2g
The Sunshine Offering
Serving: 2
Prep Time: 5 minutes
Ingredients:

- 2 cups fresh spinach
- 1 ½ cups almond milk ½ cup coconut water
- 3 cups fresh pineapple
- 2 tablespoons coconut unsweetened flakes

How To:

1. Add all the listed ingredients to your blender.
2. Blend until smooth.

3. Add a few ice cubes and serve the smoothie.

4. Enjoy!

Nutrition (Per Serving)
Calories: 200
Fat: 10g
Carbohydrates: 14g
Protein 2g

The Sleepy Bug Smoothie
Serving: 2
Prep Time: 5 minutes
Ingredients:

- 1 cup fennel tea infusion
- 1 cup almond milk
- 1 cup watermelon, chopped
- 1 green apple
- ½ cup pomegranate
- ½ inch ginger
- Stevia to sweeten

How To:

1. Add the listed ingredients to your blender.
2. Blend until smooth.
3. Add a bit of stevia if you want more sweetness.
4. Serve chilled and enjoy!

Nutrition (Per Serving)
Calories: 200
Fat: 10g
Carbohydrates: 14g
Protein 2g

Matcha Coconut Smoothie
Serving: 2
Prep Time: 5 minutes
Cook Time: Nil
Ingredients:

- 1 whole banana, cubed
- 1 cup frozen mango, chunked
- 2 kale leaves, torn
- 3 tablespoons white beans
- 2 tablespoons shredded coconut

- ½ teaspoon Matcha green tea powder
- 1 cup water

How To:

1. Add banana, kale, mango, white beans, Matcha powder and white beans to the blender.
2. Blend until you have a nice smoothie.
3. Serve and enjoy!

Nutrition (Per Serving)
Calories: 200
Fat: 10g
Carbohydrates: 14g
Protein 2g
Ravishing Apple and Cucumber Glass
Serving: 2
Prep Time: 5 minutes
Ingredients:

- 1 green apple
- 2 cucumbers, peeled
- 1 cup almond milk
- ½ cup coconut cream (raw and organic)
- Pinch of cinnamon and nutmeg (each)
- Pinch of Himalayan salt
- 1 tablespoon coconut oil

How To:

1. Add all the listed ingredients to your blender (except oil, spices and salt).
2. Blend until smooth.
3. Mix in coconut oil, spices and salt.
4. Stir and enjoy!

Nutrition (Per Serving)
Calories: 200
Fat: 10g
Carbohydrates: 14g
Protein 2g
Creative Winter Smoothie
Serving: 2
Prep Time: 5 minutes

Ingredients:

- 3 tomatoes, peeled
- 1 celery stalk
- 2 cloves garlic, peeled
- 1-inch ginger, peeled
- 1 cucumber, peeled
- Juice of 1 lemon
- 1 cup alkaline water
- Salt as needed
- Pepper as needed
- Pinch of turmeric
- Olive oil/avocado oil

How To:

1. Add tomatoes, celery, garlic, cucumber and water to your blender.
2. Blend well until smooth.
3. Add lemon juice, salt and oil.
4. Stir.
5. Season with pepper and turmeric.
6. Stir.
7. Serve chilled and enjoy!

Nutrition (Per Serving)
Calories: 200
Fat: 10g
Carbohydrates: 14g
Protein 2g
Feisty Mango and Coconut Smoothie
Serving: 2
Prep Time: 5 minutes
Ingredients:

- 1 teaspoon spirulina
- 1 cup frozen mango
- 1 cup unsweetened coconut milk
- ½ cup spinach

How To:

1. Cut mangoes and dice them.
2. Add mango, cup of unsweetened coconut milk, teaspoon of
   Spirulina and spinach to the blender.

3. Blend on low to medium until smooth.
4. Check the texture and serve chilled!

Nutrition (Per Serving)
Calories: 200
Fat: 10g
Carbohydrates: 14g
Protein 2g

Mexican Chocolate Stand-Off
Serving: 2
Prep Time: 5 minutes
Ingredients:

- 2 bananas
- 1 tablespoon hemp seeds
- 1 bag frozen blueberries
- ½ teaspoon liquid stevia
- Pure water
- 2 teaspoons raw chocolate
- 1 teaspoon raw carob powder
- ½ teaspoon green powder
- ½ teaspoon cinnamon powder
- Pinch of cayenne pepper

How To:

1. Add all the listed ingredients to your blender.
2. Blend until smooth.
3. Add a few ice cubes and serve the smoothie.
4. Enjoy!

Nutrition (Per Serving)
Calories: 200
Fat: 10g
Carbohydrates: 14g
Protein 2g

The Awesome Cleanser
Serving: 2
Prep Time: 5 minutes
Ingredients:

- 2 grapefruits, juiced
- 2 lemons, juiced
- Half cup alkaline water/filtered water

- 2 tablespoons olive oil
- 2 cucumbers, peeled
- 1 avocado, peeled and pitted
- 2 cloves fresh garlic
- 1-inch ginger
- Pinch of Himalayan salt
- Pinch of cayenne pepper

How To:

1. Add cucumber, ginger, avocado, grapefruit and lemon to your blender.
2. Blend until smooth.
3. Add alkaline water, spices and oil.
4. Stir well and drink chilled.
5. Enjoy!

Nutrition (Per Serving)
Calories: 200
Fat: 10g
Carbohydrates: 14g
Protein 2g
Gentle Tropical Papaya Smoothie
Serving: 2
Prep Time: 5 minutes
Ingredients:

- 1 papaya, cut into chunks
- 1 cup fat free plain yogurt
- ½ cup pineapple chunks
- ½ cup crushed ice
- 1 teaspoon coconut extract
- 1 teaspoon flaxseed

How To:

1. Add the listed ingredients to your blender and blend until smooth.
2. Serve chilled!

Nutrition (Per Serving)
Calories: 200
Fat: 10g
Carbohydrates: 14g
Protein 2g

Kale and Apple Smoothie
Serving: 2
Prep Time: 5 minutes
Ingredients:

- ¾ of a kale, chopped, ribs and stem removed
- 1 small stalk celery, chopped
- ½ banana
- ½ cup apple juice
- 1 tablespoon lemon juice

How To:

1. Add the listed ingredients to your blender and blend until smooth.
2. Serve chilled!

Nutrition (Per Serving)
Calories: 200
Fat: 10g
Carbohydrates: 14g
Protein 2g

Mango and Lime Generous Smoothie
Serving: 2
Prep Time: 5 minutes
Ingredients:

- 2 tablespoons lime juice
- 2 cups spinach, chopped and stemmed
- 1 ½ cups frozen mango, cubed
- 1 cup green grapes

How To:

1. Add the listed ingredients to your blender and blend until smooth
2. Serve chilled!

Nutrition (Per Serving)
Calories: 200
Fat: 10g
Carbohydrates: 14g
Protein 2g

The Pear and Chocolate Catastrophe
Serving: 2
Prep Time: 5 minutes

Ingredients:

- 1 banana (freckled skin)
- 2-3 pears
- 2 tablespoons hulled hemp seeds
- 1 bag frozen raspberries
- 2 ½ cups coconut water
- 1 teaspoon raw chocolate
- Small bunch arugula lettuce leaves
- Liquid stevia

How To:

1. Add all the listed ingredients to your blender.
2. Blend until smooth.
3. Add a few ice cubes and serve the smoothie.
4. Enjoy!

Nutrition (Per Serving)
Calories: 200
Fat: 10g
Carbohydrates: 14g
Protein 2g
The Avocado Paradise
Serving: 2
Prep Time: 5 minutes
Ingredients:

- ½ avocado, cubed
- 1 cup coconut milk
- Half a lemon
- ¼ cup fresh spinach leaves
- 1 pear
- 1 tablespoon hemp seed powder

Toppings:

- Handful of macadamia nuts
- Handful of grapes
- 2 lemon slices

How To:

1. Blend all the ingredients until smooth.

2. Add a few ice cubes to make it chilled.
3. Add your desired toppings.
4. Enjoy!

Nutrition (Per Serving)
Calories: 200
Fat: 10g
Carbohydrates: 14g
Protein 2g
The Authentic Vegetable Medley
Serving: 2
Prep Time: 5 minutes
Ingredients:

- 1 cup broccoli, steamed
- 1 bunch asparagus, steamed
- 2 cups coconut milk
- 2 tablespoons coconut oil
- 2 carrots, peeled
- Few inches of horseradish
- Himalayan salt
- Pinch of chili powder
- ½ onion
- 2 garlic cloves

How To:

1. Add all the listed ingredients to your blender except coconut oil, salt and chili powder.
2. Blend until smooth.
3. Add salt, coconut oil and chili powder.
4. Stir well and serve chilled!

Nutrition (Per Serving)
Calories: 200
Fat: 10g
Carbohydrates: 14g
Protein 2g
The Original Power Producer
Serving: 2
Prep Time: 5 minutes
Ingredients:

- ½ cup spinach

- 1 avocado, diced
- 1 cup coconut milk
- 1 tablespoon flaxseed
- 2 nori sheets, roasted and crushed
- 1 garlic clove Salt to taste

Toppings:
Handful of pistachios

- 3 tablespoons bell pepper, finely chopped
- Handful of parsley leaves

How To:

1. Blend all the ingredients until smooth.
2. Add a few ice cubes to make it chilled.
3. Add your desired toppings.
4. Enjoy!

Nutrition (Per Serving)

- Calories: 200
- Fat: 10g
- Carbohydrates: 14g
- Protein 2g

The Dreamy Cherry Mix
Serving: 2
Prep Time: 5 minutes
Ingredients:

- ½ cup ripe cherries
- Juice of 1 lemon
- 1 cup coconut milk
- 1 avocado, cubed
- ¼ cup spinach
- Few slices of cucumber, peeled

Toppings:

- Handful of pistachios
- Handful of raisins
- 1 slice lemon

How To:

1. Blend all the ingredients until smooth.
2. Add a few ice cubes to make it chilled.
3. Add your desired toppings.
4. Enjoy!

Nutrition (Per Serving)

- Calories: 200
- Fat: 10g
- Carbohydrates: 14g
- Protein 2g

Better Than Your Favorite Restaurant "Lemon Smoothie"
Serving: 2
Prep Time: 5 minutes
Ingredients:

- 2 cups organic rice milk, gluten free
- 1 cup melon, chopped
- ½ avocado, cubed
- ½ cucumber, peeled and sliced
- Ice cubes
- 2 limes, juiced
- 1 tablespoon coconut oil
- Few banana slices to taste

How To:

1. Add the listed ingredients to your blender (except coconut oil) and blend well.
2. Blend until you have a smooth texture.
3. Add coconut oil and stir.
4. Enjoy!

Nutrition (Per Serving)
Calories: 200
Fat: 10g
Carbohydrates: 14g
Protein 2g
The "One" with The Watermelon
Serving: 2
Prep Time: 5 minutes

Ingredients:

- 1 cup watermelon, sliced
- ½ cup coconut, shredded
- 1 grapefruit, cubed
- ½ cup coconut milk
- 2 tablespoons almond butter

Toppings:

- Handful of crushed almonds
- Handful of raisins
- 2 tablespoons coconut powder

How To:

1. Blend all the ingredients until smooth.
2. Add a few ice cubes to make it chilled.
3. Add your desired toppings.
4. Enjoy!

Nutrition (Per Serving)

- Calories: 200
- Fat: 10g
- Carbohydrates: 14g
- Protein 2g

Strawberry and Rhubarb Smoothie
Serving: 1
Prep Time: 5 minutes
Cook Time: 3 minutes
Ingredients:

- 1 rhubarb stalk, chopped
- 1 cup fresh strawberries, sliced
- ½ cup plain Greek yoghurt
- Pinch of ground cinnamon
- 3 ice cubes

How To:

1. Take a small saucepan and fill with water over high heat.
2. Bring to boil and add rhubarb, boil for 3 minutes.

3. Drain and transfer to a blender.
4. Add strawberries, honey, yogurt, cinnamon and pulse mixture until smooth.
5. Add ice cubes and blend until thick and has no lumps.
6. Pour into glass and enjoy chilled.

Nutrition (Per Serving)

- Calories: 295
- Fat: 8g
- Carbohydrates: 56g
- Protein: 6g

Chapter Nine

VEGAN SNAKE RECIPES

*I*t is mid-morning, and you're feeling a little peckish - what will you eat? You feel a bit deprived because you are on the vegan diet, and you can't think of any tasty and quick snack ideas. Or perhaps you've just come home from work and are craving a yummy treat, but you are tired. You, therefore, want your vegan food to be easy, hassle-free, and not one of the most complicated time-consuming recipes on the planet, even better - preferably just something that you can throw together in under 5 or 10 minutes.

Below is a list of some tasty, fast, and easy vegan food and snack recipe ideas to help make your life a little easier.

Popcorn

It's a tasty, rather low-calorie snack that can be ready to eat in under 10 minutes. It's perfect if you're craving something a little salty.

Nutritional Facts
servings per container
5

Prep Total
10 min
Serving Size
8
Amount per serving
Calories
0%

% DAILY VALUE

Total Fat 3g
20%
Saturated Fat 4g
32%
Trans Fat 2g
2%
Cholesterol
2%
Sodium 110mg
0.2%
Total Carbohydrate 21g
50%
Dietary Fiber 9g
1%
Total Sugar 1g
1%
Protein 1g

Vitamin C 7mcg
17%
Calcium 60mg
1%
Iron 7mg
10%
Potassium 23mg
21%

Ingredient & Process

Place 2 tablespoons of olive oil and ¼ Cup popcorn in a large saucepan.

Cover with a lid, and cook the popcorn over a medium flame, ensuring that you are shaking constantly. Just when you think that it's not working, keep on enduring for another minute or two, and the popping will begin.

When the popping stops, take off from the heat and place in a large bowl.

Add plenty of salt to taste, and if desired, dribble in ¼ Cup to ½ Cup of melted coconut oil. If you are craving sweet popcorn, add some maple syrup to the coconut oil, about ½ Cup, or to taste.

5 Minutes or Less Vegan Snacks

Here's a list of basically 'no-preparation required' vegan snack ideas that you can munch on anytime:

Nutritional Facts

servings per container

5

Prep Total

10 min
Serving Size
8
Amount per serving
Calories
0%

% DAILY VALUE
Total Fat 20g
190%
Saturated Fat 2g
32%
Trans Fat 1g
2%
Cholesterol
2%
Sodium 70mg
0.2%
Total Carbohydrate 32g
150%
Dietary Fiber 8g
1%
Total Sugar 1g
1%
Protein 3g

Vitamin C 7mcg
17%
Calcium 210mg
1%
Iron 4mg
10%
Potassium 25mg
20%

Ingredients and Process
Trail mix: nuts, dried fruit, and vegan chocolate pieces.
Fruit pieces with almond butter, peanut butter or vegan chocolate spread
Frozen vegan cake, muffin, brownie or slice that you made on the weekend
Vegetable sticks (carrots, celery, and cucumber etc.) with a Vegan Dip (homemade or store-bought) such as hummus or beetroot dip. (Careful of the store-bought ingredients though).
Smoothie - throw into the blender anything you can find (within limits!)

such as soy milk, coconut milk, rice milk, almond milk, soy yogurt, coconut milk yogurt, cinnamon, spices, sea salt, berries, bananas, cacao powder, vegan chocolate, agave nectar, maple syrup, chia seeds, flax seeds, nuts, raisins, sultanas... What you put into your smoothie is up to you, and you can throw it all together in less than 5 minutes!

Crackers with avocado, soy butter, and tomato slices, or hummus spread.

Packet chips (don't eat them too often). There are many vegan chip companies that make kale chips, corn chips, potato chips, and vegetable chips, so enjoy a small bowl now and again.

Fresh Fruit

The health benefits of eating fresh fruit daily should not be minimized. So, make sure that you enjoy some in-season fruit as one of your daily vegan snacks.

Nutritional Facts

servings per container

10

Prep Total

10 min

Serving Size

5/5

Amount per serving

Calories

1%

% DAILY VALUE

Total Fat 24g

2%

Saturated Fat 8g

3%

Trans Fat 4g

2%

Cholesterol

2%

Sodium 10mg

22%

Total Carbohydrate 7g

54%

Dietary Fiber 4g

1%

Total Sugar 1g

1%

Protein 1g

24

Vitamin C 2mcg
17%
Calcium 270mg
15%
Iron 17mg
20%
Potassium 130mg
2%

Ingredients:
Chop your favorite fruit and make a fast and easy fruit salad, adding some squeezed orange juice to make a nice juicy dressing.

Serve with some soy or coconut milk yogurt or vegan ice-cream if desired, and top with some tasty walnuts or toasted slithered almonds to make it a sustaining snack.

Vegan Brownie
Nutritional Facts
servings per container
3
Prep Total
10 min
Serving Size
7
Amount per serving
Calories
20%

% Daily Value
Total Fat 3g
22%
Saturated Fat 22g
8%
Trans Fat 17g
21%
Cholesterol
20%
Sodium 120mg
70%
Total Carbohydrate 30g
57%
Dietary Fiber 4g
8%
Total Sugar 10g
8%

Protein 6g

Vitamin C 1mcg
1%
Calcium 20mg
31%
Iron 2mg
12%
Potassium 140mg
92%

Ingredients:

- 1/2 cup non-dairy butter melted
- 5 tablespoons cocoa
- 1 cup granulated sugar
- 3 teaspoons Ener-G egg replacer
- 1/4 cup water
- 1 teaspoon vanilla
- 3/4 cup flour
- 1 teaspoon baking powder
- 1/2 teaspoon salt
- 1/2 cup walnuts (optional)

Instructions:

1. Heat oven to 350°. Prepare an 8" x 8" baking pan with butter or canola oil.
2. Combine butter, cocoa, and sugar in a large bowl.
3. Mix the egg replacer and water in a blender until frothy.
4. Add to the butter mixture with vanilla. Add the flour, baking powder, and salt, and mix thoroughly.
5. Add the walnuts if desired. Pour the batter into the pan, and spread evenly.
6. Bake for 40 to 45 minutes, or until a toothpick inserted comes out clean.

Spinach Dip
Serving: 2
Prep Time: 4 minutes
Cook Time: 0 minutes
Ingredients:

- 5 ounces Spinach, raw

- 1 cup Greek yogurt
- 1/2 tablespoon onion powder
- 1/4 teaspoon garlic sunflower seeds
- Black pepper to taste
- 1/4 teaspoon Greek Seasoning

How To:

1. Add the listed ingredients in a blender.
2. Emulsify.
3. Season and serve.

Nutrition (Per Serving)
Calories: 101
Fat: 4g
Carbohydrates: 4g
Protein: 10g
Cauliflower Rice
Serving: 2
Prep Time: 5 minutes
Cook Time: 6 minutes
Ingredients:

- 1 head grated cauliflower head
- 1 tablespoon coconut aminos
- 1 pinch of sunflower seeds
- 1 pinch of black pepper
- 1 tablespoon Garlic Powder
- 1 tablespoon Sesame Oil

How To:

1. Add cauliflower to a food processor and grate it.
2. Take a pan and add sesame oil, let it heat up over medium heat.
3. Add grated cauliflower and pour coconut aminos.
4. Cook for 4-6 minutes.
5. Season and enjoy!

Nutrition (Per Serving)
Calories: 329
Fat: 28g
Carbohydrates: 13g
Protein: 10g
Grilled Sprouts and Balsamic Glaze

Serving: 2
Prep Time: 10 minutes
Cook Time: 30 minutes
Ingredients:

- ½ pound Brussels sprouts, trimmed and halved
- Fresh cracked black pepper
- 1 tablespoon olive oil
- Sunflower seeds to taste
- 2 teaspoons balsamic glaze
- 2 wooden skewers

How To:

1. Take wooden skewers and place them on a largely sized foil.
2. Place sprouts on the skewers and drizzle oil, sprinkle sunflower seeds and pepper.
3. Cover skewers with foil.
4. Pre-heat your grill to low and place skewers (with foil) in the grill.
5. Grill for 30 minutes, making sure to turn after every 5-6 minutes.
6. Once done, uncovered and drizzle balsamic glaze on top.
7. Enjoy!

Nutrition (Per Serving)
Calories: 440
Fat: 27g
Carbohydrates. 33g
Protein: 26g
Amazing Green Creamy Cabbage
Serving: 4
Prep Time: 10 minutes
Cook Time: 10 minutes
Ingredients:

- 2 ounces almond butter
- 1 ½ pounds green cabbage, shredded
- 1 ¼ cups coconut cream
- Sunflower seeds and pepper to taste
- 8 tablespoons fresh parsley, chopped

How To:

1. Take a skillet and place it over medium heat, add almond butter and let it melt.

2. Add cabbage and sauté until brown.
3. Stir in cream and lower the heat to low.
4. Let it simmer.
5. Season with sunflower seeds and pepper.
6. Garnish with parsley and serve.
7. Enjoy!

Nutrition (Per Serving)
Calories: 432
Fat: 42g
Carbohydrates: 8g
Protein: 4g

Simple Rice Mushroom Risotto
Serving: 4
Prep Time: 5 minutes
Cook Time: 15 minutes
Ingredients:

- 4 ½ cups cauliflower, riced
- 3 tablespoons coconut oil
- 1-pound Portobello mushrooms, thinly sliced
- 1-pound white mushrooms, thinly sliced
- 2 shallots, diced
- ¼ cup organic vegetable broth
- Sunflower seeds and pepper to taste
- 3 tablespoons chives, chopped
- 4 tablespoons almond butter
- ½ cup kite ricotta/cashew cheese, grated

How To:

1. Use a food processor and pulse cauliflower florets until riced.
2. Take a large saucepan and heat up 2 tablespoons oil over medium-high flame.
3. Add mushrooms and sauté for 3 minutes until mushrooms are tender.
4. Clear saucepan of mushrooms and liquid and keep them on the side.
5. Add the rest of the 1 tablespoon oil to skillet.
6. Toss shallots and cook for 60 seconds.
7. Add cauliflower rice, stir for 2 minutes until coated with oil.
8. Add broth to riced cauliflower and stir for 5 minutes.
9. Remove pot from heat and mix in mushrooms and liquid.
10. Add chives, almond butter, parmesan cheese.

11. Season with sunflower seeds and pepper.
12. Serve and enjoy!

Nutrition (Per Serving)
Calories: 438
Fat: 17g
Carbohydrates: 15g
Protein: 12g
Hearty Green Bean Roast
Serving: 4
Prep Time: 10 minutes
Cook Time: 20 minutes
Ingredients:

- 1 whole egg
- 2 tablespoons olive oil
- Sunflower seeds and pepper to taste
- 1-pound fresh green beans
- 5 ½ tablespoons grated parmesan cheese

How To:

1. Pre-heat your oven to 400 degrees F.
2. Take a bowl and whisk in eggs with oil and spices.
3. Add beans and mix well.
4. Stir in parmesan cheese and pour the mix into baking pan (lined with parchment paper).
5. Bake for 15-20 minutes.
6. Serve warm and enjoy!

Nutrition (Per Serving)
Calories: 216
Fat: 21g
Carbohydrates: 7g
Protein: 9g
Almond and Blistered Beans
Serving: 4
Prep Time: 10 minutes
Cook Time: 20 minutes
Ingredients:

- 1-pound fresh green beans, ends trimmed
- 1 ½ tablespoon olive oil
- ¼ teaspoon sunflower seeds

- 1 ½ tablespoons fresh dill, minced
- Juice of 1 lemon
- ¼ cup crushed almonds
- Sunflower seeds as needed

How To:

1. Pre-heat your oven to 400 degrees F.
2. Add the green beans with your olive oil and also the sunflower seeds.
3. Then spread them in one single layer on a large sized sheet pan.
4. Roast it for 10 minutes and stir, then roast for another 8-10 minutes.
5. Remove from the oven and keep stirring in the lemon juice alongside the dill.
6. Top it with crushed almonds and some flaked sunflower seeds and serve.

Nutrition (Per Serving)
Calories: 347
Fat: 16g
Carbohydrates: 6g
Protein: 45g
Tomato Platter
Serving: 8
Prep Time: 10 minutes + Chill time
Cook Time: Nil
Ingredients:

- 1/3 cup olive oil
- 1 teaspoon sunflower seeds
- 2 tablespoons onion, chopped
- ¼ teaspoon pepper
- ½ a garlic, minced
- 1 tablespoon fresh parsley, minced
- 3 large fresh tomatoes, sliced
- 1 teaspoon dried basil
- ¼ cup red wine vinegar

How To:

1. Take a shallow dish and arrange tomatoes in the dish.
2. Add the rest of the ingredients in a mason jar, cover the jar and shake it well.

3. Pour the mix over tomato slices.
4. Let it chill for 2-3 hours.
5. Serve!

Nutrition (Per Serving)
Calories: 350
Fat: 28g
Carbohydrates: 10g
Protein: 14g
Lemony Sprouts
Serving: 4
Prep Time: 10 minutes
Cook Time: Nil
Ingredients:

- 1 pound Brussels sprouts, trimmed and shredded
- 8 tablespoons olive oil
- 1 lemon, juice and zested
- Sunflower seeds and pepper to taste
- ¾ cup spicy almond and seed mix

How To:

1. Take a bowl and mix in lemon juice, sunflower seeds, pepper and olive oil.
2. Mix well.
3. Stir in shredded Brussels sprouts and toss.
4. Let it sit for 10 minutes.
5. Add nuts and toss.
6. Serve and enjoy!

Nutrition (Per Serving)
Calories: 382
Fat: 36g
Carbohydrates: 9g
Protein: 7g
Cool Garbanzo and Spinach Beans
Serving: 4
Prep Time: 5-10 minutes
Cook Time: Nil
Ingredients:

- 1 tablespoon olive oil
- ½ onion, diced

- 10 ounces spinach, chopped
- 12 ounces garbanzo beans
- ½ teaspoon cumin

How To:

1. Take a skillet and add olive oil, let it warm over medium-low heat.
2. Add onions, garbanzo and cook for 5 minutes.
3. Stir in spinach, cumin, garbanzo beans and season with sunflower seeds.
4. Use a spoon to smash gently.
5. Cook thoroughly until heated, enjoy!

Nutrition (Per Serving)
Calories: 90
Fat: 4g
Carbohydrates:11g
Protein:4g
Delicious Garlic Tomatoes
Serving: 4
Prep Time: 10 minutes
Cook Time: 50 minutes
Ingredients:

- 4 garlic cloves, crushed
- 1 pound mixed cherry tomatoes
- 3 thyme sprigs, chopped
- Pinch of sunflower seeds
- Black pepper as needed
- ¼ cup olive oil

How To:

1. Preheat your oven to 325 degrees F.
2. Take a baking dish and add tomatoes, olive oil and thyme.
3. Season with sunflower seeds and pepper and mix.
4. Bake for 50 minutes.
5. Divide tomatoes and pan juices and serve.
6. Enjoy!

Nutrition (Per Serving)
Calories: 100
Fat: 0g
Carbohydrates: 1g

Protein: 6g
Mashed Celeriac
Serving: 4
Prep Time: 10 minutes
Cook Time: 20 minutes
Ingredients:

- 2 celeriac, washed, peeled and diced
- 2 teaspoons extra-virgin olive oil
- 1 tablespoon honey
- ½ teaspoon ground nutmeg
- Sunflower seeds and pepper as needed

How To:

1. Pre-heat your oven to 400 degrees F.
2. Line a baking sheet with aluminum foil and keep it on the side.
3. Take a large bowl and toss celeriac and olive oil.
4. Spread celeriac evenly on a baking sheet.
5. Roast for 20 minutes until tender.
6. Transfer to a large bowl.
7. Add honey and nutmeg.
8. Use a potato masher to mash the mixture until fluffy.
9. Season with sunflower seeds and pepper.
10. Serve and enjoy!

Nutrition (Per Serving)
Calories: 136
Fat: 3g
Carbohydrates: 26g
Protein: 4g
Spicy Wasabi Mayonnaise
Serving: 4
Prep Time: 15 minutes
Cook Time: Nil
Ingredients:

- 1 cup mayonnaise
- ½ tablespoon wasabi paste

How To:

1. Take a bowl and mix wasabi paste and mayonnaise.
2. Mix well.

3. Let it chill and use as needed.

Nutrition (Per Serving)
Calories: 388
Fat: 42g
Carbohydrates: 1g

- Protein: 1g

Mediterranean Kale Dish
Serving: 6
Prep Time: 15 minutes
Cook Time: 10 minutes
Ingredients:

- 12 cups kale, chopped
- 2 tablespoons lemon juice
- 1 tablespoon olive oil
- 1 teaspoon coconut aminos
- Sunflower seeds and pepper as needed

How To:

1. Add a steamer insert to your saucepan.
2. Fill the saucepan with water up to the bottom of the steamer.
3. Cover and bring water to boil (medium-high heat).
4. Add kale to the insert and steam for 7-8 minutes.
5. Take a large bowl and add lemon juice, olive oil, sunflower seeds, coconut aminos, and pepper.
6. Mix well and add the steamed kale to the bowl.
7. Toss and serve.
8. Enjoy!

Nutrition (Per Serving)
Calories: 350
Fat: 17g
Carbohydrates: 41g
Protein: 11g
Spicy Kale Chips
Serving: 4
Prep Time: 10 minutes
Cook Time: 25 minutes
Ingredients:

- 3 cups kale, stemmed and thoroughly washed, torn in 2-inch pieces
- 1 tablespoon extra-virgin olive oil
- ½ teaspoon chili powder
- ¼ teaspoon sea sunflower seeds

How To:

1. Pre-heat your oven to 300 degrees F.
2. Line 2 baking sheets with parchment paper and keep it on the side.
3. Dry kale entirely and transfer to a large bowl.
4. Add olive oil and toss.
5. Make sure each leaf is covered.
6. Season kale with chili powder and sunflower seeds, toss again.
7. Divide kale between baking sheets and spread into a single layer.
8. Bake for 25 minutes until crispy.
9. Cool the chips for 5 minutes and serve.
10. Enjoy!

Nutrition (Per Serving)

- Calories: 56

Fat: 4g
Carbohydrates: 5g
Protein: 2g

Seemingly Easy Portobello Mushrooms
Serving. 4
Prep Time: 10 minutes
Cook Time: 10 minutes
Ingredients:

- 12 cherry tomatoes
- 2 ounces scallions
- 4 portabella mushrooms
- 4 ¼ ounces almond butter
- Sunflower seeds and pepper to taste

How To:

1. Take a large skillet and melt almond butter over medium heat.
2. Add mushrooms and sauté for 3 minutes.
3. Stir in cherry tomatoes and scallions.
4. Sauté for 5 minutes. 5. Season accordingly.
5. Sauté until veggies are tender.

6. Enjoy!

Nutrition (Per Serving)
Calories: 154
Fat: 10g
Carbohydrates: 2g
Protein: 7g
The Garbanzo Bean Extravaganza
Serving: 5
Prep Time: 10 minutes
Cook Time: Nil
Ingredients:

- 1 can garbanzo beans, chickpeas
- 1 tablespoon olive oil
- 1 teaspoon sunflower seeds
- 1 teaspoon garlic powder
- ½ teaspoon paprika

How To:

1. Pre-heat your oven to 375 degrees F.
2. Line a baking sheet with a silicone baking mat.
3. Drain and rinse garbanzo beans, pat garbanzo beans dry and put into a large bowl.
4. Toss with olive oil, sunflower seeds, garlic powder, paprika and mix well.
5. Spread over a baking sheet.
6. Bake for 20 minutes.
7. Turn chickpeas so they are roasted well.
8. Place back in oven and bake for another 25 minutes at 375 degrees F.
9. Let them cool and enjoy!

Nutrition (Per Serving)
Calories: 395
Fat: 7g
Carbohydrates: 52g
Protein: 35g
Classic Guacamole
Serving: 6
Prep Time: 15 minutes
Cook Time: Nil
Ingredients:

- 3 large ripe avocados
- 1 large red onion, peeled and diced
- 4 tablespoons freshly squeezed lime juice
- Sunflower seeds as needed
- Freshly ground black pepper as needed
- Cayenne pepper as needed

How To:

1. Halve the avocados and discard stone.
2. Scoop flesh from 3 avocado halves and transfer to a large bowl.
3. Mash using a fork.
4. Add 2 tablespoons of lime juice and mix.
5. Dice the remaining avocado flesh (remaining half) and transfer to another bowl.
6. Add remaining juice and toss.
7. Add diced flesh with the mashed flesh and mix.
8. Add chopped onions and toss.
9. Season with sunflower seeds, pepper and cayenne pepper.
10. Serve and enjoy!

Nutrition (Per Serving)
Calories: 172
Fat: 15g
Carbohydrates: 11g
Protein: 2g
Apple Slices
Serving: 4
Prep Time: 10 minutes
Cook Time: 10 minutes
Ingredients:

- 1 cup of coconut oil
- ¼ cup date paste
- 2 tablespoons ground cinnamon
- 4 granny smith apples, peeled and sliced, cored

How To:

1. Take a large sized skillet and place it over medium heat.
2. Add oil and allow the oil to heat up.
3. Stir in cinnamon and date paste into the oil.
4. Add cut up apples and cook for 5-8 minutes until crispy.
5. Serve and enjoy!

Nutrition (Per Serving)
Calories: 368
Fat: 23g
Carbohydrates: 44g
Protein: 1g
Elegant Cashew Sauce
Serving: 4
Prep Time: 5 minutes
Cook Time: Nil
Ingredients:

- 3 ounces cashew nuts
- ¼ cup water
- ½ cup olive oil
- 1 tablespoons lemon juice
- ½ teaspoon onion powder
- ½ teaspoon sunflower seeds
- 1 pinch cayenne pepper

How To:

- Add nuts to your blender and process.
- Add other ingredients (except oil) and process until smooth .
- Add a little bit of oil and puree .
- Serve as needed!

Nutrition (Per Serving)
Calories: 361
Fat: 37g
Carbohydrates: 6g
Protein: 3g
Lovely Japanese Cabbage Dish
Serving: 6
Prep Time: 25 minute
Cook Time: Nil
Ingredients:

- 3 tablespoons sesame oil
- 3 tablespoons rice vinegar
- 1 garlic clove, minced
- 1 teaspoon fresh ginger root, grated
- 1 teaspoon sunflower seeds
- 1 teaspoon pepper
- ½ large head cabbage, cored and shredded

- 1 bunch green onions, thinly sliced
- 1 cup almond slivers
- ¼ cup toasted sesame seeds

How To:

1. Add all listed ingredients to a large bowl, making sure to add the wet ingredients first, followed by the dried ingredients.
2. Toss well to ensure that the cabbages are coated well.
3. Let it chill and enjoy!

Nutrition (Per Serving)
Calories: 126
Fat: 10g
Carbohydrates: 9g
Protein: 4g
Almond Buttery Green Cabbage
Serving: 4
Prep Time: 10 minutes
Cook Time: 15 minutes
Ingredients:

- 1 ½ pounds shredded green cabbage
- 3 ounces almond butter
- Sunflower seeds and pepper to taste
- 1 dollop, whipped cream

How To:

1. Take a large skillet and place it over medium heat.
2. Add almond butter and melt.
3. Stir in cabbage and sauté for 15 minutes.
4. Season accordingly.
5. Serve with a dollop of cream.
6. Enjoy!

Nutrition (Per Serving)
Calories: 199
Fat: 17g
Carbohydrates: 10g
Protein: 3g
Mesmerizing Brussels and Pistachios
Serving: 4
Prep Time: 15 minutes

Cook Time: 15 minutes

Ingredients:

- 1-pound Brussels sprouts, tough bottom trimmed and halved lengthwise
- 1 tablespoon extra-virgin olive oil
- Sunflower seeds and pepper as needed
- ½ cup roasted pistachios, chopped Juice of ½ lemon

How To:

1. Pre-heat your oven to 400 degrees F.
2. Line a baking sheet with aluminum foil and keep it on the side.
3. Take a large bowl and add Brussels sprouts with olive oil and coat well.
4. Season sea sunflower seeds, pepper, spread veggies evenly on sheet.
5. Bake for 15 minutes until lightly caramelized.
6. Remove from oven and transfer to a serving bowl.
7. Toss with pistachios and lemon juice.
8. Serve warm and enjoy!

Nutrition (Per Serving)
Calories: 126
Fat: 7g
Carbohydrates: 14g
Protein: 6g
Brussels's Fever
Serving: 4
Prep Time: 10 minutes
Cook Time: 20 minutes
Ingredients:

- 2 tablespoons olive oil
- 1 yellow onion, chopped
- 2 pounds Brussels sprouts, trimmed and halved
- 4 cups vegetable stock
- ¼ cup coconut cream

How To:

1. Take a pot and place it over medium heat.
2. Add oil and let it heat up.
3. Add onion and stir-cook for 3 minutes.
4. Add Brussels sprouts and stir, cook for 2 minutes.

5. Add stock and black pepper, stir and bring to a simmer.
6. Cook for 20 minutes more.
7. Use an immersion blender to make the soup creamy.
8. Add coconut cream and stir well.
9. Ladle into soup bowls and serve.
10. Enjoy!

Nutrition (Per Serving)
Calories: 200
Fat: 11g
Carbohydrates: 6g
Protein: 11g
Hearty Garlic and Kale Platter
Serving: 4
Prep Time: 5 minutes
Cook Time: 10 minutes
Ingredients:

- 1 bunch kale
- 2 tablespoons olive oil
- 4 garlic cloves, minced

How To:

1. Carefully tear the kale into bite sized portions, making sure to remove the stem.
2. Discard the stems.
3. Take a large sized pot and place it over medium heat.
4. Add olive oil and let the oil heat up.
5. Add garlic and stir for 2 minutes.
6. Add kale and cook for 5-10 minutes.
7. Serve!

Nutrition (Per Serving)
Calories: 121
Fat: 8g
Carbohydrates: 5g
Protein: 4g
Acorn Squash with Mango Chutney
Serving: 4
Prep Time: 10 minutes
Cook Time: 3 hours 10 minutes
Ingredients:

- 1 large acorn squash
- ¼ cup mango chutney
- ¼ cup flaked coconut
- Salt and pepper as needed

How To:

1. Cut the squash into quarters and remove the seeds, discard the pulp.
2. Spray your cooker with olive oil.
3. Transfer the squash to the Slow Cooker and place lid.
4. Take a bowl and add coconut and chutney, mix well and divide the mixture into the center of the Squash.
5. Season well.
6. Place lid on top and cook on LOW for 2-3 hours.
7. Enjoy !

Nutrition (Per Serving)
Calories: 226
Fat: 6g
Carbohydrates: 24g
Protein: 17g
Satisfying Honey and Coconut Porridge
Serving: 8
Prep Time: 10 minutes
Cook Time: 8 hours
Ingredients:

- 4 cups light coconut milk
- 3 cups apple juice
- 2 ¼ cups coconut flour
- 1 teaspoon ground cinnamon
- ¼ cup honey

How To:

1. In a Slow Cooker, add the coconut milk, apple juice, flour, cinnamon and honey.
2. Stir well.
3. Close lid and cook on LOW for 8 hours.
4. Open lid and stir.
5. Serve with an additional seasoning of fresh fruits.
6. Enjoy!

Nutrition (Per Serving)
Calories: 372
Fat: 14g
Carbohydrates: 56g
Protein: 8g

Pure Maple Glazed Carrots
Serving: 6
Prep Time: 10 minutes
Cook Time: 8 hours

Ingredients:

- ¼ cup pure maple syrup
- ½ teaspoon ground ginger
- ¼ teaspoon ground nutmeg
- ½ teaspoon salt
- Juice of 1 orange
- 1-pound baby carrots

How To:

1. Take a small bowl and whisk in syrup, nutmeg, ginger, salt, orange juice.
2. Add carrots to your Slow Cooker and pour the maple syrup.
3. Toss to coat.
4. Close lid and cook on LOW for 8 hours.
5. Serve and enjoy!

Nutrition (Per Serving)
Calories: 76
Fat: 1g
Carbohydrates: 19g
Protein: 76g

Ginger and Orange "Beets"
Serving: 6
Prep Time: 20 minutes
Cook Time: 8 hours

Ingredients:

- 2 pounds beets, peeled and cut into wedges
- Juice of 2 oranges
- Zest of 1 orange
- 1 teaspoon fresh ginger, grated
- 1 tablespoon honey
- 1 tablespoon apple cider vinegar

- 1/8 teaspoon fresh ground black pepper Sea salt

How To:

1. Add beets, zest, orange juice, ginger, honey, pepper, salt and vinegar to your Slow Cooker.
2. Stir well.
3. Close lid and cook on LOW for 8 hours.
4. Serve and enjoy!

Nutrition (Per Serving)
Calories: 108
Fat: 1g
Carbohydrates: 25g
Protein: 3g
Pineapple Rice
Serving: 2
Prep Time: 10 minutes
Cook Time: 2 hours
Ingredients:

- 1 cup rice
- 2 cups water
- 1 small cauliflower, florets separated and chopped
- ½ small pineapple, peeled and chopped
- Salt and pepper as needed
- 1 teaspoon olive oil

How To:

1. Add rice, cauliflower, pineapple, water, oil, salt and pepper to your Slow Cooker.
2. Gently stir.
3. Place lid and cook on HIGH for 2 hours.
4. Fluff the rice with fork and season with more salt and pepper if needed.
5. Divide between serving platters and enjoy!

Nutrition (Per Serving)
Calories: 152
Fat: 4g
Carbohydrates: 18g
Protein: 4g
Creative Lemon and Broccoli Dish

Serving: 6
Prep Time: 10 minutes
Cook Time: 15 minutes
Ingredients:

- 2 heads broccocli, separated into florets
- 2 teaspoons extra virgin olive oil
- 1 teaspoon sunflower seeds
- ½ teaspoon black pepper
- 1 garlic clove, minced
- ½ teaspoon lemon juice

How To:

1. Pre-heat your oven to 400 degrees F.
2. Take a large sized bowl and add broccoli florets.
3. Drizzle olive oil and season with pepper, sunflower seeds and garlic.
4. Spread broccoli out in a single even layer on a baking sheet.
5. Bake for 15-20 minutes until fork tender.
6. Squeeze lemon juice on top.
7. Serve and enjoy!

Nutrition (Per Serving)
Calories: 49
Fat: 1.9g
Carbohydrates: 7g
Protein: 3g
Baby Potatoes
Serving: 4
Prep Time: 10 minutes
Cook Time: 35 minutes
Ingredients:

- 2 pounds new yellow potatoes, scrubbed and cut into wedges
- 2 tablespoons extra virgin olive oil
- 2 teaspoons fresh rosemary, chopped
- 1 teaspoon garlic powder
- ½ teaspoon freshly ground black pepper and sunflower seeds

How To:

1. Pre-heat your oven to 400 degrees F.
2. Line a baking sheet with aluminum foil and set it aside.

3. Take a large bowl and add potatoes, olive oil, garlic, rosemary, sea sunflower seeds and pepper.
4. Spread potatoes in a single layer on a baking sheet and bake for 35 minutes.
5. Serve and enjoy!

Nutrition (Per Serving)
Calories: 225
Fat: 7g
Carbohydrates: 37g
Protein: 5g
Cauliflower Cakes
Serving: 4
Prep Time: 10 minutes
Cook Time: 10 minutes
Ingredients:

- 4 cups cauliflowers, cut into florets
- 1 cup kite ricotta/cashew cheese, grated
- 2 eggs, lightly beaten
- 1 teaspoon paprika
- 1 teaspoon chili powder
- Sunflower seeds and pepper to taste
- ½ cup fresh parsley, chopped
- 1 tablespoon olive oil

How To:

1. Add cauliflower, cheese, paprika, eggs, chili, sunflower seeds, pepper and parsley into a large sized bowl.
2. Mix well.
3. Drizzle olive oil into frying pan and place over medium-high heat.
4. Shape cauliflower mixture into 12 even patties.
5. Once oil is hot, fry cakes until both sides are golden brown.
6. Serve hot and enjoy!

Nutrition (Per Serving)
Calories: 180
Fat: 8g
Carbohydrates: 6g
Protein: 8g
Tender Coconut and Cauliflower Rice with Chili
Serving: 4
Prep Time: 20 minutes

Cook Time: 20 minutes
Ingredients:

- 3 cups cauliflower, riced
- 2/3 cups full-fat coconut almond milk
- 1-2 teaspoons sriracha paste
- ¼- ½ teaspoon onion powder
- Sunflower seeds as needed
- Fresh basil for garnish

How To:

1. Take a pan and place it over medium low heat.
2. Add all of the ingredients and stir them until fully combined.
3. Cook for about 5-10 minutes, making sure that the lid is on.
4. Remove the lid and keep cooking until any excess liquid is absorbed.
5. Once the rice is soft and creamy, enjoy!

Nutrition (Per Serving)

- Calories: 95
- Fat: 7g
- Carbohydrates: 4g
- Protein: 1g

Apple Slices
Serving: 4
Prep Time: 10 minutes
Cook Time: 10 minutes
Ingredients:

- 1 cup of coconut oil
- ¼ cup date paste
- 2 tablespoons ground cinnamon
- 4 Granny Smith apples, peeled and sliced, cored

How To:

1. Take a large sized skillet and place it over medium heat.
2. Add oil and allow the oil to heat up.
3. Stir cinnamon and date paste into the oil.
4. Add sliced apples and cook for 5-8 minutes until crispy.
5. Serve and enjoy!

Nutrition (Per Serving)
Calories: 368
Fat: 23g
Carbohydrates: 44g
Protein: 1g

The Exquisite Spaghetti Squash
Serving: 6
Prep Time: 5 minutes
Cooking Time: 7-8 hours

Ingredients:

- 1 spaghetti squash
- 2 cups water

How To:

1. Wash squash carefully with water and rinse it well.
2. Puncture 5-6 holes in the squash using a fork.
3. Place squash in Slow Cooker.
4. Place lid and cook on LOW for 7-8 hours.
5. Remove squash to cutting board and let it cool.
6. Cut squash in half and discard seeds.
7. Use two forks and scrape out squash strands and transfer to bowl.
8. Serve and enjoy!

Nutrition (Per Serving)
Calories: 52
Fat: 0g
Carbohydrates: 12g
Protein: 1g

The Hearty Garlic and Mushroom Crunch
Serving: 6
Prep Time: 10 minutes
Cooking Time: 8 hours

Ingredients:

- ¼ cup vegetable stock
- 2 tablespoons extra virgin olive oil
- 1 tablespoon Dijon mustard
- 1 teaspoon dried thyme
- 1 teaspoon sea salt
- ½ teaspoon dried rosemary
- ¼ teaspoon fresh ground black pepper
- 2 pounds cremini mushrooms, cleaned

- 6 garlic cloves, minced
- ¼ cup fresh parsley, chopped

How To:

1. Take a small bowl and whisk in vegetable stock, mustard, olive oil, salt, thyme, pepper and rosemary.
2. Add mushrooms, garlic and stock mix to your Slow Cooker.
3. Close lid and cook on LOW for 8 hours.
4. Open lid and stir in parsley.
5. Serve and enjoy!

Nutrition (Per Serving)
Calories: 92
Fat: 5g
Carbohydrates: 8g
Protein: 4g
Easy Pepper Jack Cauliflower
Serving: 6
Prep Time: 10 minutes
Cooking Time: 3 hours 35 minutes
Ingredients:

- 1 head cauliflower
- ¼ cup whipping cream 4 ounces cream cheese
- ½ teaspoon pepper
- 1 teaspoon salt
- 2 tablespoons butter
- 4 ounces pepper jack cheese

How To:

1. Grease slow cooker and add listed ingredients.
2. Stir and place lid, cook on LOW for 3 hours.
3. Remove lid and add cheese, stir.
4. Place lid and cook for 1 hour more.
5. Enjoy!

Nutrition (Per Serving)
Calories: 272
Fat: 21g
Carbohydrates: 5g
Protein: 10g
The Brussels Platter

Serving: 4
Prep Time: 15 minutes
Cooking Time: 4 hours
Ingredients:

- 1 pound Brussels sprouts, bottoms trimmed and cut
- 1 tablespoon olive oil
- 1 ½ tablespoons Dijon mustard
- Salt and pepper to taste
- ½ teaspoon dried tarragon

How To:

1. Add Brussels sprouts, mustard, water, salt and pepper to your Slow Cooker
2. Add dried tarragon. 3. Stir well and cover.
3. Cook on LOW for 5 hours, making sure to keep cooking until the Brussels sprouts are tender.
4. Stir well and arrange.
5. Add Dijon over the Brussels sprouts.
6. Enjoy!

Nutrition (Per Serving)
Calories: 83
Fat: 4g
Carbohydrates: 11g
Protein: 4g
The Crazy Southern Salad
Serving: 2
Prep Time: 10 minutes
Cook Time: nil
Ingredients:

- 5 cups Romaine lettuce
- ½ cup sprouted black beans
- 1 cup cherry tomatoes, halved
- 1 avocado, diced
- ¼ cup almonds, chopped
- ½ cup of fresh cilantro
- ½ cup of Salsa Fresca

How To:

1. Take a large sized bowl and add lettuce, tomatoes, beans, almonds, cilantro, avocado, Salsa Fresco
2. Toss everything well and mix them
3. Divide the salad into serving bowls and serve!
4. Enjoy!

Nutrition (Per Serving)
Calories: 211
Fat: 16g
Carbohydrates: 6g
Protein: 10g

Kale and Carrot with Tahini Dressing
Serving: 1
Prep Time: 15 minutes
Cook Time: nil
Ingredients:

- Handful of kale
- 1 tablespoon tahnini
- ½ head lettuce
- Pinch of garlic powder
- 1 tablespoon olive oil
- Juice of ½ lime
- 1 carrot, grated

How To:

1. Add kale and roughly chopped lettuce to a bowl.
2. Add grated carrots to the greens and mix.
3. Take a small bowl and add the remaining ingredients, mix well.
4. Pour dressing on top of greens and toss.
5. Enjoy!

Nutrition (Per Serving)
Calories: 249
Fat: 11g
Carbohydrates: 35g
Protein: 10g

Crispy Kale
Serving: 4
Prep Time: 10 minutes
Cook Time: 25 minutes
Ingredients:

- 3 cups kale, stemmed and thoroughly washed, torn in 2-inch pieces
- 1 tablespoon extra-virgin olive oil
- ½ teaspoon chili powder
- ¼ teaspoon sea salt

How To:

1. Prepare your oven by pre-heating to 300 degrees F.
2. Line 2 baking sheets with parchment paper and keep them on the side.
3. Dry kale and transfer to a large bowl.
4. Add olive oil and toss, making sure to cover the leaves well.
5. Season kale with salt, chili powder and toss.
6. Divide kale between baking sheets and spread into single layer.
7. Bake for 25 minutes until crispy.
8. Let them cool for 5 minutes, serve.
9. Enjoy!

Nutrition (Per Serving)
Calories: 56
Fat: 4g
Carbohydrates: 5g
Protein: 2g
Juicy Summertime Veggies
Serving: 6
Prep Time: 10 minutes
Cooking Time: 3 hours 5 minutes
Ingredients:

- 1 cup grape tomatoes
- 2 cups okra
- 1 cup mushrooms
- 2 cups yellow bell peppers
- 1 ½ cup red onions
- 2 ½ cups zucchini
- ½ cup olive oil
- ½ cup balsamic vinegar
- 1 tablespoon fresh thyme, chopped
- 2 tablespoons fresh basil, chopped

How To:

1. Slice and chop okra, onions, tomatoes, zucchini, mushrooms.
2. Add veggies to a large container and mix.

3. Take another dish and add oil and vinegar, mix in thyme and basil.
4. Toss the veggies into the Slow Cooker and pour marinade.
5. Stir well.
6. Close lid and cook on 3 hours on HIGH, making sure to stir after every hour.

Nutrition (Per Serving)
Calories: 233
Fat: 18g
Carbohydrates: 14g
Protein: 3g
Crazy Caramelized Onion
Serving: 4
Prep Time: 10 minutes
Cooking Time: 9-10 hours
Ingredients:

- 6 onions, sliced
- 2 tablespoons oil
- ½ teaspoon salt

How To:

1. Add onions, oil and salt to your Slow Cooker.
2. Close lid and cook on LOW for 8 hours.
3. Open lid and keep simmering for 1-2 hours until any excess water has evaporated.
4. Serve and enjoy!

Nutrition (Per Serving)
Calories: 126
Fat: 15g
Carbohydrates: 15g
Protein: 2g
Kidney Beans and Cilantro
Serving: 6
Prep Time: 5 minutes
Cook Time: nil
Ingredients:

- 1 can (15 ounces) kidney beans, drained and rinsed
- ½ English cucumber, chopped
- 1 medium heirloom tomato, chopped
- 1 bunch fresh cilantro, stems removed and chopped

- 1 red onion, chopped
- Juice of 1 large lime
- 3 tablespoons Dijon mustard
- ½ teaspoon fresh garlic paste
- 1 teaspoon Sumac
- Salt and pepper as needed

How To:

1. Take a medium-sized bowl and add kidney beans, chopped up veggies and cilantro.
2. Take a small bowl and make the vinaigrette by adding lime juice, oil, fresh garlic, pepper, mustard and Sumac.
3. Pour the vinaigrette over the salad and give it a gentle stir.
4. Add some salt and pepper.
5. Cover and allow to chill for half an hour.
6. Serve!

Nutrition (Per Serving)
Calories: 74
Fat: 0.7g
Carbohydrates: 16g
Protein: 21g
Broccoli Crunchies
Serving: 4
Prep Time: 10 minutes
Cooking Time: 3 hours
Ingredients:

- 2 cups broccoli florets
- 2 ounces cream of celery soup
- **2 tablespoons cheddar cheese, shredded**
- 1 small yellow onion, chopped
- ¼ teaspoon Worcestershire sauce
- Salt and pepper as needed
- ½ tablespoon butter

How To:

1. Add broccoli, cream, cheese, onion, cheddar to Slow Cooker.
2. Stir and season with salt and pepper.
3. Place lid and cook on LOW for 3 hours.
4. Serve and enjoy!

Nutrition (Per Serving)
Calories: 162
Fat: 11g
Carbohydrates: 11g
Protein: 5g
Ultimate Buffalo Cashews
Serving: 4
Prep Time: 10 minutes
Cook Time: 55 minutes
Ingredients:

- 2 cups raw cashews
- ¾ cup red hot sauce
- 1/3 cup avocado oil
- ½ teaspoon garlic powder
- ¼ teaspoon turmeric

How To:

1. Take a bowl, mix the wet ingredients in a bowl and stir in seasoning.
2. Add cashews to the bowl and mix.
3. Soak cashews in hot sauce mix for 2-4 hours.
4. Pre-heat your oven to 325 degrees F.
5. Spread cashews onto baking sheet.
6. Bake for 35-55 minutes, turning after every 10-15 minutes.
7. Let them cool and serve!

Nutrition (Per Serving)
Calories: 268
Fat: 16g
Carbohydrates: 20g
Protein: 14g
A Green Bean Mixture
Serving: 2
Prep Time: 10 minutes
Cooking Time: 2 hours
Ingredients:

- 4 cups green beans, trimmed
- 2 tablespoons butter, melted
- 1 tablespoon date paste
- Salt and pepper as needed
- ¼ teaspoon coconut aminos

How To:

1. Add green beans, date paste, pepper, salt, coconut aminos to the Slow Cooker, gently stir.
2. Toss and place lid.
3. Cook on LOW for 2 hours.
4. Serve and enjoy!

Nutrition (Per Serving)
Calories: 236
Fat: 6g
Carbohydrates: 10g
Protein: 6g

Decisive Cauliflower and Mushroom Risotto
Serving: 4
Prep Time: 10 minutes
Cook Time: 20 minutes

Ingredients:

- 1 cup vegetable stock
- head cauliflower, grated
- 9 ounces mushroom, chopped
- tablespoons almond butter
- Sunflower seeds and black pepper, to taste
- 1 cup coconut cream

How To:

1. Take a saucepan and pour stock into it.
2. Bring it to boil and set it aside.
3. Then take a skillet and melt almond butter over medium heat.
4. Add mushroom to sauté until it turns golden brown.
5. Stir in stock and grated cauliflower.
6. Bring the mixture to a simmer and add cream.
7. Cook until liquid is reduced and cauliflower is al dente.
8. Serve warm and enjoy!

Nutrition (Per Serving)
Calories: 186
Fat: 16.5g
Carbohydrates: 6.7g
Protein: 2.8g

Authentic Zucchini Boats
Serving: 4

Prep Time: 10 minutes
Cook Time: 25 minutes
Ingredients:

- 4 medium zucchini
- ½ cup marinara sauce
- ¼ red onion, sliced
- ¼ cup kalamata olives, chopped
- ½ cup cherry tomatoes, sliced
- 2 tablespoons fresh basil

How To:

1. Pre-heat your oven to 400 degrees F.
2. Cut the zucchini half-lengthwise and shape them in boats.
3. Take a bowl and add tomato sauce, spread 1 layer of sauce on top of each of the boat.
4. Top with onion, olives, and tomatoes.
5. Bake for 20-25 minutes.
6. Top with basil and enjoy!

Nutrition (Per Serving)
Calories: 278
Fat: 20g
Carbohydrates: 10g
Protein: 15g
Roasted Onions and Green Beans
Serving: 6
Prep Time: 10 minutes
Cook Time: 15 minutes
Ingredients:

- 1 yellow onion, sliced into rings
- ½ teaspoon onion powder
- 2 tablespoons coconut flour
- 1 1/3 pounds fresh green beans, trimmed and chopped

How To:

1. Take a large bowl and mix sunflower seeds with onion powder and coconut flour.
2. Add onion rings.
3. Mix well to coat.
4. Spread the rings in the baking sheet, lined with parchment paper.

5. Drizzle with some oil.
6. Bake for 10 minutes at 400 degrees F.
7. Parboil the green beans for 3 to 5 minutes in the boiling water.
8. Drain and serve the beans with baked onion rings.
9. Serve warm and enjoy!

Nutrition (Per Serving)
Calories: 214
Fat: 19.4g
Carbohydrates:3.7g
Protein: 8.3g

Chapter Ten

BREAKFASTS RECIPES

Poached Eggs with Hollandaise and Bacon
With this slimmed-down hollandaise, it is easy to enjoy a version of eggs Benedict that is SmartPoints-friendly. The sauce also makes an excellent combination with steamed asparagus or grilled salmon fillets.

SmartPoints value: Green plan – 7SP, Blue plan – 5SP, Purple plan – 5SP

Total Time: 26 min, **Prep time**: 12 min, **Cooking time**: 14 min, **Serves**: 4

Nutritional value: Calories – 677.3, Carbs – 29.2g, Fat – 47.8g, Protein - 31.4g

Ingredients

- Plain fat-free yogurt - ¼ cup(s)
- Reduced-calorie mayonnaise - ¼ cup(s)
- Dijon Mustard - 1 tsp
- Uncooked Canadian bacon - 4 slice(s)
- Lemon zest - ½ tsp
- Egg(s) - 4 item(s), large
- Fresh lemon juice - 1 tsp
- Fresh tomato(es) - 4 slice(s), thick
- Unsalted butter - 2 tsp, softened
- Chives - 2 Tbsp, chopped fresh (optional)
- English muffin - 2 item(s), multigrain or whole wheat variety, split and toasted
- White wine vinegar - 1 Tbsp

Instructions

1. To prepare the sauce, get a small microwavable bowl and whisk yogurt, mayonnaise, mustard, and lemon zest and juice together in the bowl.
2. Set the microwave to High, and allow the mixture to heat up for about 30 seconds. Remove the bowl from the microwave carefully using your mitts.
3. Scoop a tablespoon of butter and stir it in until melted. Cover the bowl to keep your sauce warm.
4. Poach eggs by filling a large, deep skillet with water and allow to boil; add vinegar.
5. Reduce the heat to a bare simmer. Carefully break the eggs into a custard cup, one at a time, and slip into the hot water.
6. Cook the eggs until the whites are firm, but the yolks are still soft. This process should take about 5 minutes.
7. Transfer the eggs, one at a time, with a slotted spoon to a paper towel-lined plate to drain. Cover the plate to keep the eggs warm.
8. Wipe the skillet dry with a paper towel.
9. Add four slices of Canadian bacon and cook over medium-high heat until they brown in spots, about 60 seconds per side.
10. Place one half each of the English muffins on four plates.
11. Top each with one slice of bacon, one slice of tomato, one poached egg, and about two tablespoons sauce. Speckle with chives, if using.

Note: You can keep the hollandaise sauce warm for up to 40 minutes before serving.

Nut-crusted Mahi-mahi

This recipe sounds fantastic and preparing it is super easy; it only takes about 20 minutes. It works well with just about any thin fish fillet and any kind of nuts. I will like you to add macadamia nuts here for their rich and buttery flavor and because they pair well together with the panko. Also, the mahi-mahi is firm enough to withstand the dredging and roasting. You are free to experiment with whatever you have in your fridge.

SmartPoints value: Green plan - 3SP, Blue plan - 2SP, Purple plan - 2SP

Total Time: 20 min, **Prep time**: 8 min, **Cooking time**: 12 min, **Serves**: 4

Nutritional value: Calories - 234.1, Carbs - 13.9g, Fat - 9.8g, Protein - 24.7g

Ingredients

- Cooking spray - 2 spray(s)
- Egg white(s) (whipped) - 1 large
- Macadamia nuts (dry roasted, salted) - 3 Tbsp, chopped
- Mahi-mahi fillet(s) (uncooked) - 1 pound(s), no skin
- Parsley (fresh) - 2 Tbsp, or cilantro (fresh, minced)

- Plain breadcrumbs (dried) - ¼ cup(s), panko (Japanese variety)
- Table salt - ¾ tsp (divided)

Instructions

1. Prepare the oven by preheating to 450°F. Coat a baking pan with cooking spray and place the container in the oven to heat.
2. Place some nuts, parsley (or cilantro), panko, and 1/4 tsp of salt in a small blender, then blend all together.
3. Pour the crumbs into a shallow bowl or plate and set the plate aside.
4. With the fish placed on a plate, rub 1/2 teaspoon of salt all over it.
5. Dip the fish into the egg white and turn it to coat. After that, dip the fish into the blended nut mixture and turn to coat.
6. Remove the pan from the oven and place the coated fish on it.
7. Roast the fish until the center of the fish is no longer translucent; about 10 to 12 minutes. Serve it immediately once it is ready.

Note: If you desire it, you can garnish with salt and pepper, but that could affect the Smart Points value.

Pan-Fried Flounder

You can serve this dish with homemade fries, or you can add freshly sliced tomatoes alongside. Bear in mind that the cooking time will be different depending on the size of your fillets.

SmartPoints value: Green plan - 4SP, Blue plan - 3SP, Purple plan - 3SP

Total Time: 20 min, **Prep time**: 14 min, **Cooking time**: 6 min, **Serves**: 4

Nutritional value: Calories - 441.2, Carbs - 14.8g, Fat - 30.3g, Protein - 8.3g

Ingredients

- Black pepper (freshly ground) - ½ tsp (or to taste)
- Cornmeal (yellow) - ¼ cup(s)
- Dijon mustard - 1 Tbsp
- Egg white(s) (whipped) - 1 large
- Lemon(s) - ½ medium, cut into four wedges
- Olive oil cooking spray - 2 spray(s)
- Olive oil - 1 Tbsp
- Parmesan cheese (grated) - 2 Tbsp
- Thyme (fresh) - 1 Tbsp, or 1 tsp dried thyme
- Table salt - ½ tsp (or to taste)
- Uncooked flounder fillet(s) - 1 pound(s)

Instructions

1. Wash the fish with clean water and pat it dry. Place the fish on a plate and sprinkle both sides of fish with mustard, then dip it into the egg white and set aside.
2. Mix cornmeal, thyme, Parmesan cheese, salt, and pepper in a medium bowl, then dust the fish with cornmeal-mixture. Ensure that to cover both sides.
3. Get a large oven-proof skillet and coat it with cooking spray, then set it over medium to medium-high heat. Apply heat to the oil until it starts shimmering.
4. Add the fish to the skillet and cook for 2 to 3 minutes on one side, then flip the fish and cook until it is ready on the other side; about 2 to 3 minutes.
5. Serve the fish with your lemon wedges.

Blueberry-Almond Oatmeal
SmartPoints value: Green plan - 3SP, Blue plan - 3SP, Purple plan - 1SP
Total time: 10 min, **Prep time**: 2 min, **Cooking time**: 5 min, **Serves**: 1
Nutritional value: Calories - 340, Carbs - 54g Fat - 8g, Protein - 16g
Ingredients

- Blueberries (fresh) - ¼ cup(s)
- Almond milk (unsweetened) - 2 Tbsp
- Slivered almonds - 2 tsp (toasted)
- Old-fashioned rolled oats (such as Quaker Oats) - 1 cup
- Milk - 1 cup
- Water - 1 cup
- Kosher salt - 1/8 tsp
- Ground cinnamon - 1/2 tsp
- Honey - 1 tsp

Instructions

1. To prepare oatmeal, combine oats, water, milk, salt, and cinnamon in a medium-sized saucepan. Get it to boil on medium-high heat, and reduce heat to low; about 4-5 min.
2. Simmer it uncovered until it thickens, occasionally stirring. Remove it from the heat and allow to cool slightly.
3. Stir blueberries and milk into the oatmeal, then sprinkle it with almonds and cinnamon. Add artificial sweetener to taste if you desire.

Toasted Blueberry Muffin with Warm Citrus Compote
SmartPoints value: Green plan - 4SP, Blue plan - 4SP, Purple plan - 4SP

Total Time: 20 min, **Prep time**: 10 min, **Cooking time**: 10 min, **Serves**: 6

Nutritional value: Calories - 231, Carbs - 36.3g Fat - 7.7g, Protein - 5.2g

Ingredients

- Brown sugar (Splenda) blend - 1 tsp
- Cornstarch - 1 Tbsp
- Water - 2 Tbsp
- Orange juice (fresh) - ½ cup(s)
- Orange sections - 1 cup(s), divided
- Vanilla extract - ⅛ teaspoon
- Lemon zest - ⅛ teaspoon
- Lime zest - ⅛ teaspoon
- WW Blueberry muffin - 3 item(s)

Instructions

1. Prepare the oven by preheating to 350°F.
2. Whisk cornstarch, brown sugar, and water together in a medium-sized saucepan.
3. Whip the mixture in orange juice. While whipping constantly, bring the mixture to a boil over medium heat; about 2 minutes. The mixture will thicken rapidly, so make sure to whisk continuously to prevent lumps.
4. Whisk the thick mixture in half cup of orange segments and continue to simmer over medium-low heat for another 6 to 8 minutes, stirring it regularly. The orange sections should break down, and the sauce should become thick, but it should not stiffen up.
5. Drop the thick sauce from the heat and stir in vanilla extract, lemon zest, and lime zest. Allow it to cool off for about 10 minutes.
6. While the sauce is getting cooled, cut each muffin in half and toast them in the oven lightly on both sides.
7. Serve each person half a muffin topped with two tablespoons of compote. Garnish them with the remaining half cup of orange segments.

Notes: You can also use leftover compote as a delicious breakfast marmalade. Spread it on whole-wheat toast, apple slices, or stir it into fat-free plain yogurt. Preserve the leftover compote in an airtight container inside a refrigerator for up to 3 days.

Cuban Black Beans and Rice

SmartPoints value: Green plan - 7SP, Blue plan - 4SP, Purple plan - 4SP

Total Time: 35 min, Prep time: 10 min, Cooking time: 25 min, Serves: 6

Nutritional value: Calories - 333.5, Carbs - 54.8g Fat - 5.1g, Protein - 16.1g

Ingredients

- Water - 2½ cup(s), divided
- Uncooked white rice (long grain-variety) - 1 cup(s)
- Olive oil - 2 tsp
- Banana pepper(s) - 1 medium
- Black beans (canned) - 31 oz, two 15.5 oz cans (undrained)
- Cilantro (fresh, chopped, divided) - ⅔ cup(s)
- Minced garlic - 1½ Tbsp
- Ground cumin - 1 tsp
- Uncooked red onion(s) (chopped) - 1¾ cup(s)
- Oregano (dried) - 1 tsp
- Table salt - 1 tsp (or to taste)
- Red wine vinegar - 1 Tbsp
- Lime(s) (fresh) - 1 medium, cut into six wedges

Instructions

1. Bring two cups of water to a boil in a small saucepan and add the rice, then cook as package directs.
2. Heat some oil in a large nonstick skillet over medium-high heat.
3. Add a cup of chopped onions and all of the pepper, then cook, occasionally stirring, until it is tender; about 7 minutes.
4. Toss in garlic, cumin, and oregano, then cook, stirring until fragrant; about 30 seconds.
5. Stir in the beans and their liquid, the remaining half cup of water and salt, then bring to a simmer.
6. Reduce the heat to low and simmer for the flavors to blend in about 5 minutes.
7. Remove the dish from heat, then stir in vinegar and 1/3 cup of cilantro.
8. To serve, use a spoon to put beans over rice and sprinkle it with 1/4 cup of the remaining onion and 1/3 cup of the remaining cilantro, then squeeze fresh lime juice over the top.

Note: If you desire, sprinkle the dish with salt before serving.

Spaghetti Squash With Fresh Tomato-Basil Sauce

SmartPoints value: Green plan - 2SP, Blue plan - 2SP, Purple plan - 2SP

Total time: 30 min, **Prep time**: 15 min, **Cooking time**: 15 min, **Serves:** 4

Nutritional value: Calories - 216.2, Carbs - 14.2g Fat - 17.2g, Protein - 5.0g

Enjoy this recipe with its taste of summer. Ensure to cook it with very ripe tomatoes and fresh basil to get the best flavour.

Ingredients

- Tomato(es) (fresh) - 2¼ pound(s)
- Olive oil (extra virgin) - 2 Tbsp
- Minced garlic - 1¼ tsp, finely minced
- Basil (fresh, sliced) - ½ cup(s)
- Kosher salt - ½ tsp (or to taste)
- Black pepper (freshly ground) - ¼ tsp (or to taste)
- Spaghetti squash (uncooked) - 2½ pound(s)

Instructions

1. Toss tomatoes, oil, garlic, basil, salt and pepper together in a large bowl and let it stand, occasionally tossing, until the tomatoes release their juices and the mixture is quite juicy; about 10 to 15 minutes.
2. Cut the spaghetti squash in half and scoop out the seeds, then place the squash in a covered microwave-safe container.
3. Cook the spaghetti squash on high power until strands of squash separate when you scrape the flesh with a fork; about 15 minutes. Alternatively, you can also roast the squash for about 20 minutes in the oven.
4. Scrape the spaghetti squash from the peel with a fork to form strands and add it to the bowl with tomatoes and toss to coat.
5. **Notes:** It would be delicious to add chunks of fresh mozzarella or freshly grated Parmesan cheese to this meal. However, it might affect the Smart Points value.

Barley, Grape Tomato And Arugula Sauté
SmartPoints value: Green plan - 3SP, Blue plan - 3SP, Purple plan - 1SP
Total time: 50 min, **Prep time**: 10 min, **Cooking time**: 40 min, **Serves**: 4
Nutritional value: Calories - 82.8, Carbs - 4.8g Fat - 7.2g, Protein - 1.2g
This grain and vegetable side dish is colourful and sweet with a peppery bite. Toss in some yellow grape tomatoes to add even more colour.

Ingredients

- Water - 1¼ cup(s)
- Table salt - ¾ tsp, divided
- Pearl barley (uncooked) - ½ cup(s)
- Olive oil (extra-virgin) - 1½ tsp, divided
- Tomatoes (grape) - 1½ cup(s), halved

- Minced garlic - 1½ tsp
- Black pepper (freshly ground) - ¼ tsp
- Arugula (baby leaves) - 3 cup(s)
- Lemon zest (finely grated) - ¼ tsp (or to taste)

Instructions

1. Stir half tsp of salt into a small saucepan of water and bring it to a boil. Add barley to it and cover; reduce the heat to low and cook until the water is absorbed and the barley is tender but still has a nice bite to it; about 30-35 minutes. Remove the saucepan from the heat and set it aside.
2. Apply heat to one teaspoon of oil in a medium nonstick skillet over medium-high heat. Add the tomatoes and garlic, then sauté it until the tomatoes start to soften and release their juices; about 1-2 minutes.
3. Put in more barley, the remaining one-quarter teaspoon of salt and pepper, and reduce the heat to medium and cook, stirring it until the tomatoes soften further and the grain absorbs tomato liquid; about 2-3 minutes.
4. Stir in the arugula and toss it over medium heat until it wilts; about 30 seconds.
5. Remove the dish from the heat and stir in the remaining half teaspoon of oil and lemon zest.

Note: You can reheat this recipe the next day, and it will still taste great. Alternatively, you can serve it as a cold salad. Allow it come to room temperature and then toss it, adding just a bit of red wine or balsamic vinegar.

Creamy Mushroom And Chicken Stew Crockpot
SmartPoints value: Green plan - 2SP, Blue plan - 2SP, Purple plan - 2SP
Total Time: 4hr 20min, **Prep time**: 10 min, **Cooking time**: 4hr 10mins,
Serves: 4
Nutritional value: Calories – 278, Carbs – 24.2g, Fat – 4.2g, Protein – 32g
The mushroom and chicken stew crockpot is a fantastic low-calorie dinner idea. It's a healthy and easy slow cooker recipe with great taste.

Ingredients

- Chicken breast (skinless) - 1 lb
- Baby portabella mushroom (sliced) - 8 oz
- Onion (finely chopped) - 1 piece
- Carrots (cut into matchsticks) - 1/2 cup
- Peas (fresh or frozen) - 1/2 cup
- Celery (chopped) - 2 stalks
- Mushroom seasoning (powdered) - 2 tbsp

- Chicken broth (fat-free) - 2 cups
- Sour cream (fat-free, at room temp) - 1 cup
- Garlic (minced) - 3 cloves
- Salt (1 tsp)
- Pepper (1/2 tsp)

Instructions

1. Combine all ingredients in a crockpot except the sour cream.
2. For 4- 6 hrs., cook on low heat.
3. For about 5 minutes, stir in sour cream, and warm until it is thoroughly heated. Serve immediately.

Smashed Avocado And Egg Toast
SmartPoints value: Green plan – 6SP, Blue plan – 4SP, Purple plan - 4SP
Total Time: 7 min, Prep time: 5 min, Cooking time: 2 min, Serves: 1
Nutritional value: Calories – 214.0, Carbs - 16.4g, Fat – 14.2g, Protein - 8.4g
Ingredients

- Avocado - ¼ item(s), medium-sized, ripe but still a touch firm
- Light whole-grain bread - 1 slice(s)
- Whole hard-boiled egg(s) - 1 item(s), sliced
- Table salt - 1 pinch
- Crushed red pepper flakes - 1 pinch
- Black pepper - 1 pinch

Instructions

1. Place one slice of bread on a clean plate.
2. Top with a portion of peeled avocado and gently smash with a knife or fork.
3. Cut hard-boiled egg in half and place each half on the bread.
4. Gently smash egg and mix with smashed avocado. Season the bread to taste with salt, pepper, and red pepper flakes.
5. Cover with another slice of bread and place in a flat-sitting electric bread toaster.
6. Remove smashed avocado and egg toast from the toaster once the "ready" light comes on.

Sweet Pineapple and Strawberry Salsa with Yogurt
The best salsas sometimes don't contain tomatoes, and this sweet pineapple and strawberry salsa with yogurt recipe is a good example.

I've added coconut flakes to this recipe to give a pleasant taste of fresh fruit.

SmartPoints value: Green plan – 3SP, Blue plan – 2SP, Purple plan - 2SP

Total Time: 8 min, Prep time: 4 min, Cooking time: 4 min

Serves: 1

Nutritional value: Calories - 30.9, Carbs - 7.4g, Fat - 0.4g, Protein - 0.4g

Ingredients

- Strawberries - 3 medium-sized, diced - fresh mint leaves - 1 tsp (chopped)
- Pineapple - ½ cup(s), Golden species (diced)
- Plain fat-free Greek yogurt - ½ cup(s)
- Lime zest - ⅛ tsp (grated)
- Unsweetened coconut flakes - 1 Tbsp (toasted)
- Coconut flakes – 3 Tbsp

Instructions

Dice strawberries, pineapple, mint, and lime zest into a small bowl, all mixed.

Add yogurt and speckle with coconut. You can also spoon the yogurt into a glass dish and top it with fruit and coconut.

Creamy Banana French Toast Casserole

You can give a bright flavor to this creamy casserole and also keep the banana from turning black by adding a small quantity of lemon juice.

SmartPoints value: Green plan – 7SP, Blue plan – 6SP, Purple plan - 6SP

Total Time: 55 min, **Prep time**: 20 min, **Cooking time**: 35 min,

Serves: 12

Nutritional value:

Calories - 489, Carbs - 68.7g, Fat - 18g, Protein - 15.4g

Ingredients

- Cooking spray - 5 spray(s)
- Whole wheat/oatmeal bread - 12 slice(s), cut into quarters (about 1 oz per slice)
- Neufchâtel cheese - 4 oz, (1/3-less-fat cream cheese)
- 2% reduced-fat milk - 1 cup(s)
- Maple syrup - ½ cup(s)
- Egg(s) - 6 large
- Banana(s) - 4 medium-sized, ripe (divided)
- Fresh lemon juice - 2 tsp
- Rum - 1 Tbsp
- Ground cinnamon - ½ tsp
- Vanilla extract - 1 tsp
- Ground nutmeg - ½ tsp

- Table salt - ¼ tsp
- Powdered sugar - 3 Tbsp

Instructions

1. Get a clean 13 inches by 9 inches baking dish and coat it with cooking spray.
2. Stand quarter portions of bread up in the prepared dish, so it lines the sides and bottom in a single layer — Preheat the oven to 350°F.
3. Place the cheese, milk, and syrup in a blender.
4. Add eggs, two bananas, rum, vanilla, juice, nutmeg, cinnamon, and salt to the blender.
5. Allow the blending process to Dash until the mixture is smooth.
6. Gently pour the mixture over the bread and press those on the sides of the baking dish into the egg mixture, making sure it is completely submerged.
7. Refrigerate the dish for 30 minutes after covering with foil.
8. Preheat the oven again to 350°F. Just before baking, thinly slice the remaining two bananas and put the slices in between pieces of bread.
9. Cover the dish with new foil and bake for 25 minutes. Remove the foil and continue baking until the color is golden brown. Set for about 10 minutes more, then sprinkle the top with powdered sugar. Slice the casserole into 12 pieces and serve immediately.

Note: You can serve with fresh berries if you desire.

Fried Egg With Asparagus-Potato Hash

Eggs look great with asparagus in this fantastic breakfast recipe. To effortlessly prepare asparagus so that the cooking will be fast and be tender, bend the spears near the tail until the woody part breaks off. You can also use the points of the spears and reserve the middle of the asparagus stalks for another preparation like a veggie stir-fry or steamed in a green salad. You should microwave the potato and then sauté it. Microwaving ensures that the interior is soft, with a crisped, browned exterior, a perfectly hashed topping to your egg.

SmartPoints value: Green plan – 7SP, Blue plan – 5SP, Purple plan - 1SP

Total Time: 22 min, **Prep time**: 12 min, **Cooking time**: 10 min, **Serves**: 1

Nutritional value: Calories - 319, Carbs - 38.4g, Fat - 8g, Protein - 11.5g

Ingredients

- Uncooked red potato(es) - 1 medium-sized, pierced severally with a fork

- Uncooked asparagus - 4 spear(s), medium-sized, trimmed, diagonally sliced 1/2-inch thick (1/2 cup)
- Uncooked scallion(s) - 1 small (sliced)
- Olive oil - 1 tsp
- Table salt - ¼ tsp
- Fresh thyme - 1 tsp (chopped)
- Egg(s) - 1 large, cooked sunny-side up
- Black pepper - 1 pinch

Instructions

1. Microwave potato for about 3-4 minutes and cut into small dice.
2. Heat the oil in a medium-sized, nonstick skillet over a medium to high heat.
3. Add the asparagus and diced potato to the oil
4. Cook, occasionally stirring, until the diced potatoes are browned, and asparagus is crisp-tender, about 4 minutes.
5. Add the scallion and thyme; keep stirring until scallion wilts, about 30 seconds.
6. Season with salt and pepper, then serve with egg.

Greek-Style Scrambled Eggs
If you need a quick and easy weeknight dish, you can prepare these scrambled eggs within 20 minutes. These eggs make a perfect one-dish meal, loaded with various flavors that include butter beans, chicken chorizo sausage, grape tomatoes, and onions.

To make this meal vegetarian, add soy-based breakfast sausage. You can use lentils in place of butter beans if you can't find them.

Prevent overcooking by turning off the heat before the eggs are all the way cooked.

SmartPoints value: Green plan – 8SP, Blue plan – 3SP, Purple plan - 3SP

Total Time: 20 min, **Prep time**: 12 min, **Cooking time**: 8 min, **Serves**: 1

Nutritional value: Calories - 221, Carbs - 5.1g, Fat - 10.3g, Protein - 21.0g

Ingredients

- Cooked chicken chorizo sausage - 1½ oz (diced)
- Cooking spray - 5 spray(s)
- Canned butter beans - ¼ cup(s), rinsed and drained
- Crumbled feta cheese - 1 Tbsp
- Uncooked onion(s) - ¼ cup(s) (chopped)
- Grape tomatoes - 6 medium-sized (halved)
- Egg(s) - 2 large
- Black pepper - 1 pinch, or add to taste

- Table salt - 1 pinch, or add to taste
- Dill - 1 Tbsp, chopped

Instructions

1. Coat a medium-sized nonstick skillet with nonstick spray.
2. Add chicken chorizo and onion, then cook over medium heat, occasionally stirring, until lightly browned, about 5 minutes.
3. Add tomatoes and beans, then stir until the tomatoes start to soften, about 1 minute.
4. Push the mixture to one side of the skillet and add eggs to the other side.
5. Scramble the eggs until softly set, 1-2 minutes.
6. Turn in the chorizo mixture and season with salt and pepper, then sprinkle with dill and feta.

Italian Turkey Sausage And Vegetable Omelet

You can prepare this hearty 20-minute entrée for breakfast, lunch, or dinner, and it is perfect for one-person cooking.

The omelet fills with chicken sausage, onion, mushrooms, and roasted red peppers, then finished with salty Pecorino Romano cheese, which is chopped parsley. This addition injects freshness and color. Italian sausages come in several varieties that are sweet and spicy, so use your favorite in this recipe. When preparing omelets, it's good to practice to cook all the fillings and get them ready to go before you start cooking the eggs, since the cooking process is a quick one that takes only a couple minutes per omelet.

SmartPoints value: Green plan - 6SP, Blue plan - 2SP, Purple plan - 2SP

Total Time: 20 min, **Prep time**: 10 min, **Cooking time**: 10 min, **Serves**: 1

Nutritional value: Calories - 292.3, Carbs - 5.1g, Fat - 21.4g, Protein - 22.9g

Ingredients

- Cooked chicken or turkey sausage(s) - 1½ oz, Italian-variety, chopped
- Fresh edible mushroom(s) - ¾ cup(s), chopped
- Fresh parsley - ½ Tbsp, chopped
- Uncooked onion(s) - ¼ cup(s), chopped
- Cooking spray - 4 spray(s)
- Egg(s) - 2 large, beaten with a pinch of salt and pepper
- Grated Pecorino Romano cheese - 1½ Tbsp
- Chopped and roasted red peppers (packed in water) - ¼ cup(s)

Instructions

1. Coat a small-sized omelet pan with cooking spray and heat over medium flame.
2. Add the sausage, mushroom, and onion, then cook, frequently stirring, until the onions soften, 5 minutes. Remove the cooked omelet from pan to a bowl and stir in roasted pepper, then set aside.
3. Wipe the pan clean with a paper towel.
4. Put off heat, coat the pan again with cooking spray, and heat over medium flame.
5. Add the beaten eggs and swirl to spread egg over the pan.
6. Cook it until the bottom is done and the top is nearly cooked for about 3 minutes.
7. Top the omelet with chicken sausage mixture and sprinkle with cheese.
8. Fold the omelet over and cook for 1-2 minutes more. Serve it sprinkled with parsley.

Chinese-Style Zucchini With Ginger
Servings per container - 10
Prep Total - 10 min
Serving Size 2/3 cup (55g)

Nutritional Facts

- Total Fat 8g
- Total Carbohydrate 37g
- Protein 3g
- Sodium 160mg

Ingredients:

- 1 teaspoon oil
- 1 lb. zucchini cut into 1/4-inch slices
- 1/2 cup vegetarian broth
- 2 teaspoon light soy sauce
- 1 teaspoon dry sherry
- 1 teaspoon toasted sesame oil

Instructions:

1. Heat a large wok or heavy skillets over high heat until very hot then add the oil. When the oil is hot, add the zucchini and ginger.
2. Stir-fry 1 minute.
3. Add the broth, soy sauce, and sherry.
4. Stir-fry over high heat until the broth cooks down a bit and the zucchini is crisp-tender.
5. Remove from the heat, sprinkle with sesame oil and serve.

Breakfast Super Antioxidant Berry Smoothie
servings per container - 5
Prep Total - 10 min
Serving Size - 4 cup (20g)
Nutritional Facts

- Total Fat 2g
- Sodium 7mg
- Total Carbohydrate 20g
- Protein 3g

Ingredients

- 1 cup of filtered water
- 1 whole orange, peeled, de-seeded & cut into chunks
- 2 cups frozen raspberries or blackberries
- 1 Tablespoon goji berries
- 1 1/2 Tablespoons hemp seeds or plant-based protein powder
- 2 cups leafy greens (parsley, spinach, or kale)

Instructions:
Blend on high until smooth
Serve and drink immediately
Cucumber Tomato Surprise
servings per container - 5
Prep Total - 10 min
Serving Size 2/3 cup (55g)

Nutritional Facts

- Total Fat 20g
- Total Carbohydrate 14g
- Total Sugar 2g
- Protein 7g

Ingredients

- Chopped 1 medium of tomato
- 1 small cucumber peeled in stripes and chopped
- 1 large avocado cut into cubes
- 1 half of a lemon or lime squeezed
- ½1 tsp. Himalayan or Real salt
- 1 Teaspoon of original olive oil, MCT or coconut oil

Instructions:

1. Mix everything together and enjoy
2. This dish tastes even better after sitting for 40 – 60 minutes
3. Blend into a soup if desired.

Avocado Nori Rolls
Nutritional Facts
servings per container
10
Prep Total
10 min
Serving Size 2/3 cup (70g)

AMOUNT PER SERVING
Calories
15

% DAILY VALUE
Total Fat 2g
10%
Saturated Fat 1g
9%
Trans Fat 10g
-

Cholesterol

1%
Sodium 70mg
5%
Total Carbohydrate 22g
40%
Dietary Fiber 4g
2%
Total Sugar 12g
-

Protein 3g

Vitamin C 2mcg
2%
Calcium 260mg
7%
Iron 8mg
2%
Potassium 235mg
4%

Ingredients

- 2 sheets of raw or toasted sushi nori
- 1 large Romaine leaf cut in half down the length of the spine
- 2 Teaspoon of spicy miso paste
- 1 avocado, peeled and sliced
- ¼ red, yellow or orange bell pepper, julienned
- ½ cucumber, peeled, seeded and julienned
- ½ cup raw sauerkraut
- ½ carrot, beet or zucchini, shredded
- 1 cup alfalfa or favorite green sprouts
- 1 small bowl of water for sealing roll

Instructions:

1. Place a sheet of nori on a sushi rolling mat or washcloth, lining it up at the end closest to you.
2. Place the Romaine leaf on the edge of the nori with the spine closest to you.
3. Spread Spicy Miso Paste on the Romaine
4. Line the leaf with all ingredients in descending order, placing sprouts on last
5. Roll the Nori sheet away from you, tucking the ingredients in with your fingers, and seal the roll with water or Spicy Miso Paste. Slice

the roll into 6 or 8 rounds.

Maple Ginger Pancakes
Nutritional Facts
servings per container
4
Prep Total
10 min
Serving Size 2/3 cup (20g)

AMOUNT PER SERVING
Calories
20

% DAILY VALUE
Total Facts 10g
10%
Saturated Fat 0g
7%
Trans **Fat** 2g
-

Cholesterol
3%
Sodium 10mg
2%
Total Carbohydrate 7g
3%
Dietary Fiber 2g
4%
Total Sugar 1g
-

Protein 3g

Vitamin C 2mcg
10%
Calcium 260mg
20%
Iron 8mg
30%
Potassium 235mg
6%

Ingredients

- 1 or 2 cup flour
- 1 tablespoonful baking powder
- 1/2 tablespoonful kosher salt
- 1/4 tablespoonful ground ginger
- 1/4 table spoonful pumpkin pie spice
- 1/3 cup maple syrup
- 2/4 cup water
- minced 1/4 cup + 1 tablespoonful crystallized ginger slices together

Instructions:

1. In a neat bowl mix together the first five recipes
2. Add flour with syrup with water and stir together, after that add in the chopped ginger & stir until-just-combined.
3. Heat your frying pan and coat with a nonstick cooking spray
4. Pour in 1/4 cup of the batter and allow to heat until it form bubbles. Allow to cook until browned
5. Serve warm & topped with a slathering of vegan butter, a splash of maple syrup, and garnished with chopped candied ginger.

Chewy Chocolate Chip Cookies
Nutritional Facts
servings per container
10
Prep Total
10 min
Serving Size 2/3 cup (40g)

AMOUNT PER SERVING
Calories
10

% DAILY VALUE
Total Fat 10g
2%
Saturated Fat 1g
5%
Trans Fat 0g
-

Cholesterol

15%
Sodium 120mg
8%
Total Carbohydrate 21g
10%
Dietary Fiber 4g
1%
Total Sugar 1g
0%
Protein 6g

Vitamin C 2mcg
7%
Calcium 210mg
51%
Iron 8mg
1%
Potassium 235mg
10%

Ingredients

- 1 cup vegan butter, softened
- ½ cup white sugar
- ½ cup brown sugar
- ¼ cup dairy-free milk
- 1 teaspoon vanilla
- 2 ¼ cups flour
- ½ teaspoon salt
- 1 teaspoon baking soda
- 12 ounces dairy-free chocolate chips

Instructions:

1. Preheat oven to 350°F.
2. In a large bowl, mix the butter, white sugar, and brown sugar until light and fluffy. Slowly stir in the dairy-free milk and then add the vanilla to make a creamy mixture.
3. In a separate bowl, combine the flour, salt, and baking soda.
4. You need to add this dry mixture to the liquid mixture and stir well. Fold in the chocolate chips.
5. Drop small spoonful of the batter onto non-stick cookie sheets and bake for 9 minutes.

Fudge Brownies
Nutritional Facts
servings per container
9
Prep Total
10 min
Serving Size 2/3 cup (70g)

Calories
10

Total Fat 20g
2%
Saturated Fat 2g
10%
Trans Fat 4g
-
Cholesterol
10%
Sodium 50mg
12%
Total Carbohydrate 7g
20%
Dietary Fiber 4g
7%
Total Sugar 12g
-

Protein 3g

Vitamin C 2mcg
19%
Calcium 260mg
20%
Iron 8mg
8%
Potassium 235mg
6%
Ingredients

- 2 cups flour
- 2 cups of sugar
- ½ cup of cocoa powder
- 1 teaspoon baking powder
- ½ teaspoon salt
- 1 cup of vegetable oil
- 1 cup of water
- 1 teaspoon vanilla
- 1 cup dairy-free chocolate chips (optional)
- ½ cup chopped walnuts (optional)

Instructions:

1. Preheat oven to 350°F and grease a 9 x 13-inch baking pan.
2. Add dry ingredients in a mixing bowl. Whisk together wet ingredients and fold into the dry ingredients.
3. If desired, add half the chocolate chips and chopped walnuts to the mix. Pour mixture into the prepared pan and sprinkle with remaining chocolate chips and walnuts, if using.
4. For fudge-like brownies, bake for 20-25 minutes. For cake-like brownies, bake 25-30 minutes. Let the brownies cool slightly before serving.

Pomegranate Quinoa Porridge
Nutritional Facts
servings per container
4
Prep Total
10 min
Serving Size 2/3 cup (40g)

AMOUNT PER SERVING
Calories
22

% DAILY VALUE
Total Fat 12g
20%
Saturated Fat 2g
4%
Trans Fat 01g
1.22%

**Cholesterol
22%
Sodium 170mg
10%
Total Carbohydrate 34g
22%**
Dietary Fiber 5g
14%
Total Sugar 7g
-

Protein 3g

Vitamin C 2mcg
10%
Calcium 260mg
20%
Iron 0mg
40%
Potassium 235mg
6%
Ingredients

- 1 1/2 cup quinoa flakes
- 2 1/2 teaspoons cinnamon
- 1 teaspoon vanilla extract
- 10 organic pDashes, pitted and cut into 1/4's
- 1 pomegranate pulp
- 1/4 cup desiccated coconut
- Stewed apples
- Coconut flakes to garnish

Instructions:

1. Gently place quinoa & almond milk into saucepan, & stir on medium to low heat for 9 minutes, until it smooth
2. Include cinnamon, desiccated coconut & vanilla extract & taste
3. Pit pDashes & cut into quarters include to porridge stir in well
4. Serve into individual bowls
5. Add a scoop of stewed apple (kindly view recipe below), pomegranates, pDashes & coconut flakes
6. Ready to eat!

Stewed apples

1. Peel, core, slice apples and place into a saucepan with water
2. Cook apples on medium heat, until extremely soft
3. Remove from heat, drain & mash apples
4. Ready to serve and enjoy your breakfast!

Cinnamon and Coconut Porridge
Serving: 4
Prep Time: 5 minutes
Cook Time: 5 minutes
Ingredients:

- 1 cup water
- 1/2 cup 36-percent low-fat cream
- ½ cup unsweetened dried coconut, shredded
- 1 tablespoon oat bran
- 1 tablespoon flaxseed meal
- 1/2 tablespoon almond butter
- 1 ½ teaspoons stevia
- ½ teaspoon cinnamon
- Toppings, such as blueberries or banana slices

How To:

1. Add the ingredients to alittle pot and blend well until fully incorporated
2. Transfer the pot to your stove over medium-low heat and convey the combination to a slow boil.
3. Stir well and take away from the warmth .
4. Divide the mixture into equal servings and allow them to sit for 10 minutes.
5. Top together with your desired toppings and enjoy!

Nutrition (Per Serving)
Calories: 171
Fat: 16g
Protein: 2g
Carbohydrates: 8g
Coconut Porridge
Serving: 2
Prep Time: 15 minutes
Cook Time: Nil
Ingredients:

- 2 tablespoons coconut flour

- 2 tablespoons vanilla protein powder
- 3 tablespoons Golden Flaxseed meal
- 1 ½ cups almond milk, unsweetened
- Powdered Erythritol

How To:

1. Take a bowl and blend within the flaxseed meal, protein powder, coconut flour and blend well.
2. Add the combination to the saucepan (placed over medium heat).
3. Add almond milk and stir, let the mixture thicken.
4. Add your required amount of sweetener and serve.
5. Enjoy!

Nutrition (Per Serving)
Calories: 259
Fat: 13g
Carbohydrates: 5g
Protein: 16g
Cinnamon Pear Oatmeal
Serving: 2
Prep Time: 10 minutes
Cook Time: 15 minutes
Ingredients:

- 3 cups water
- 1 cup steel-cut oats
- 1 tablespoon cinnamon powder
- 1 cup pear, cored and peeled, cubed

How To:

1. Take a pot and add the water, oats, cinnamon, pear and toss well.
2. Bring it to simmer over medium heat.
3. Let it cook for quarter-hour , and divide into two bowls.
4. Enjoy!

Nutrition (Per Serving)
Calories: 171
Fat: 5g
Carbohydrates: 11g
Protein: 6g
Banana and Walnut Bowl
Serving: 4

Prep Time: 10 minutes
Cook Time: 15 minutes
Ingredients:

- 2 cups water
- 1 cup steel-cut oats
- 1 cup almond milk
- ¼ cup walnuts, chopped
- 2 tablespoons chia seeds
- 2 bananas, peeled and mashed
- 1 teaspoon vanilla flavoring

How To:

1. Take a pot and add all ingredients, toss well.
2. Bring it to simmer over medium heat.
3. Let it cook for quarter-hour , and divide into 4 bowls.
4. Enjoy!

Nutrition (Per Serving)
Calories: 162
Fat: 4g
Carbohydrates: 11g
Protein: 4g
Scrambled Pesto Eggs
Serving: 2
Prep Time: 5 minutes
Cook Time: 5 minutes
Ingredients:

- 2 large whole eggs
- 1/2 tablespoon almond butter
- 1/2 tablespoon pesto
- 1 tablespoon creamed coconut
- almond milk
- Sunflower seeds and pepper as needed

How To:

1. Take a bowl and crack open your eggs.
2. Season with a pinch of sunflower seeds and pepper.
3. Pour eggs into a pan.
4. Add almond butter and introduce heat.
5. Cook on low heat and gently add pesto.

6. Once the eggs are cooked and scrambled, remove from the warmth.
7. Spoon in coconut milk and blend well.
8. activate the warmth and cook on LOW for a short time until you've got a creamy texture.
9. Serve and enjoy!

Nutrition (Per Serving)
Calories: 467
Fat: 41g
Carbohydrates: 3g
Protein: 20g
Barley Porridge
Serving: 4
Prep Time: 5 minutes
Cook Time: 25 minutes
Ingredients:

- 1 cup barley
- 1 cup wheat berries
- 2 cups unsweetened almond milk
- 2 cups water
- Toppings, such as hazelnuts, honey, berry, etc.

How To:

1. Take a medium saucepan and place it over medium-high heat.
2. Place barley, almond milk, wheat berries, water and convey to a boil.
3. Lower the warmth to low and simmer for 25 minutes.
4. Divide amongst serving bowls and top together with your desired toppings.
5. Serve and enjoy!

Nutrition (Per Serving)
Calories: 295
Fat: 8g
Carbohydrates: 56g
Protein: 6g
Olive Cherry Bites
Serving: 30
Prep Time: 15 minutes
Cook Time: Nil
Ingredients:

- 24 cherry tomatoes, halved

- 24 black olives, pitted
- 24 feta cheese cubes
- 24 toothpick/decorative skewers

How To:

1. Use a toothpick or skewer and thread feta cheese, black olives, cherry tomato halves therein order.
2. Repeat until all the ingredients are used.
3. Arrange during a serving platter.
4. Serve and enjoy!

Nutrition (Per Serving)
Calories: 57
Fat: 5g
Carbohydrates: 2g
Protein: 2g
Roasted Herb Crackers
Serving: 75 Crackers
Prep Time: 10 minutes
Cook Time: 120 minutes
Ingredients:

- ¼ cup avocado oil
- 10 celery sticks
- 1 sprig fresh rosemary, stem discarded
- 2 sprigs fresh thyme, stems discarded
- 2 tablespoons apple cider vinegar
- 1 teaspoon Himalayan sunflower seeds
- 3 cups ground flaxseeds

How To:

1. Preheat your oven to 225 degrees F.
2. Line a baking sheet with parchment paper and keep it on the side.
3. Add oil, herbs, celery, vinegar, sunflower seeds to a kitchen appliance and pulse until you've got a good mixture.
4. Add flax and puree.
5. Let it sit for 2-3 minutes.
6. Transfer batter to your prepared baking sheet and spread evenly, dig cracker shapes.
7. Bake for hour , flip and bake for hour more.
8. Enjoy!

Nutrition (Per Serving)
Calories: 34
Fat: 5g
Carbohydrates: 1g
Protein: 1.3g
Banana Steel Oats
Serving: 3
Prep Time: 10 minutes
Cook Time: 15 minutes
Ingredients:

- 1 small banana
- 1 cup almond milk
- ¼ teaspoon cinnamon, ground
- ½ cup rolled oats
- 1 tablespoon honey

How To:

1. Take a saucepan and add half the banana, whisk in almond milk, ground cinnamon.
2. Season with sunflower seeds.
3. Stir until the banana is mashed well, bring the mixture to a boil and stir in oats.
4. Reduce heat to medium-low and simmer for 5-7 minutes until the oats are tender.
5. Dice the remaining half banana and placed on the highest of the oatmeal.
6. Enjoy!

Nutrition (Per Serving)
Calories: 358
Fat: 6g
Carbohydrates: 76g
Protein: 7g
Swiss Chard Omelet
Serving: 2
Prep Time: 5 minutes
Cook Time: 5 minutes
Ingredients:

- 2 eggs, lightly beaten
- 2 cups Swiss chard, sliced
- 1 tablespoon almond butter

- ½ teaspoon sunflower seeds Fresh pepper

How To:

1. Take a non-stick frypan and place it over medium-low heat.
2. Once the almond butter melts, add Swiss chard and stir-cook for two minutes.
3. Pour the eggs into the pan and gently stir them into Swiss chard.
4. Season with garlic sunflower seeds and pepper.
5. Cook for two minutes.
6. Serve and enjoy!

Nutrition (Per Serving)
Calories: 260
Fat: 21g
Carbohydrates: 4g
Protein: 14g
Hearty Pineapple Oatmeal
Serving: 5
Prep Time: 10 minutes
Cook Time: 4-8 hours
Ingredients:

- 1 cup steel-cut oats
- 4 cups unsweetened almond milk
- 2 medium apples, sliced
- 1 teaspoon coconut oil
- 1 teaspoon cinnamon
- ¼ teaspoon nutmeg
- 2 tablespoons maple syrup, unsweetened
- A drizzle of lemon juice

How To:

1. Add listed ingredients to a pan and blend well.
2. Cook on very low flame for 8 hours/or on high flame for 4 hours.
3. Gently stir.
4. Add your required toppings.
5. Serve and enjoy!
6. Store within the fridge for later use; confirm to feature a splash of almond milk after re-heating for added flavor.

Nutrition (Per Serving)
Calories: 180

Fat: 5g
Carbohydrates: 31g
Protein: 5g
Zingy Onion and Thyme Crackers
Serving: 75 crackers
Prep Time: 15 minutes
Cooking Time: 120 minutes
Ingredients:

- 1 garlic clove, minced
- 1 cup sweet onion, coarsely chopped
- 2 teaspoons fresh thyme leaves
- ¼ cup avocado oil
- ¼ teaspoon garlic powder
- Freshly ground black pepper
- ¼ cup sunflower seeds
- 1 ½ cups roughly ground flax seeds

How To:

1. Preheat your oven to 225 degrees F.
2. Line two baking sheets with parchment paper and keep it on the side.
3. Add garlic, onion, thyme, oil, sunflower seeds, and pepper to a kitchen appliance .
4. Add sunflower and flax seeds, pulse until pureed.
5. Transfer the batter to prepared baking sheets and spread evenly, dig crackers
6. Bake for hour .
7. Remove parchment paper and flip crackers, bake for an additional hour.
8. If crackers are thick, it'll take longer .
9. Remove from oven and allow them to cool.
10. Enjoy!

Nutrition (Per Serving)
Total Carbs: 0.8g
Fiber: 0.2g
Protein: 0.4g
Fat: 2.7g
Crunchy Flax and Almond Crackers
Serving: 20-24 crackers
Prep Time: 15 minutes
Cooking Time: 60 minutes

Ingredients:

- ½ cup ground flaxseeds
- ½ cup almond flour
- 1 tablespoon coconut flour
- 2 tablespoons shelled hemp seeds
- ¼ teaspoon sunflower seeds
- 1 egg white
- 2 tablespoons unsalted almond butter, melted

How To:

1. Preheat your oven to 300 degrees F.
2. Line a baking sheet with parchment paper, keep it on the side.
3. Add flax, almond, coconut flour, hemp seed, seeds to a bowl and blend .
4. Add albumen and melted almond butter, mix until combined.
5. Transfer dough to a sheet of parchment paper and canopy with another sheet of paper.
6. Roll out dough.
7. dig crackers and bake for hour .
8. allow them to cool and enjoy!

Nutrition (Per Serving)
Total Carbs: 1.2
Fiber: 1g
Protein: 2g
Fat: 6g
Basil and Tomato Baked Eggs
Serving: 2
Prep Time: 10 minutes
Cook Time: 15 minutes
Ingredients:

- 1/2 garlic clove, minced
- 1/2 cup canned tomatoes
- ¼ cup fresh basil leaves, roughly chopped
- 1/4 teaspoon chili powder
- 1/2 tablespoon olive oil
- 2 whole eggs
- Pepper to taste

How To:

1. Preheat your oven to 375 degrees F.
2. Take alittle baking dish and grease with vegetable oil .
3. Add garlic, basil, tomatoes chili, vegetable oil into a dish and stir.
4. Crack eggs into a dish, keeping space between the 2 .
5. Sprinkle the entire dish with sunflower seeds and pepper.
6. Place in oven and cook for 12 minutes until eggs are set and tomatoes are bubbling.
7. Serve with basil on top.

Enjoy!
Nutrition (Per Serving)
Calories: 235
Fat: 16g
Carbohydrates: 7g
Protein: 14g
Cool Mushroom Munchies
Serving: 2
Prep Time: 5 minute
Cook Time: 10 minutes
Ingredients:

- 4 Portobello mushroom caps
- 3 tablespoons coconut aminos
- 2 tablespoons sesame oil
- 1 tablespoon fresh ginger, minced
- 1 small garlic clove, minced

How To:

1. Set your broiler to low, keeping the rack 6 inches from the heating source.
2. Wash mushrooms under cold water and transfer them to a baking sheet (top side down).
3. Take a bowl and blend in vegetable oil , garlic, coconut aminos, ginger and pour the mixture over the mushrooms tops .
4. Cook for 10 minutes.
5. Serve and enjoy!

Nutrition (Per Serving)
Calories: 196
Fat: 14g
Carbohydrates: 14g
Protein: 7g
Banana and Buckwheat Porridge

Serving: 2
Prep Time: 10 minutes
Cook Time: 15 minutes
Ingredients:

- 1 cup of water
- 1 cup buckwheat groats
- 2 big grapefruits, peeled and sliced
- 1 tablespoon ground cinnamon
- 3-4 cups almond milk
- 2 tablespoons natural almond butter

How To:

1. Take a medium-sized saucepan and add buckwheat and water.
2. Place the pan over medium heat and convey to a boil.
3. Keep cooking until the buckwheat absorbs the water.
4. Reduce heat to low and add almond milk, stir gently.
5. Add the remainder of the ingredients (except the grapefruits).
6. Stir and take away from the warmth .
7. Transfer into cereal bowls and add grapefruit chunks.
8. Serve and enjoy!

Nutrition (Per Serving)
Calories: 223
Fat: 4g
Carbohydrates: 4g
Protein: 7g
Delightful Berry Quinoa Bowl
Serving: 4
Prep Time: 5 minutes
Cook Time: 15 minutes
Ingredients:

- 1 cup quinoa
- 2 cups of water
- 1 piece, 2-inch sized cinnamon stick
- 2-3 tablespoons of maple syrup
- Flavorful Toppings
- ½ cup blueberries, raspberries or strawberries
- 2 tablespoons raisins
- 1 teaspoon lime
- ¼ teaspoon nutmeg, grated
- 3 tablespoons whipped coconut cream

- 2 tablespoon cashew nuts, chopped

How To:

1. Take a metal strainer and pass your grain through them to strain them well.
2. Rinse the grains under cold water thoroughly.
3. Take a medium-sized saucepan and pour within the water.
4. Add the strained grains and convey the entire mixture to a boil.
5. Add cinnamon sticks and canopy the saucepan.
6. Lower the warmth and let the mixture simmer for quarter-hour to permit the grain to soak up the liquid.
7. Remove the warmth and plump up the mixture employing a fork.
8. Add syrup if you would like additional flavor.
9. Also, if you're looking to form things a touch more interesting, just add any of the abovementioned ingredients.

Nutrition (Per Serving)
Calories: 202
Fat: 5g
Carbohydrates: 35g
Protein: 6g
Protein: 1.4g
Fantastic Bowl of Steel Oats
Serving: 4
Prep Time: 5 minutes
Cook Time: 25 minutes
Ingredients:

- 3 ¾ cup water
- 1 ¼ cup steel-cut oats
- ¼ teaspoon salt
- Flavorful Toppings
- 1 teaspoon cinnamon
- ½ teaspoon nutmeg
- ½ teaspoon lemon pepper
- 1 teaspoon Garam masala
- Mixed berries as needed
- Diced mangos as needed
- Sliced bananas as needed
- Dried fruits as needed
- Nuts as needed
- Flavorful Toppings
- 1 tablespoon coconut milk

How To:

1. Take a medium-sized saucepan and convey it over high heat.
2. Add water and permit the water to heat up.
3. Add the steel-cut oats with some salt and lower the warmth to medium-low.
4. Let the mixture simmer for about 25 minutes, ensuring to stay stirring it all the way.
5. Add coconut milk or almond butter for a few extra flavor.
6. Once done, serve with some berries or nuts.
7. Enjoy!

Nutrition (Per Serving)
Calories: 125
Fat: 3g
Carbohydrates: 20g
Protein: 7g
Quinoa and Cinnamon Bowl
Serving: 2
Prep Time: 10 minutes
Cook Time: 15 minutes
Ingredients:

- 1 cup uncooked quinoa
- 1½ cups water
- ½ teaspoon ground cinnamon
- ½ teaspoon sunflower seeds
- A drizzle of almond/coconut milk for serving

How To:

1. Rinse quinoa thoroughly underwater.
2. Take a medium-sized saucepan and add quinoa, water, cinnamon, and seeds.
3. Stir and place it over medium-high heat.
4. Bring the combination to a boil.
5. Reduce heat to low and simmer for 10 minutes.
6. Once cooked, remove from the warmth and let it cool.
7. Serve with a drizzle of almond or coconut milk.
8. Enjoy!

Nutrition (Per Serving)
Calories: 255
Fat: 13g

Carbohydrates: 33g
Protein: 5g

Awesome Breakfast Parfait

Serving: 2
Prep Time: 5 minutes
Cook Time: Nil

Ingredients:

- 1 teaspoon sunflower seeds
- ½ cup low-fat milk
- 1 cup all-purpose flour
- 1 teaspoon vanilla
- 3 eggs, beaten
- 1 teaspoon baking soda
- 2 cups non-fat Greek yogurt

How To:

1. Hack pretzels into small-sized portions and slice the strawberries.
2. Add yogurt to rock bottom of the glass and top with pretzel pieces and strawberries.
3. Add more yogurt and keep repeating until you've got spent all the ingredients.
4. Enjoy!

Nutrition (Per Serving)

Calorie: 304
Fat: 1g
Carbohydrates: 58g
Protein: 15g

Amazing and Healthy Granola Bowl

Serving: 6
Prep Time: 5 minutes
Cook Time: 25 minutes

Ingredients:

- 1-ounce Porridge oats
- 2 teaspoons maple syrup
- Cooking spray as needed
- 4 medium bananas
- 4 pots of Caramel
- Layered Fromage Frais
- 5 ounce fresh fruit salad, such as strawberries, blueberries, and raspberries

- ¼ ounce pumpkin seeds
- ¼ ounce sunflower seeds
- ¼ ounce dry chia seeds
- ¼ ounce desiccated coconut

How To:

1. Preheat your oven to 300 degrees F.
2. Take a baking tray and line with baking paper.
3. Take an outsized bowl and add oats, syrup , and seeds.
4. Spread mix on a baking tray.
5. Spray copra oil on top and bake for 20 minutes, ensuring to stay stirring from time to time.
6. Sprinkle coconut after the primary quarter-hour .
7. Remove from oven and let it cool.
8. Take a bowl and layer sliced bananas on top of the Fromage Fraise.
9. Spread the cooled granola mix on top and serve with a topping of berries.
10. Enjoy!

Nutrition (Per Serving)
Calories: 446
Fat: 29g
Carbohydrates: 37g
Protein: 13g
Cinnamon and Pumpkin Porridge Medley
Serving: 2
Prep Time: 10 minutes
Cook Time: 15 minutes
Ingredients:

- 1 cup unsweetened almond/coconut milk
- 1 cup of water
- 1 cup uncooked quinoa
- ½ cup pumpkin puree
- 1 teaspoon ground cinnamon
- 2 tablespoons ground flaxseed meal
- Juice of 1 lemon

How To:

1. Take a pot and place it over medium-high heat.
2. Whisk in water, almond milk and convey the combination to a boil.
3. Stir in quinoa, cinnamon, and pumpkin.

4. Reduce heat to low and simmer for 10 minutes until the liquid has evaporated.
5. Remove from the warmth and stir in flaxseed meal.
6. Transfer porridge to small bowls.
7. Sprinkle juice and add pumpkin seeds on top.
8. Serve and enjoy!

Nutrition (Per Serving)
Calories: 245
Fat: 1g
Carbohydrates: 59g
Protein: 4g
Quinoa and Date Bowl
Serving: 2
Prep Time: 10 minutes
Cook Time: 15 minutes
Ingredients:

- 1 date, pitted and chopped finely
- ½ cup red quinoa, dried
- 1 cup unsweetened almond milk
- 1/8 teaspoon vanilla extract
- ¼ cup fresh strawberries, hulled and sliced
- 1/8 teaspoon ground cinnamon

How To:

1. Take a pan and place it over low heat.
2. Add quinoa, almond milk, cinnamon, vanilla, and cook for about quarter-hour , ensuring to stay stirring from time to time.
3. Garnish with strawberries and enjoy!

Nutrition (Per Serving)
Calories: 195
Fat: 4.4g
Carbohydrates: 32g
Protein: 7g
Crispy Tofu
Serving: 8
Prep Time: 5 minutes
Cook Time: 20-30 minutes
Ingredients:

- 1 pound extra-firm tofu, drained and sliced

- 2 tablespoons olive oil
- 1 cup almond meal
- 1 tablespoons yeast
- ½ teaspoon onion powder ½ teaspoon garlic powder
- ½ teaspoon oregano

How To:

1. Add all ingredients except tofu and vegetable oil during a shallow bowl.
2. Mix well.
3. Preheat your oven to 400 degrees F.
4. during a wide bowl, add the almond meal and blend well.
5. Brush tofu with vegetable oil , read the combination and coat well.
6. Line a baking sheet with parchment paper.
7. Transfer coated tofu to the baking sheet.
8. Bake for 20-30 minutes, ensuring to flip once until golden brown.
9. Serve and enjoy!

Nutrition (Per Serving)
Calories: 282
Fat: 20g
Carbohydrates: 9g
Protein: 12g
Hearty Pumpkin Oats
Serving: 3
Prep Time: 5 minutes
Cook Time: 8 minutes
Ingredients:

- 1 cup quick-cooking rolled oats
- ¾ cup almond milk
- ½ cup canned pumpkin puree
- ¼ teaspoon pumpkin pie spice
- 1 teaspoon ground cinnamon

How To:

1. Take a secure microwave bowl and add oats, almond milk, and microwave on high for 1-2 minutes.
2. Add more almond milk if needed to realize your required consistency.
3. Cook for 30 seconds more.
4. Stir in pumpkin puree, pie spice, ground cinnamon.

5. Heat gently and enjoy!

Nutrition (Per Serving)
Calories: 229
Fat: 4g
Carbohydrates: 38g
Protein:10g
Wholesome Pumpkin Pie Oatmeal
Serving: 2
Prep Time: 10 minutes
Cook Time: 10 minutes
Smart Points: 6
Ingredients:

- ½ cup canned pumpkin, low sodium
- Mashed banana as needed
- ¾ cup unsweetened almond milk
- ½ teaspoon pumpkin pie spice
- 1 cup oats

How To:

1. Mash banana employing a fork and blend within the remaining ingredients (except oats) and blend well.
2. Add oats and finely stir.
3. Transfer mixture to a pot and let the oats cook until it's absorbed the liquid and is tender.
4. Serve and enjoy!

Nutrition (Per Serving)
Calories: 264
Fat: 4g
Carbohydrates: 52g
Protein: 7g
Power-Packed Oatmeal
Serving: 2
Prep Time: 10-15 minutes
Cook Time: 5 minutes
Ingredients:

- ¼ cup quick-cooking oats
- ¼ cup almond milk
- 2 tablespoons low fat Greek yogurt
- ¼ banana, mashed

- 2-1/4 tablespoons flaxseed meal

How To:

1. Whisk altogether of the ingredients during a bowl.
2. Transfer the bowl to your fridge and let it refrigerate for quarter-hour .
3. Serve and enjoy!

Nutrition (Per Serving)
Calories:
Fat: 11g
Carbohydrates: 27g
Protein: 10g
Chia Porridge
Serving: 2
Prep Time: 10 minutes
Cook Time: 5-10 minutes
Ingredients:

- 1 tablespoon chia seeds
- 1 tablespoon ground flaxseed
- 1/3 cup coconut cream
- ½ cup water
- 1 teaspoon vanilla extract
- 1 tablespoon almond butter

How To:

1. Add chia seeds, coconut milk , flaxseed, water and vanilla to alittle pot.
2. Stir and let it sit for five minutes.
3. Add almond butter and place pot over low heat.
4. Keep stirring as almond butter melts.
5. Once the porridge is hot/not boiling, pour into bowl.
6. Enjoy!
7. Add a couple of berries or a touch of cream for extra flavor.

Nutrition (Per Serving)
Calories: 410
Fat: 38g
Carbohydrates: 10g
Protein: 6g
Mouthwatering Chicken Porridge

Serving: 4
Prep Time: 1 hour
Cook Time: 10-20 minutes
Ingredients:

- 1 cup jasmine rice
- 1 pound steamed/cooked chicken legs
- 5 cups chicken broth
- 4 cups water
- 1 ½ cups fresh ginger
- Green onions
- Toasted cashew nuts

How To:

1. Place the rice in your fridge and permit it to relax 1 hour before cooking.
2. Take the rice out and add it to your Instant Pot.
3. Pour in chicken stock and water.
4. Lock the lid and cook on PORRIDGE mode, using the default settings and parameters.
5. Release the pressure naturally over 10 minutes.
6. Open the lid.
7. Remove the meat from the chicken legs and add the meat to your soup.
8. Stir overflow Sauté mode.
9. Season with a touch of flavored vinegar and luxuriate in with a garnish of nuts and onion.

Nutrition (Per Serving)
Calories: 206
Fat: 8g
Carbohydrates: 8g
Protein: 23g
Simple Blueberry Oatmeal
Serving: 4
Prep Time: 10 minutes
Cooking Time: 8 hours
Ingredients:

- 1 cup blueberries
- 1 cup steel-cut oats1 cup coconut milk
- 2 tablespoons agave nectar
- ½ teaspoon vanilla extract Coconut flakes, garnish

How To:

1. Grease Slow Cooker with cooking spray.
2. Add oats, milk, nectar, blueberries, and vanilla.
3. Toss well.
4. Place lid and cook on LOW for 8 hours.
5. Divide between serving bowls and serve.
6. Enjoy!

Nutrition (Per Serving)
Calories: 202
Fat: 6g
Carbohydrates: 12g
Protein: 6g
The Decisive Apple "Porridge"
Serving: 2
Prep Time: 10 minutes
Cook Time: 5 minutes
Ingredients:

- 1 large apple, peeled, cored and grated
- 1 cup unsweetened almond milk
- 1 ½ tablespoons sunflower seeds
- 1/8 cup fresh blueberries
- ¼ teaspoon fresh vanilla bean extract

How To:

1. Take an outsized pan and add sunflower seeds, vanilla, almond milk, apples, and stir.
2. Place over medium-low heat.
3. Cook for five minutes, ensuring to stay the mixture stirring.
4. Transfer to a serving bowl.
5. Serve and enjoy!

Nutrition (Per Serving)
Calories: 123
Fat: 1.3g
Carbohydrates:23g
Protein: 4g
The Unique Smoothie Bowl
Serving: 2
Prep Time: 10 minutes
Cook Time: Nil

Ingredients:

- 2 cups baby spinach leaves
- 1 cup coconut almond milk
- ¼ cup low fat cream
- 2 tablespoons flaxseed oil
- 2 tablespoons chia seeds
- 2 tablespoons walnuts, roughly chopped A handful of fresh berries

How To:

1. Add spinach leaves, coconut almond milk, cream and linseed oil to a blender.
2. Blitz until smooth.
3. Pour smoothie into serving bowls.
4. Sprinkle chia seeds, berries, walnuts on top.
5. Serve and enjoy!

Nutrition (Per Serving)
Calories: 380
Fat: 36g
Carbohydrates: 12g
Protein: 5g
Cinnamon and Coconut Porridge
Serving: 4
Prep Time: 5 minutes
Cook Time:5 minutes
Ingredients:

- 2 cups water
- 1 cup coconut cream
- ½ cup unsweetened dried coconut, shredded
- 2 tablespoons flaxseed meal
- 1 tablespoon almond butter
- 1 ½ teaspoons stevia
- 1 teaspoon cinnamon
- Toppings as blueberries

How To:

1. Add the listed ingredients to alittle pot, mix well.
2. Transfer pot to stove and place over medium-low heat.
3. bring back mix to a slow boil.
4. Stir well and take away from the warmth .

5. Divide the combination into equal servings and allow them to sit for 10 minutes.
6. Top together with your desired toppings and enjoy!

Nutrition (Per Serving)
Calories: 171
Fat: 16g
Carbohydrates: 6g
Protein: 2g
Morning Porridge
Serving: 2
Prep Time: 15 minutes
Cook Time: Nil
Ingredients:

- 2 tablespoons coconut flour
- 2 tablespoons vanilla protein powder
- 3 tablespoons Golden Flaxseed meal
- 1 ½ cups almond milk, unsweetened Powdered erythritol

How To:

1. Take a bowl and blend in flaxseed meal, protein powder, coconut flour and blend well.
2. Add mix to the saucepan (place over medium heat).
3. Add almond milk and stir, let the mixture thicken .
4. Add your required amount of sweetener and serve.
5. Enjoy!

Nutrition (Per Serving)
Calories: 259
Fat: 13g
Carbohydrates: 5g
Protein: 16g
Vanilla Sweet Potato Porridge
Serving: 5
Prep Time: 10 minutes
Cook Time: 8 hours
Ingredients:

- 6 sweet potatoes, peeled and cut into 1-inch cubes
- 1 ½ cups light coconut milk
- 1 teaspoon ground cinnamon
- 1 teaspoon ground cardamom

- 1 teaspoon pure vanilla extract
- 1 cup raisins Pinch of salt

How To:

1. Add sweet potatoes coconut milk, vanilla, cardamom, cinnamon to your Slow Cooker.
2. Close lid and cook on LOW for 8 hours.
3. Open the lid and mash the entire mixture using potato masher to mash the sweet potatoes, stir well.
4. Stir in raisins, salt and serve.
5. Serve and enjoy!

Nutrition (Per Serving)

- Calories: 317
- Fat: 4g
- Carbohydrates: 71g
- Protein: 4g

A Nice German Oatmeal
Serving: 3
Prep Time: 10 minutes
Cook Time: 8 hours
Ingredients:

- 1 cup steel-cut oats
- 3 cups water
- 6 ounces coconut milk
- 2 tablespoons cocoa powder
- 1 tablespoon brown sugar
- 1 tablespoon coconut, shredded

How to

1. Grease the Slow Cooker well.
2. Add the listed ingredients to your Cooker and stir.
3. Place lid and cook on LOW for 8 hours.
4. Divide amongst serving bowls and enjoy!

Nutrition (Per Serving)
Calories: 200
Fat: 4g
Carbohydrates: 11g

Protein: 5g
Very Nutty Banana Oatmeal
Serving: 4
Prep Time: 15 minutes
Cook Time: 7-9 hours
Ingredients:

- 1 cup steel-cut oats
- 1 ripe banana, mashed
- 2 cups unsweetened almond milk
- 1 cup water
- 1 ½ tablespoons honey
- ½ teaspoon vanilla extract
- ¼ cup almonds, chopped
- 1 teaspoon ground cinnamon
- ¼ teaspoon ground nutmeg

How To:

1. Grease the Slow Cooker well.
2. Add the listed ingredients to your Slow Cooker and stir.
3. Cover with lid and cook on LOW for 7-9 hours.
4. Serve and enjoy!

Nutrition (Per Serving)
Calories: 230
Fat: 7g
Carbohydrates: 40g
Protein: 5g
Cool Coconut Flatbread
Serving: 4
Prep Time: 15 minutes
Cooking Time: 10 minutes
Ingredients:

- 1 ½ tablespoons coconut flour
- ¼ teaspoon baking powder
- 1/8 teaspoon sunflower seeds
- 1 tablespoon coconut oil, melted
- 1 whole egg

How To:

1. Preheat your oven to 350 degrees F.

2. Add coconut flour, leaven , sunflower seeds.
3. Add copra oil , eggs and stir well until mixed.
4. Leave the batter for several minutes.
5. Pour half the batter onto the baking pan.
6. Spread it to make a circle, repeat with remaining batter.
7. Bake within the oven for 10 minutes.
8. Once you get a golden-brown texture, let it cool and serve.
9. Enjoy!

Nutrition (Per Serving)
Total Carbs: 9 (%)
Fiber: 3g
Protein: 8g (%)
Fat: 20g (%)

Perfect Homemade Pickled Ginger Gari
Serving: 8
Prep Time: 40 minute
Cook Time: 5 minutes
Ingredients:

- About 8 ounces of fresh ginger root, completely peeled
- 1 teaspoon and extra ½ teaspoon of fine sunflower seeds
- 1 cup vinegar, rice
- 1/3 cup sugar, white

How To:

1. Cut your ginger into small-sized chunks and transfer them to a bowl.
2. Season with sunflower seeds and stir, let the mixture sit for a minimum of half-hour .
3. Take a saucepan and add sugar and vinegar, heat it up, bring the mixture to a boil and keep boiling until the sugar has completely dissolved.
4. Pour the liquid over your ginger pieces.
5. Let it cool and wait until the water changes color.
6. Enjoy!
7. Alternatively, store in jars and use as required .

Nutrition (Per Serving)
Calories: 14
Fat: 0.1g
Carbohydrates: 3g
Protein: 0.1g

Avocado and Blueberry Medley

Serving: 4
Prep Time: 5 minutes
Cook Time: Nil
Ingredients:

- 1 frozen banana
- 2 avocados, quartered
- 2 cups berries
- Maple syrup as needed

How To:

1. Take your blender and add all ingredients except syrup.
2. Add drinking water and blend.
3. Garnish with syrup and pour in smoothie glasses.
4. Enjoy!

Nutrition (Per Serving)

Calories: 250
Fat: 13g
Carbohydrates: 40g
Protein 4g

Healthy Zucchini Stir Fry

Serving: 4
Prep Time: 10 minutes
Cook Time: 10 minutes
Ingredients:

- 2 heaped tablespoons olive oil
- 1 medium-sized onion, sliced thinly
- 2 medium-sized zucchini, cut up into thin sized strips
- 2 heaped tablespoons teriyaki flavored sauce, low sodium
- 1 tablespoon coconut aminos
- 1 tablespoon sesame seed, toasted
- Ground pepper (black) as much as needed

How To:

1. Take a skillet and place it over medium level heat.
2. Add onions, and stir-cook for five minutes.
3. Add your zucchini and stir-cook for 1 minute more.
4. Gently add the sauces alongside the sesame seeds.
5. Cook for five minutes more until the zucchini are soft.

6. Finally, add the pepper and enjoy!

Nutrition (Per Serving)
Calories: 110
Fat: 9g
Carbohydrates: 8g
Protein: 3g

Herbed Parmesan Walnuts
Serving: 4
Prep Time: 5 minutes
Cook Time: 30 minutes

Ingredients:

- ½ cup kite ricotta/cashew cheese
- ½ teaspoon Italian herb seasoning and garlic sunflower seeds
- 1 teaspoon parsley flakes
- 2 cups walnuts
- 1 egg white

How To:

1. Preheat your oven to 250 degrees F.
2. Take a bowl and add all ingredients except the albumen and walnuts.
3. Whisk within the albumen , stir in halved walnuts and blend well.
4. Transfer the mixture to a greased baking sheet and bake for half-hour .
5. Serve and enjoy!

Nutrition (Per Serving)
Calories: 220
Fat: 21g
Carbohydrates: 4g
Protein 8g

Amazing Scrambled Turkey Eggs
Serving: 2
Prep Time: 15 minutes
Cook Time: 15 minutes

Ingredients:

- 1 tablespoon coconut oil
- 1 medium red bell pepper, diced
- ½ medium yellow onion, diced
- ¼ teaspoon hot pepper sauce

- 3 large free-range eggs
- ¼ teaspoon black pepper, freshly ground
- ¼ teaspoon salt

How To:

1. Set a pan to medium-high heat, add copra oil , let it heat up.
2. Add onions and sauté.
3. Add turkey and red pepper .
4. Cook until the turkey is cooked.
5. Take a bowl and beat eggs, stir in salt and pepper.
6. Pour eggs within the pan with turkey and gently cook and scramble eggs.
7. Top with sauce and enjoy!

Nutrition (Per Serving)
Calories: 435
Fat: 30g
Carbohydrates: 34g
Protein: 16g
Egg and Bacon Cups
Serving: 6
Prep Time: 10 minutes
Cook Time: 15 minutes
Ingredients:

- 2 bacon strips
- 2 large eggs
- A handful of fresh spinach
- ¼ cup cheese
- Salt and pepper to taste

How To:

1. Preheat your oven to 400 degrees F.
2. Fry bacon during a skillet over medium heat, drain the oil and keep them on the side.
3. Take muffin tin and grease with oil.
4. Line with a slice of bacon, depress the bacon well, ensuring that the ends are protruding (to be used as handles).
5. Take a bowl and beat eggs.
6. Drain and pat the spinach dry.
7. Add the spinach to the eggs.
8. Add 1 / 4 of the mixture in each of your muffin tins.

9. Sprinkle cheese and season.
10. Bake for quarter-hour .
11. Enjoy!

Nutrition (Per Serving)
Calories: 101
Fat: 7g
Carbohydrates: 2g
Protein: 8g
Fiber: 1g
Net Carbs: 1g
Pepperoni Omelet
Serving: 2
Prep Time: 5 minutes
Cook Time: 20 minutes
Ingredients:

- 3 eggs
- 7 pepperoni slices
- 1 teaspoon coconut cream
- Salt and freshly ground black pepper, to taste
- 1 tablespoons butter

How To:

1. Take a bowl and whisk eggs with all the remaining ingredients in it.
2. Then take a skillet and warmth the butter.
3. Pour ¼ of the egg mixture into your skillet.
4. After that, cook for two minutes per side.
5. Repeat to use the whole batter.
6. Serve warm and enjoy!

Nutrition (Per Serving)
Calories: 141
Fat: 11.5g
Carbohydrates: 0.6g

- Protein: 8.9g

Cinnamon Baked Apple Chips
Serving: 2
Prep Time: 5 minutes
Cook Time: 2 hours
Ingredients:

- 1 teaspoon cinnamon
- 1-2 apples

How To:

1. Preheat your oven to 200 degrees F.
2. Take a pointy knife and slice apples into thin slices.
3. Discard seeds.
4. Line a baking sheet with parchment paper and arrange apples thereon .
5. Confirm they are doing not overlap.
6. Once done, sprinkle cinnamon over apples.
7. Bake within the oven for 1 hour.
8. Flip and bake for an hour more until not moist.
9. Serve and enjoy!

Nutrition (Per Serving)
Calories: 147
Fat: 0g
Carbohydrates: 39g
Protein: 1g

Herb and Avocado Omelet
Serving: 2
Prep Time: 2 minutes
Cook Time: 10 minutes

Ingredients:

- 3 large free-range eggs
- ½ medium avocado, sliced
- ½ cup almonds, sliced
- Salt and pepper as needed

How To:

1. Take a non-stick skillet and place it over medium-high heat.
2. Take a bowl and add eggs, beat the eggs.
3. Pour into the skillet and cook for 1 minute.
4. Reduce heat to low and cook for 4 minutes.
5. Top the omelet with almonds and avocado.
6. Sprinkle salt and pepper and serve.
7. Enjoy!

Nutrition (Per Serving)
Calories: 193

Fat: 15g
Carbohydrates: 5g
Protein: 10g
Classic Apple and Cinnamon Oatmeal
Serving: 4
Prep Time: 15 minutes
Cook Time: 7-9 hours
Ingredients:

- 1 apple, cored, peeled and diced
- 1 cup steel-cut oats
- 2 ½ cups unsweetened vanilla almond milk
- 2 tablespoons honey
- ½ teaspoon vanilla extract
- 1 teaspoon ground cinnamon

How To:

1. Grease the Slow Cooker well.
2. Add the listed ingredients to your Slow Cooker and stir.
3. Cover with lid and cook on LOW for 7-9 hours.
4. Serve and enjoy!

Nutrition (Per Serving)
Calories: 126
Fat: 3g
Carbohydrates. 25g
Protein: 3g
Carrot and Zucchini Oatmeal
Serving: 3
Prep Time: 10 minutes
Cook Time: 8 hours
Ingredients:

- ½ cup steel cut oats
- 1 cup coconut milk
- 1 carrot, grated
- ¼ zucchini, grated
- Pinch of nutmeg
- ½ teaspoon cinnamon powder
- 2 tablespoons brown sugar
- ¼ cup pecans, chopped

How To:

1. Grease the Slow Cooker well.
2. Add oats, zucchini, milk, carrot, nutmeg, cloves, sugar, cinnamon and stir well.
3. Place lid and cook on LOW for 8 hours.
4. Divide amongst serving bowls and enjoy!

Nutrition (Per Serving)
Calories: 200
Fat: 4g
Carbohydrates: 11g
Protein: 5g
Blueberry and Walnut "Steel" Oatmeal
Serving: 8
Prep Time: 5 minutes
Cook Time: 7-8 hours
Ingredients:

- 2 cups steel-cut oats
- 6 cups water
- 2 cups low-fat milk
- 2 cups fresh blueberries
- 1 ripe banana, mashed
- 1 teaspoon vanilla extract
- 2 teaspoons ground cinnamon
- 2 tablespoons brown sugar
- Pinch of salt
- ½ cup walnuts, chopped

How To:

1. Grease the within of your Slow Cooker.
2. Add oats, milk, water, blueberries, banana, vanilla, sugar , cinnamon and salt to your Slow Cooker.
3. Stir.
4. Place lid and cook on LOW for 7-8 hours.
5. Serve warm with a garnish of chopped walnuts.
6. Enjoy!

Nutrition (Per Serving)
Calories: 372
Fat: 14g
Carbohydrates: 56g
Protein: 8g
Shrimp and Egg Medley

Serving: 4
Prep Time: 15 minutes
Cook Time: nil
Ingredients:

- 4 hardboiled eggs, peeled and chopped
- 1-pound cooked shrimp, peeled and de-veined, chopped
- 1 sprig fresh dill, chopped
- ¼ cup mayonnaise
- 1 teaspoon Dijon mustard
- 4 fresh lettuce leaves

How To:

1. Take an outsized serving bowl and add the listed ingredients (except lettuce.)
2. Stir well.
3. Serve over bet of lettuce leaves.
4. Enjoy!

Nutrition (Per Serving)
Calories: 292
Fat: 17g
Carbohydrates: 1.6g
Protein: 30g
Crispy Walnut Crumbles
Serving: 10
Prep Time: 10 minutes
Cook Time: 8 minutes
Ingredients:

- 6 ounces kite ricotta/cashew cheese, grated
- 2 tablespoons walnuts, chopped
- 1 tablespoon almond butter
- ½ tablespoon fresh thyme chopped

How To:

1. Preheat your oven to 350 degrees F.
2. Take two large rimmed baking sheets and line with parchment.
3. Add cheese, almond butter to a kitchen appliance and blend.
4. Add walnuts to the combination and pulse.
5. Take a tablespoon and scoop mix onto a baking sheet.
6. Top them with chopped thymes.

7. Bake for 8 minutes, transfer to a cooling rack.
8. Let it cool for half-hour .
9. Serve and enjoy!

Nutrition (Per Serving)
Calories: 80
Fat: 3g
Carbohydrates: 7g
Protein: 7g

Cheesy Zucchini Omelette
Serving: 3
Prep Time: 10 minutes
Cook Time: 20 minutes

Ingredients:

- 4 large eggs
- 2-3 medium zucchinis
- 1-2 garlic cloves, crushed
- 4 tablespoons grated cheese Season as needed

How To:

1. Take a bowl and add grated zucchinis, confirm to peel them because the skin is bitter.
2. Take a bowl and break within the eggs, crushed garlic and cheese.
3. Pour the mixture during a hot frypan with a touch little bit of oil and place it over medium heat, keep a lid on.
4. Once the egg is cooked nicely, and therefore the bottom is crispy and golden, serve and luxuriate in with a garnish of chopped parsley.
5. Enjoy!

Nutrition (Per Serving)
Calories: 289
Fat: 20g
Carbohydrates: 7g
Protein: 21g

Old Fashioned Breakfast Oatmeal
Serving: 4
Prep Time: 10 minutes
Cook Time: 5 minutes

Ingredients:

- 2 ½ cups water

- 1 cup old fashioned oats
- 1 cup apple, peeled, cored and chopped
- 3 tablespoons low-fat butter
- 2 tablespoons palm sugar
- ½ teaspoon cinnamon powder

How To:

1. Add water, oats, apple, butter, cinnamon, and sugar to a moment Pot.
2. Toss well and lock the lid.
3. Cook on high for five minutes.
4. Release the pressure naturally over 10 minutes.
5. Stir oats and divide into bowls.
6. Enjoy!

Nutrition (Per Serving)
Calories: 191
Fat: 2g
Carbohydrates: 9g
Protein: 5g
Healthy Peach Oatmeal
Serving: 8
Prep Time: 10 minutes
Cook Time: 10 minutes
Ingredients:

- 4 cups old fashioned rolled oats
- 3 ½ cups low-fat milk
- 3 ½ cups water
- 1 teaspoon cinnamon powder
- 1/3 cup palm sugar
- 4 peaches, chopped

How To:

1. Add oats, milk, cinnamon, water, sugar, and peaches to your Instant Pot.
2. Toss well.
3. Lock the lid and cook for 10 minutes on high .
4. Release the pressure naturally over 10 minutes .
5. Divide the combination in bowls and serve!

Nutrition (Per Serving)

Calories: 192
Fat: 3g
Carbohydrates: 12g
Protein: 4g

Fancy Banana Oatmeal

Serving: 4
Prep Time: 10 minutes
Cook Time: 10 minutes

Ingredients:

- 2 cups water
- 1 cup steel-cut oats
- 1 cup almond milk
- ¼ cup walnuts, chopped
- 2 tablespoons flaxseeds, ground
- 2 tablespoons chia seeds
- 2 bananas, peeled and mashed
- 1 teaspoon vanilla extract
- 1 teaspoon cinnamon powder

How To:

1. Add water, oats, almond milk, flaxseed, walnuts, chia seeds, vanilla, bananas, cinnamon to your Instant Pot and provides it a pleasant toss.
2. Lock the lid and cook on high for 10 minutes.
3. Release the pressure naturally and open the lid.
4. Divide the combination amongst bowls and serve.
5. Enjoy!

Nutrition (Per Serving)

Calories: 200
Fat: 4g
Carbohydrates: 11g
Protein: 4g

Traditional Frittata

Serving: 6
Prep Time: 10 minutes
Cook Time: 5 minutes

Ingredients:

- 2 tablespoons almond milk
- Just a pinch pepper
- 6 eggs, cracked and whisked

- 2 tablespoons parsley, chopped
- 1 tablespoon low-fat cheese, shredded
- 1 cup of water

How To:

1. Take a bowl and add the eggs, almond milk, pepper, cheese, and parsley. Whisk well.
2. Take a pan that might slot in your Instant Pot and grease with cooking spray.
3. Pour the egg mix into the pan.
4. Add a cup of water to your pot and place a steamer basket.
5. Add the pan within the basket.
6. Lock the lid and cook on high for five minutes.
7. Release the pressure naturally over 10 minutes.
8. Remove the lid and divide the frittata amongst serving plates.
9. Enjoy!

Nutrition (Per Serving)
Calories: 200
Fat: 4g
Carbohydrates: 17g
Protein: 6g
Pepperoni Omelet
Serving: 2
Prep Time: 5 minutes
Cook Time: 20 minutes
Ingredients:

- 3 eggs
- 7 pepperoni slices
- 1 teaspoon coconut cream
- Salt and freshly ground black pepper, to taste
- 1 tablespoon butter

How To:

1. Take a bowl and whisk eggs with all the remaining ingredients in it.
2. Then take a skillet and warmth butter.
3. Pour quarter of the egg mixture into your skillet.
4. After that, cook for two minutes per side.
5. Repeat to use the whole batter.
6. Serve warm and enjoy!

Nutrition (Per Serving)
Calories: 141
Fat: 11.5g
Carbohydrates: 0.6g
Protein: 8.9g

Eggy Tomato Scramble
Serving: 2
Prep Time: 10 minutes
Cook Time: 5 minutes
Ingredients:

- 2 whole eggs
- ½ cup fresh basil, chopped
- 2 tablespoons olive oil
- ½ teaspoon red pepper flakes, crushed
- 1 cup grape tomatoes, chopped
- Salt and pepper to taste

How To:

1. Take a bowl and whisk in eggs, salt, pepper, red pepper flakes and blend well.
2. Add tomatoes, basil, and mix.
3. Take a skillet and place over medium-high heat.
4. Add the egg mixture and cook for five minutes until cooked and scrambled.
5. Enjoy!

Nutrition (Per Serving)
Calories: 130
Fat: 10g
Carbohydrates: 8g
Protein: 1.8g

Breakfast Fruit Pizzas
Ingredients

- Two whole-wheat pita flatbreads
- 7 ounces Arla Original Cream Cheese
- 1-2 teaspoons honey
- 1/2 teaspoon pure vanilla extract
- Three kiwi skin removed and sliced
- 1/2 cup sliced strawberries
- 1/2 cup blackberries
- 1/4 cup blueberries

- Two raspberries for the center

Instructions

1. Preheat the oven to broil. Put the entire wheat pita flatbreads within the oven. Broil for 1 minute and switch over. Broilfor one minute more. you'll also toast the entire pita bread during a kitchen appliance . Set the dough aside to chill.
2. Take a bowl and blend the cheese , honey, and vanilla. Spread the cheese on the pita bread.
3. Decorate the fruit on top of the cheese . dig slices and serve immediately.
4. Note-you can use your favorite fruit. Bananas, peaches, pineapple, oranges, nectarines would even be good!

Peanut Butter Overnight Oats
Ingredients

- Oats
- Half of cup unsweetened plain almond milk (or sub other dairy-free milk, such as coconut, soy, or hemp!)
- 3/4 Tbsp of chia seed
- 2 Tbsp of natural salted peanut butter or almond butter (creamy or crunchy // or sub other nut or seed butter)
- 1 Tbsp of maple syrup (or sub coconut sugar, natural brown sugar, or stevia to taste) half of cup gluten-loose rolled oats (rolled oats are best, vs. Steel-cut or quick-cooking)
- Toppings optional
- Sliced banana, strawberries, or raspberries
- Flaxseed meal or additional chia seed
- Granola

Instructions

1. Take alittle bowl with a lid, add almond milk, chia seeds, spread , and syrup (or every othersweetener) and stir with a spoon to mix . The spread doesn't got to be alright blended with the almond milk (doing so leaves swirls of spread to enjoy the next day).
2. Add oats and stir a couple of extra times. Then depress with a spoon to form sure all oats were moistened and areimmersed in almond milk.
3. Cover tightly with a lid or seal and set within the fridge overnight (or for a minimum of 6 hours) to place/soak.

4. the next day, open and knowledge as is or garnish with preferred toppings.
5. Overnight oats will preserve within the refrigerator for 2-three days, though high-quality within the primary 12-24 hours in our experience. Not freezer friendly.

Nutrition

Calories: 452, Fat: 22.8g, Saturatedfat: 4.1g, Sodium: 229mgPotassium: 479mgCarbohydrates: 51.7g Fiber: 8.3gSugar: 15.8g Protein: 14.6g

Wedge Salad Skewers
Ingredients

- One head of iceberg lettuce (cut into wedge pieces)
- Four Roma tomatoes cut in half
- One red onion (cut into 1-inch pieces)
- Two avocados cut into 1-inch pieces
- Five slices of bacon cooked and cut into thirds
- One cucumber (sliced (peeled or unpeeled))
- Eight wooden skewers
- Two green onions (diced)
- 1 5 oz container blue cheese crumbles One bottle blue cheese dressing

Instructions

1. One skewer at a time adds an iceberg wedge, tomato, onion, avocado, two pieces of bacon, every other iceberg wedge, and then cucumber.
2. Continue till all skewers have been made, then garnish with crumbled blue cheese, blue cheese dressing, and diced leafy green onions.

Nutrition

Calories: 238kcal, Fat: 19g, Saturated fat: 6gCholesterol: 25mg Sodium: 401mgPotassium: 573mgCarbohydrates: 10gFiber: 5g Sugar: 3gProtein: 8gVitamin A: 890%Vitamin C: 13.9%Calcium: 144%Iron: 0.9%

Low Sodium Sheet Pan Chicken Fajitas
Ingredients

- Two lbs chicken breast tenderloin each sliced in half lengthwise
- One green pepper sliced
- One red bell pepper sliced
- One Vidalia onion sliced
- Olive oil spray

- One tablespoon olive oil Seasoning:
- One teaspoon chili powder
- 1/2 teaspoon smoked paprika
- 1/2 teaspoon garlic powder 1/2 teaspoon onion powder 1/2 teaspoon dried oregano
- 1/2 teaspoon dried cilantro
- 1/2 teaspoon cumin
- 1/4 teaspoon cayenne pepper

Instructions

1. Preheat oven to 350 degrees F.
2. Apply a coat on a sheet pan with vegetable oil spray.
3. Spread pepper and onion slices onto a prepared sheet pan.
4. Place chicken slices on top of vegetables.
5. Combine seasoning ingredients and stir to mix .
6. Drizzle seasoning mixture over chicken, peppers, and onion.
7. Sprinkle 1 tbsp of vegetable oil over chicken, peppers, and onion.
8. Gently toss ingredients to distribute seasoning and oil evenly. (make sure chicken strips aren't overlapping)
9. Bake for 20 min or until chicken reaches 165 deg F.
10. Serve in warm low sodium tortillas.
11. Top together with your favorite toppings! i really like cheddar and soured cream .

Nutrition Facts
Calories 168Calories from Fat 36 Fat 4g6% Sodium 140mg6% Potassium 531mg15% Carbohydrates 5g2% Fiber 1g4% Sugar 3g3% Protein 24g48% Vitamin C 34.3mg42% Calcium 17mg2% Iron 0.8mg4%

Pineapple Protein Smoothie Ingredients

- 3/4 cup milk
- 3/4 cup pineapple chunks
- 1/2 cup ice
- 3/4 cup canned chickpeas (rinsed and drained)
- 2 tbsp almond butter
- Two pitted dates
- 2 tsp ground turmeric

Directions
Blend all ingredients until smooth.
Nutrients Calories: 461
Spinach Sunshine Smoothie Bowl
Ingredients

- One packed cup baby spinach
- One banana
- 1 cup of orange juice
- 1/2 avocado
- 1/2 cup ice cubes
- Blueberries (optional)
- Diced pineapple (optional)
- Ground flaxseeds (optional)

Directions
Process the spinach, banana, fruit juice , avocado, and ice during a blender until very smooth.

Serve topped with blueberries, diced pineapple, and ground flaxseeds.

Almond Butter Berry Smoothie
Ingredients

- 1/4 cup 1% low-fat milk
- 1/2 medium ripe banana
- 1 tbsp creamy almond butter
- 1 cup fresh or frozen raspberries
- 1/2 cup crushed ice

Directions
Blend all ingredients until smooth and enjoy!

Pomegranate and Peaches Avocado Toast
Ingredients

- one slice whole-grain bread
- 1/2 avocado
- 1 tbsp ricotta
- Pomegranate seeds, a small amount like one handful
- Drizzle honey

Directions

1. Toast the entire grain bread within the oven or toaster.
2. Spread avocado onto the toast, as smooth or coarse as you favor .
3. Spread a dollop of ricotta across the avocado.
4. Drizzle a piece of honey over the avocado mixture.
5. Sprinkle pomegranate seeds on top and luxuriate in .

Breakfast in a Jar
Ingredients

- 1/4 cup of oatmeal
- 3/4 cup of kefir
- 1 tbsp of chia seeds
- 2 tbsp of raisins
- 1 tbsp of unsweetened coconut flakes

Instructions

Make Layers of elements during a 16-ounce Mason jar , close the lid and refrigerate overnight.

When it's able to eat, remove the jar from the fridge and provides it a fast stir.

Avocado Egg Cups
Ingredients

- Two avocados, ripe
- 1/4 tsp coarse salt
- 1/4 tsp pepper
- 1/2 tsp olive oil
- Four medium eggs
- 1 tbsp grated cheese, such as Parmesan, cheddar, or Swiss
- Assorted toppings: herbs, scallions, salsa, diced tomato, crumbled bacon, Sriracha, paprika, crumbled feta

Directions

1. Heat oven to 375°F. Halve avocados lengthwise and pit. Cut a thin slice from bottom of every avocado half so that it sits level. Where Hell was, scoop out only enough of the flesh (about ½ tbsp) to form room for an egg.
2. Place avocados on a foil-lined rimmed baking sheet. Season each with salt and pepper, and rub with vegetable oil .
3. Crack an egg into each cavity (some of the albumen will run over the side, but don't be concerned about it). Sprinkle with cheese, if using. Cover loosely with foil.
4. Bake almost 20 to 25 min, or until eggs are set to your liking. Sprinkle with toppings.

Sugar Break Apple and Peanut Butter Oatmeal
Ingredients

- 1 cup steel-cut oats
- Three medium-large Granny Smith apples, cored and sliced into 1-2" chunks
- A swirl of peanut butter

- pinch ground cinnamon
- 1 tbsp butter (optional)
- 4 cups of water
- pinch salt

Directions

Cook the oats till they reach the specified texture and creaminess.
Cut apples, toss them into the oats, and stir.
Then add spread into it and stir until melted and spread throughout.
Top with a touch of cinnamon and butter (optional) and enjoy!

Nutrient Calories: 453
Sweet Potato Toast
Ingredients

- One potato (sweet)

Instructions

1. Divide the sweet potato into 1/4-inch slices and pop into the toaster.
2. Top with anything you select . Popular combinations include spread with fruit, avocado, hummus, eggs,cheese, and tuna fish salad .

Nutrient Calories: 112
Ulli'sGranelli
Ingredients

- 4 cups rolled oats
- 2 cups raw cashews
- 2 cups raw walnuts
- 2 cups of raw almonds
- 2 cups of fresh sunflower seed
- 2 cups of raw pumpkin seeds
- 3 cups unsweetened coconut flakes
- 1/2 cup of maple liquid syrup
- 1/4 cup of unrefined coconut oil, plus 2 tsp for oiling the baking sheet
- pinch of sea salt
- 1/3 cup of pure orange oil
- 2 cups of organic raisins
- 2 cups of dried cherries or cranberries

Directions

1. Set the oven to 300°F.
2. during a considerable bowl, mix the oats, nuts, seeds, and coconut flakes.
3. Take alittle bowl, stir together the syrup , copra oil , salt, and orange oil till well combined, then pourover the oat-nut combination and blend nicely.
4. Spread granola on an outsized oiled baking sheet (do it in batches if needed) and bake for 35-forty minutes untilgolden brown (rotate the baking sheet halfway via for even baking).
5. Remove from oven and permit refreshing absolutely before mixing with raisins and dried cherries or cranberries.
6. Store in airtight place within the fridge to stay extra crispiness.

Tofu Turmeric Scramble
Ingredients

- One 8-ounce block of firm or extra-firm tofu, drained
- 1 tbsp extra virgin olive oil
- ¼ red onion, chopped
- One green or purple bell pepper, chopped
- 2 cups of clean spinach, loosely chopped
- ½ cup sliced button mushrooms
- ½ tsp every salt and pepper
- 1 tsp garlic powder
- ½ tbsp turmeric
- ¼ cup nutritional yeast

Directions

1. Drain the tofu and squeeze lightly to try to to away with extra water. Crumble tofu right into a bowl with the help ofhand - the smaller the pieces, the higher .
2. Prep vegetables and region an outsized skillet at medium temperature. Once ready, then add vegetable oil , onions, and bellpeppers. Mix during a pinch of the salt and pepper and prepare dinner for about five minutes to melt the vegetables. Then add mushrooms and sauté for two mins. Then upload tofu. Sauté for about three minutes, a touch more if the tofu is watery.
3. Add the remainder of the salt, pepper, garlic turmeric, and nutritional yeast and blend with a spatula, ensuring the spicescombo well. Cook for an additional 5 to eight mins till tofu is lightly browned.
4. Add the spinach and canopy the pan so as to steam for 2 minutes. Serve immediately with facets of yourchoice.

5. Nutrient CALORIES: 158

Whole Grain Cheese Pancakes
Ingredients

- 1 cup of oat flour
- 1/2 cup of sorghum flour
- 2 tbsp of teff flour
- 1/3 cup of plus 1 tbsp, tapioca starch
- 1 tbsp of baking powder
- 1/2 of tsp salt
- 3 1/2 of tsp sugar
- 1/2 tsp of flax meal
- 3/4 cup of buttermilk
- 1/3 cup of cottage cheese
- Three eggs
- half tsp vanilla extract
- 4 tsp canola oil
- 1-pint blueberries
- 1/2 cup maple syrup
- 3 tbsp water
- 1 tsp lemon juice
- pinch of salt

Instructions

1. Combine all of your dry elements during a huge bowl and stir to combine evenly.
2. Whisk all of your wet ingredients in another bowl collectively.
3. Make a hole within the center of your dry substances and start to slowly pour within the wet materials, a few quartercup at a time. this may confirm that no lumps form when whisking.
4. Continue including your wet components to the flour base till a smooth batter forms. Let the batter relax for quarter-hour at an equivalent time as you preheat your grill.
5. While the grill is warming up, make a warm maple blueberry compote. Mix blueberries, syrup , water,lemon juice, and a pinch salt during a small pot. Stir frivolously to combine .
6. Gently heat the pot over medium-low warmth till the blueberries start to pop and release their natural juices. Setaside, but maintain heat.
7. Once the grill is preheated to a medium-hot temperature, lightly oil the restaurant employing a nonstick spray or asmall amount of neutral-flavored oil.

8. Ladle the batter on to the skillet, ensuring you are doing not overload it.
9. Give time to the pancakes to cook undisturbed until the looks of the sides dry and bubbles come to thesurface without breaking. This has got to take roughly minutes.
10. Flip the pancakes over and cook at the opposite facet for an additional two minutes.
11. Keep heat or serve immediately with the sweet and comfy maple-blueberry compote.

Nutrient Calories: 511
Red Pepper, Kale, and Cheddar Frittata
Ingredients

- 1 tsp olive oil
- 5 oz baby kale and spinach
- One red pepper, diced
- 1/3 cup sliced scallions
- 12 eggs
- 3/4 cup milk
- 1 cup sharp shredded cheddar cheese
- 1/4 tsp salt
- 1/4 tsp pepper

Directions

1. Preheat oven to 3/5 °F .
2. Spray an eight 1/2-inch by using 12-inch glass or casserole dish with vegetable oil or nonstick spray.
3. Heat oil during a large frypan . Add crimson peppers on low and cook until tender. Add kale and spinach, onoccasion stirring till vegetables are wilted, or for about three min.
4. Transfer peppers and greens to the plate, spreading evenly. Add sliced scallions.
5. Beat eggs with milk, salt, and pepper. Pour the egg aggregate over the pan. Sprinkle cheese on top.
6. Bake about 35-40 mins or till the mixture is totally set and starting to lightly brown. For extra color, place under broiler for an extra 1 to 3 minutes, watching to make sure the highest doesn't burn. Let cool about five mins before cutting it.
7. Serve it as warm or refrigerate for a fast breakfast during the week — microwave for 1-2 minutes to reheat.

Nutrient CALORIES: 77

Scrambled Eggs with Bell Pepper and Feta
Ingredients

- Olive oil-Salad or cooking-1 tsp-4.5 grams
- Green bell pepper-Sweet, green, raw-2 medium (approx 2-3/4" long, 2-1/2" dia)-238 grams
- Egg-Whole, fresh eggs-Four large-200 grams
- Feta cheese-1 oz-28.4 grams

Directions

1. Heat the oil during a skillet on medium heat. Add chopped peppers and cook till tender.
2. Stir the eggs and increase the skillet with the peppers. Stir slowly over medium-low heat till they attain your preferred doneness. Sprinkle inside the feta cheese and stir to combine and soften the cheese. Serve directly and luxuriate in it!

Nutrient
Calories 448 Carbs 14g Fat 30g Protein 31g Fiber 4g Net carbs 10g Sodium 551mg Cholesterol 769mg

Devilled Egg Toast
Ingredients

- Egg-Whole, fresh eggs-Two large-100 grams
- Mustard-Prepared, yellow-2 tbsp-30 grams
- Light mayonnaise-Salad dressing, Kraft brand-2 tbsp-30 grams
- Whole-wheat bread-Commercially prepared-Four slice-112 grams

Directions

1. Place egg during a bowl and canopy with water. Boil the water, remove from heat, cover, and let sit 10 minutes. Drain under cold water, peel, and mash.
2. Combine egg with the mustard and mayonnaise. Mix well.
3. Toast bread and top with egg mixture. Enjoy!

Nutrition
Calories 543 Carbs 53g Fat 24g Protein 28g Fiber 8g Net carbs 45g Sodium 1173mg Cholesterol 382mg

Basic scrambled eggs
Ingredients

- Egg-Whole, fresh eggs-Six large-300 grams

- Butter-Unsalted-1 tbsp-14.2 grams
- Chives-Raw-1 tbsp chopped-3 grams
- Tarragon-Spices, dried-1 tbsp, ground-4.8 grams
- Table-One dash-0.40 grams
- Pepper-Spices, black-One dash-0.10 grams

Directions

1. Beat the eggs during a bowl and till damaged up. Sprinkle with a pinch each of salt and pepper and beat to include .Place tablespoons of the eggs during a small bowl; put aside .
2. Heat a 10-inch nonstick frypan over medium-low warmth until hot, approximately 2 minutes. Add butter to the pan and therefore the usage of a rubber spatula, swirl until it's melted and foamy, and therefore the box is flippantly coated. Pour within the massive a part of the eggs, sprinkle with chives and tarragon (if the usage of), and let sit down undisturbed till eggs just start to line round the edges, about 1 to 2 minutes. Using the rubber spatula, push the eggs from the edges into the center . After30 seconds repeat pushing the eggs from the sides into the middle every 30 seconds till simply set, for a complete cooking time of about 5 minutes.
3. Add the last word tablespoons raw egg and stir till eggs not look wet. Remove from warmness and season with salt and pepper as required . Serve immediately.

Nutrition
Calories 546 Carbs 5g Fat 40g Protein 39g Fiber 0g Net carbs 4g Sodium 586mg Cholesterol 1147mg

Baked Butternut-Squash Rigatoni
Ingredients

- One large butternut squash
- Three clove garlic
- 2 tbsp. olive oil
- 1 lb. rigatoni
- 1/2 c. heavy cream
- 3 c. shredded fontina
- 2 tbsp. chopped fresh sage
- 1 tbsp. salt
- 1 tsp. freshly ground pepper
- 1 c. panko breadcrumbs

Directions

1. Set oven at 425 degrees. At an equivalent time, take an outsized bowl and toss garlic, squash, and vegetable oil for coating. Take a baking sheet and roast for about hour . Then calm for 20 minutes. Reduce oven to 350 degrees.
2. Then, boil the salted water and cook rigatoni consistent with package directions. Drain and put aside .
3. employing a blender, purée reserved squash with cream until smooth.
4. Take an outsized bowl and blend squash puree with reserved rigatoni, 2 cups fontina, sage, salt, and pepper. Apply olive oil on the edges of the baking pan. Transfer rigatoni-squash mixture to plate.
5. Take a little bowl, combine the remaining fontina and panko. Sprinkle over pasta and bake until golden brown,20 to 25 minutes.

Chapter Eleven

LUNCH RECIPES

Sweet Corn Soup

NUTRITIONAL FACTS
servings per container
4
Prep Total
10 min
Serving Size 2/3 cup (50g)

AMOUNT PER SERVING
Calories
120

% DAILY VALUE
Total Fat 2g
5%
Saturated Fat 0g
8%
Trans Fat 2g
1.20%
Cholesterol
2%

Sodium 16mg
7%
Total Carbohydrate 7g
10%
Dietary Fiber 4g
10%
Total Sugar 12g
-

Protein 3g

Vitamin C 2mcg
10%
Calcium 260mg
20%
Iron 20mg
25%
Potassium 235mg
8%
Ingredients

- 6 ears of corn
- 1 tablespoon of corn oil
- 1 small onion
- 1/2 cup grated celery root
- 7 cups water or vegetable stock
- Add salt to taste

Instructions:

1. Shuck the corn & slice off the kernels
2. In a large soup pot put in the oil, onion, celery root, and one cup of water
3. Let that mixture stew under low heat until the onion is soft
4. Include the corn, salt & remaining water and bring it to a boil
5. Cool briefly & then puree in a blender, then wait for it to cool before putting it through a food mill.
6. Reheat & add salt with pepper to taste nice.

Mexican Avocado Salad
Nutritional Facts
servings per container
6
Prep Total

10 min
Serving Size 2/3 cup (70g)

AMOUNT PER SERVING
Calories
120

% DAILY VALUE
Total Fat 8g
10%
Saturated Fat 1g
8%
Trans Fat 0g
21
Cholesterol
22%
Sodium 16mg
7%
Total Carbohydrate 7g
13%
Dietary Fiber 4g
14%
Total Sugar 1g
-
Protein 2g

Vitamin C 1mcg
1%
Calcium 260mg
20%
Iron 2mg
25%
Potassium 235mg
6%
Ingredients

- 24 cherry tomatoes, quartered
- 2 tablespoon extra-virgin olive oil
- 4 teaspoons red wine vinegar
- 2 teaspoon salt
- ¼ teaspoon freshly ground black pepper

- Gently chopped ½ medium yellow or white onion
- 1 jalapeño, seeded & finely chopped
- 2 tablespoons chopped fresh cilantro
- ¼ medium head iceberg lettuce, cut into ½-inch ribbons
- Chopped 2 ripe Hass avocados, seeded, peeled

Instructions:

1. Add tomatoes, oil, vinegar, salt, & pepper in a neat medium bowl. Add onion, jalapeño & cilantro; toss well
2. Put lettuce on a platter & top with avocado
3. Spoon tomato mixture on top and serve.

Crazy Delicious Raw Pad Thai
Nutritional Facts
servings per container
3
Prep Total
10 min
Serving Size 2/3 cup (77g)

AMOUNT PER SERVING
Calories
210

% DAILY VALUE
Total Fat 3g
10%
Saturated Fat 2g
8%
Trans Fat 7g
-

Cholesterol
0%
Sodium 120mg
7%
Total Carbohydrate 77g
10%
Dietary Fiber 4g
14%
Total Sugar 12g
-

Protein 3g

Vitamin C 1mcg
20%
Calcium 260mg
20%
Iron 2mg
41%
Potassium 235mg
1%

Ingredients

- 2 large zucchini
- Thinly sliced ¼ red cabbage
- Chopped ¼ cup fresh mint leaves
- Sliced 1 spring onion
- peeled and sliced ½ avocado
- 10 raw almonds
- 4 tablespoonful sesame seeds Dressing
- ¼ cup peanut butter
- 2 tablespoonful tahini
- 2 lemon, juiced
- 2 tablespoonful tamari / salt-reduced soy sauce and add ½ chopped green chili

Instructions:

1. Collect dressing ingredients in a container
2. Pop the top on and shake truly well to join. I like mine pleasant and smooth however you can include a dash of sifted water on the off chance that it looks excessively thick.
3. Using a mandoline or vegetable peeler, expel one external portion of skin from every zucchini and dispose of.
4. Combine zucchini strips, cabbage & dressing in a vast blending bowl and blend well
5. Divide zucchini blend between two plates or bowls
6. Top with residual fixings and appreciate!

Kale And Wild Rice Stir Fly
Nutritional Facts
servings per container

3
Prep Total

10 min
Serving Size 2/3 cup (80g)

AMOUNT PER SERVING
Calories
220

% DAILY VALUE
Total Fat 5g
22%
Saturated Fat 1g
8%
Trans Fat 0g
-

Cholesterol
0%
Sodium 200mg
7%
Total Carbohydrate 12g
2%
Dietary Fiber 1g
14%
Total Sugar 12g
-

Protein 3g

Vitamin C 2mcg
10%
Calcium 20mg
1%
Iron 2mg
2%
Potassium 235mg
6%
Ingredients

- 1 tablespoonful extra virgin olive oil
- Diced ¼ onion
- 3 carrots, cut into ½ inch slices
- 2 cups assorted mushrooms
- 2 bunch kale, chopped into bite-sized pieces

- 2 tablespoonful lemon juice
- 2 tablespoonful chili flakes, more if desired
- 1 tablespoon Braggs Liquid Aminos
- 2 cup wild rice, cooked

Instructions:

1. In a large sauté pan, heat oil over on heater. Include onion & cook until translucent, for 35 to 10 minutes.
2. Include carrots & sauté for another 2 minutes. Include mushrooms & cook for 4 minutes. Include kale, lemon juice, chili flakes & Braggs. Cook until kale is slightly wilted.
3. Serve over wild rice and enjoy your Lunch!

Creamy Avocado Pasta
Nutritional Facts
servings per container
7
Prep Total
10 min
Serving Size 2/3 cup (25g)

AMOUNT PER SERVING
Calories
19

% DAILY VALUE
Total Fat 8g
300%
Saturated Fat 1g
40%
Trans Fat 0g
20%
Cholesterol
6%
Sodium 210mg
3%
Total Carbohydrate 22g
400%
Dietary Fiber 4g
1%
Total Sugar 12g

02.20%
Protein 3g

Vitamin C 2mcg
20%
Calcium 10mg
6%
Iron 4mg
7%
Potassium 25mg
6%

Ingredients

- 340 g / 12 oz spaghetti
- 2 ripe avocados, halved, seeded & neatly peeled
- 1/2 cup fresh basil leaves
- 3 cloves garlic
- 1/3 cup olive oil
- 2-3 teaspoon freshly squeezed lemon juice
- Add sea salt & black pepper, to taste
- 1.5 cups cherry tomatoes, halved

Instructions:

1. In a large pot of boiling salted water, cook pasta according to the package. When al dente, drain and set aside.
2. To make the avocado sauce, combine avocados, basil, garlic, oil, and lemon juice in food processor. Blend on high until smooth. Season with salt and pepper to taste.
3. In a large bowl, combine pasta, avocado sauce, and cherry tomatoes until evenly coated.
4. To serve, top with additional cherry tomatoes, fresh basil, or lemon zest.
5. Best when fresh. Avocado will oxidize over time so store leftovers in a covered container in refrigerator up to one day.

Black Bean Vegan Wraps
Nutritional Facts
servings per container
5
Prep Total
10 min
Serving Size 2/3 cup (27g)

. . .

AMOUNT PER SERVING
Calories
200

% DAILY VALUE
Total Fat 8g
1%
Saturated Fat 1g
2%
Trans Fat 0g
2%
Cholesterol
2%
Sodium 240mg
7%
Total Carbohydrate 12g
2%
Dietary Fiber 4g
14%
Total Sugar 12g
01.21%
Protein 3g

Vitamin C 2mcg
2%
Calcium 20mg
1%
Iron 7mg
2%
Potassium 25mg
6%
Ingredients

- 1 1/2 half cup of beans (sprouted & cooked)
- 2 carrot
- 1 or 2 tomatoes
- 2 avocado
- 1 cob of corn
- 1 Kale
- 2 or 3 sticks of celery

- 2 persimmons
- 1 Coriander

Dressing:

- 1 hachiyapersimmon (or half a mango)
- Juice of 1 lemon
- 2 to 3 tablespoons original olive oil
- 1/4 clean cup water
- 1 or 2 teaspoons grated fresh ginger
- 1/2 teaspoon of salt

Instructions:

1. Sprout & cook the black beans
2. Chop all the ingredients & mix them in a neat bowl with the black beans
3. Mix all the ingredients for the dressing & pour into the salad
4. Serve a spoonful in a clean lettuce leaf that you can easily roll into a wrap. Most people do use iceberg or romaine lettuce.

Fascinating Spinach and Beef Meatballs

Serving: 4
Prep Time: 10 minutes
Cook Time: 20

Ingredients:

- ½ cup onion
- 4 garlic cloves
- 1 whole egg
- ¼ teaspoon oregano
- Pepper as needed
- 1 pound lean ground beef
- 10 ounces spinach

How To:

1. Preheat your oven to 375 degrees F.
2. Take a bowl and blend within the remainder of the ingredients, and using your hands, roll into meatballs.
3. Transfer to a sheet tray and bake for 20 minutes.
4. Enjoy!

Nutrition (Per Serving)

Calorie: 200
Fat: 8g
Carbohydrates: 5g
Protein: 29g

Juicy and Peppery Tenderloin

Serving: 4
Prep Time: 10 minutes
Cook Time: 20

Ingredients:

- 2 teaspoons sage, chopped
- Sunflower seeds and pepper
- 2 1/2 pounds beef tenderloin
- 2 teaspoons thyme, chopped
- 2 garlic cloves, sliced
- 2 teaspoons rosemary, chopped
- 4 teaspoons olive oil

How To:

1. Preheat your oven to 425 degrees F.
2. Take alittle knife and cut incisions within the tenderloin; insert one slice of garlic into the incision.
3. Rub meat with oil.
4. Take a bowl and add sunflower seeds, sage, thyme, rosemary, pepper and blend well.
5. Rub the spice mix over tenderloin.
6. Put rubbed tenderloin into the roasting pan and bake for 10 minutes.
7. Lower temperature to 350 degrees F and cook for 20 minutes more until an indoor thermometer reads 145 degrees F.
8. Transfer tenderloin to a chopping board and let sit for 15 minutes; slice through 20 pieces and enjoy!

Nutrition (Per Serving)
Calorie: 183
Fat: 9g
Carbohydrates: 1g
Protein: 24g

Healthy Avocado Beef Patties

Serving: 2
Prep Time: 15 minutes
Cook Time: 10 minutes

Ingredients:

- 1 pound 85% lean ground beef
- 1 small avocado, pitted and peeled
- Fresh ground black pepper as needed

How To:

1. Pre-heat and prepare your broiler to high.
2. Divide beef into two equal-sized patties.
3. Season the patties with pepper accordingly.
4. Broil the patties for five minutes per side.
5. Transfer the patties to a platter.
6. Slice avocado into strips and place them on top of the patties.
7. Serve and enjoy!

Nutrition (Per Serving)
Calories: 568
Fat: 43g
Net Carbohydrates: 9g
Protein: 38g
Ravaging Beef Pot Roast
Serving: 4
Prep Time: 10 minutes
Cook Time: 75 minutes
Ingredients:

- 3 ½ pounds beef roast
- 4 ounces mushrooms, sliced
- 12 ounces beef stock
- 1-ounce onion soup mix
- ½ cup Italian dressing, low sodium, and low fat

How To:

1. Take a bowl and add the stock, onion soup mix and Italian dressing .
2. Stir.
3. Put roast beef in pan.
4. Add mushrooms, stock mix to the pan and canopy with foil.
5. Preheat your oven to 300 degrees F.
6. Bake for 1 hour and quarter-hour .
7. Let the roast cool.
8. Slice and serve.
9. Enjoy with the gravy on top!

Nutrition (Per Serving)
Calories: 700
Fat: 56g
Carbohydrates: 10g
Protein: 70g

Lovely Faux Mac and Cheese
Serving: 4
Prep Time: 15 minutes
Cook Time: 45 minutes
Ingredients:

- 5 cups cauliflower florets
- Sunflower seeds and pepper to taste
- 1 cup coconut almond milk
- ½ cup vegetable broth
- 2 tablespoons coconut flour, sifted
- 1 organic egg, beaten
- 1 cup cashew cheese

How To:

1. Preheat your oven to 350 degrees F.
2. Season florets with sunflower seeds and steam until firm.
3. Place florets during a greased ovenproof dish.
4. Heat coconut almond milk over medium heat during a skillet, confirm to season the oil with sunflower seeds and pepper.
5. Stir in broth and add coconut flour to the combination , stir.
6. Cook until the sauce begins to bubble.
7. Remove heat and add beaten egg.
8. Pour the thick sauce over the cauliflower and blend in cheese.
9. Bake for 30-45 minutes.
10. Serve and enjoy!

Nutrition (Per Serving)
Calories: 229
Fat: 14g
Carbohydrates: 9g
Protein: 15g

Epic Mango Chicken
Serving: 4
Prep Time: 25 minutes
Cook Time: 10 minutes
Ingredients:

- 2 medium mangoes, peeled and sliced
- 10-ounce coconut almond milk
- 4 teaspoons vegetable oil
- 4 teaspoons spicy curry paste
- 14-ounce chicken breast halves, skinless and boneless, cut in cubes
- 4 medium shallots
- 1 large English cucumber, sliced and seeded

How To:

1. Slice half the mangoes and add the halves to a bowl.
2. Add mangoes and coconut almond milk to a blender and blend until you've got a smooth puree.
3. Keep the mixture on the side.
4. Take a large-sized pot and place it over medium heat, add oil and permit the oil to heat up.
5. Add curry paste and cook for 1 minute until you've got a pleasant fragrance, add shallots and chicken to the pot and cook for five minutes.
6. Pour mango puree in to the combination and permit it to heat up.
7. Serve the cooked chicken with mango puree and cucumbers.
8. Enjoy!

Nutrition (Per Serving)
Calories: 398
Fat: 20g
Carbohydrates: 32g
Protein: 26g
Chicken and Cabbage Platter
Serving: 2
Prep Time: 9 minutes
Cook Time: 14 minutes
Ingredients:

- ½ cup sliced onion
- 1 tablespoon sesame garlic-flavored oil
- 2cups shredded Bok-Choy
- 1/2 cups fresh bean sprouts
- 1 1/2 stalks celery, chopped
- 1 ½ teaspoons minced garlic
- 1/2 teaspoon stevia
- 1/2 cup chicken broth
- 1 tablespoon coconut aminos
- 1/2 tablespoon freshly minced ginger

- 1/2 teaspoon arrowroot
- 2 boneless chicken breasts, cooked and sliced thinly

How To:

1. Shred the cabbage with a knife.
2. Slice onion and increase your platter alongside the rotisserie chicken.
3. Add a dollop of mayonnaise on top and drizzle vegetable oil over the cabbage.
4. Season with sunflower seeds and pepper consistent with your taste.
5. Enjoy!

Nutrition (Per Serving)
Calories: 368
Fat: 18g
Net Carbohydrates: 8g
Protein: 42g
Fiber: 3g
Carbohydrates: 11g

Hearty Chicken Liver Stew
Serving: 2
Prep Time: 10 minutes
Cook Time: Nil
Ingredients:

- 10 ounces chicken livers
- 1-ounce onion, chopped
- 2 ounces sour cream
- 1 tablespoon olive oil
- Sunflower seeds to taste

How To:

1. Take a pan and place it over medium heat.
2. Add oil and let it heat up.
3. Add onions and fry until just browned.
4. Add livers and season with sunflower seeds.
5. Cook until livers are half cooked.
6. Transfer the combination to a stew pot.
7. Add soured cream and cook for 20 minutes.
8. Serve and enjoy!

Nutrition (Per Serving)

Calories: 146
Fat: 9g
Carbohydrates: 2g
Protein: 15g

Chicken Quesadilla

Serving: 2
Prep Time: 10 minutes
Cook Time: 35 minutes

Ingredients:

- ¼ cup ranch dressing
- ½ cup cheddar cheese, shredded
- 20 slices bacon, center-cut
- 2 cups grilled chicken, sliced

How To:

1. Re-heat your oven to 400 degrees F.
2. Line baking sheet using parchment paper.
3. Weave bacon into two rectangles and bake for half-hour .
4. Lay grilled chicken over bacon square, drizzling ranch dressing on top.
5. Sprinkle cheddar and top with another bacon square.
6. Bake for five minutes more.
7. Slice and serve.
8. Enjoy!

Nutrition (Per Serving)

Calories: 619
Fat: 35g
Carbohydrates: 2g
Protein: 79g

Mustard Chicken

Serving: 2
Prep Time: 10 minutes
Cook Time: 40 minutes

Ingredients:

- 2 chicken breasts
- 1/4 cup chicken broth
- 2 tablespoons mustard
- 1 1/2 tablespoons olive oil
- 1/2 teaspoon paprika
- 1/2 teaspoon chili powder

- 1/2 teaspoon garlic powder

How To:

1. Take alittle bowl and blend mustard, olive oil, paprika, chicken stock , garlic powder, chicken stock , and chili.
2. Add pigeon breast and marinate for half-hour .
3. Take a lined baking sheet and arrange the chicken.
4. Bake for 35 minutes at 375 degrees F.
5. Serve and enjoy!

Nutrition (Per Serving)
Calories: 531
Fat: 23g
Carbohydrates: 10g
Protein: 64g
Chicken and Carrot Stew
Serving: 4
Prep Time: 15 minutes
Cook Time: 6 hours
Ingredients:

- 4 boneless chicken breast, cubed
- 3 cups of carrots, peeled and cubed
- 1 cup onion, chopped
- 1 cup tomatoes, chopped
- 1 teaspoon of dried thyme
- 2 cups of chicken broth
- 2 garlic cloves, minced
- Sunflower seeds and pepper as needed

How To:

1. Add all of the listed ingredients to a Slow Cooker.
2. Stir and shut the lid.
3. Cook for six hours.
4. Serve hot and enjoy!

Nutrition (Per Serving)
Calories: 182
Fat: 3g
Carbohydrates: 10g
Protein: 39g
The Delish Turkey Wrap

Serving: 6
Prep Time: 10 minutes
Cook Time: 10 minutes
Ingredients:

- 1 ¼ pounds ground turkey, lean
- 4 green onions, minced
- 1 tablespoon olive oil
- 1 garlic clove, minced
- 2 teaspoons chili paste
- 8-ounce water chestnut, diced
- 3 tablespoons hoisin sauce
- 2 tablespoon coconut aminos
- 1 tablespoon rice vinegar
- 12 almond butter lettuce leaves
- 1/8 teaspoon sunflower seeds

How To:

1. Take a pan and place it over medium heat, add turkey and garlic to the pan.
2. Heat for six minutes until cooked.
3. Take a bowl and transfer turkey to the bowl.
4. Add onions and water chestnuts.
5. Stir in duck sauce , coconut aminos, vinegar and chili paste.
6. Toss well and transfer mix to lettuce leaves.
7. Serve and enjoy!

Nutrition (Per Serving)
Calories: 162
Fat: 4g
Net Carbohydrates: 7g
Protein: 23g
Almond butternut Chicken
Serving: 4
Prep Time: 15 minutes
Cook Time: 30 minutes
Ingredients:

- ½ pound Nitrate free bacon
- 6 chicken thighs, boneless and skinless
- 2-3 cups almond butternut squash, cubed
- Extra virgin olive oil
- Fresh chopped sage

- Sunflower seeds and pepper as needed

How To:

1. Prepare your oven by preheating it to 425 degrees F.
2. Take an outsized skillet and place it over medium-high heat, add bacon and fry until crispy.
3. Take a slice of bacon and place it on the side, crumble the bacon.
4. Add cubed almond butternut squash within the bacon grease and sauté, season with sunflower seeds and pepper.
5. Once the squash is tender, remove skillet and transfer to a plate.
6. Add copra oil to the skillet and add chicken thighs, cook for 10 minutes.
7. Season with sunflower seeds and pepper.
8. Remove skillet from stove and transfer to oven.
9. Bake for 12-15 minutes, top with the crumbled bacon and sage.
10. Enjoy!

Nutrition (Per Serving)
Calories: 323
Fat: 19g
Carbohydrates: 8g
Protein: 12g
Zucchini Zoodles with Chicken and Basil
Serving: 3
Prep Time: 10 minutes
Cook Time: 10 minutes
Ingredients:

- 2 chicken fillets, cubed
- 2 tablespoons ghee
- 1-pound tomatoes, diced
- ½ cup basil, chopped
- ¼ cup almond milk
- 1 garlic clove, peeled, minced
- 1 zucchini, shredded

How To:

1. Sauté cubed chicken in ghee until not pink.
2. Add tomatoes and season with sunflower seeds.
3. Simmer and reduce liquid.
4. Prepare your zucchini Zoodles by shredding zucchini during a kitchen appliance .

5. Add basil, garlic, coconut almond milk to the chicken and cook for a couple of minutes.
6. Add half the zucchini Zoodles to a bowl and top with creamy tomato basil chicken.
7. Enjoy!

Nutrition (Per Serving)
Calories: 540
Fat: 27g
Carbohydrates: 13g
Protein: 59g
Duck with Cucumber and Carrots
Serving: 8
Prep Time: 10 minutes
Cook Time: 40 minutes
Ingredients:

- 1 duck, cut up into medium pieces
- 1 chopped cucumber, chopped
- 1 tablespoon low sodium vegetable stock
- 2 carrots, chopped
- 2 cups of water
- Black pepper as needed
- 1-inch ginger piece, grated

How To:

1. Add duck pieces to your Instant Pot.
2. Add cucumber, stock, carrots, water, ginger, pepper and stir.
3. Lock up the lid and cook on low for 40 minutes.
4. Release the pressure naturally.
5. Serve and enjoy!

Nutrition (Per Serving)
Calories: 206
Fats: 7g
Carbs: 28g
Protein: 16g
Parmesan Baked Chicken
Serving: 2
Prep Time: 5 minutes
Cook Time: 20 minutes
Ingredients:

- 2 tablespoons ghee
- 2 boneless chicken breasts, skinless
- Pink sunflower seeds
- Freshly ground black pepper
- ½ cup mayonnaise, low fat
- ¼ cup parmesan cheese, grated
- 1 tablespoon dried Italian seasoning, low fat, low sodium
- ¼ cup crushed pork rinds

How To:

1. Preheat your oven to 425 degrees F.
2. Take an outsized baking dish and coat with ghee.
3. Pat chicken breasts dry and wrap with a towel.
4. Season with sunflower seeds and pepper.
5. Place in baking dish.
6. Take alittle bowl and add mayonnaise, parmesan cheese, Italian seasoning.
7. Slather mayo mix evenly over pigeon breast .
8. Sprinkle crushed pork rinds on top.
9. Bake for 20 minutes until topping is browned.
10. Serve and enjoy!

Nutrition (Per Serving)
Calories: 850
Fat: 67g
Carbohydrates: 2g
Protein: 60g

Buffalo Chicken Lettuce Wraps
Serving: 2
Prep Time: 35 minutes
Cook Time: 10 minutes

Ingredients:

- 3 chicken breasts, boneless and cubed
- 20 slices of almond butter lettuce leaves
- ¾ cup cherry tomatoes halved
- 1 avocado, chopped
- ¼ cup green onions, diced
- ½ cup ranch dressing
- ¾ cup hot sauce

How To:

1. Take a bowl and add chicken cubes and sauce , mix.
2. Place within the fridge and let it marinate for half-hour .
3. Preheat your oven to 400 degrees F.
4. Place coated chicken on a cookie pan and bake for 9 minutes.
5. Assemble lettuce serving cups with equal amounts of lettuce, green onions, tomatoes, ranch dressing, and cubed chicken.
6. Serve and enjoy!

Nutrition (Per Serving)
Calories: 106
Fat: 6g
Net Carbohydrates: 2g
Protein: 5g
Crazy Japanese Potato and Beef Croquettes
Serving: 10
Prep Time: 10 minute
Cook Time: 20 minutes
Ingredients:

- 3 medium russet potatoes, peeled and chopped
- 1 tablespoon almond butter
- 1 tablespoon vegetable oil
- 3 onions, diced
- ¾ pound ground beef
- 4 teaspoons light coconut aminos
- All-purpose flour for coating
- 2 eggs, beaten
- Panko bread crumbs for coating
- ½ cup oil, frying

How To:

1. Take a saucepan and place it over medium-high heat; add potatoes and sunflower seeds water, boil for 16 minutes.
2. Remove water and put potatoes in another bowl, add almond butter and mash the potatoes.
3. Take a frypan and place it over medium heat, add 1 tablespoon oil and let it heat up.
4. Add onions and fry until tender.
5. Add coconut aminos to beef to onions.
6. Keep frying until beef is browned.
7. Mix the meat with the potatoes evenly.
8. Take another frypan and place it over medium heat; add half a cup of oil.

9. Form croquettes using the potato mixture and coat them with flour, then eggs and eventually breadcrumbs.
10. Fry patties until golden on all sides.
11. Enjoy!

Nutrition (Per Serving)
Calories: 239
Fat: 4g
Carbohydrates: 20g
Protein: 10g
Spicy Chili Crackers
Serving: 30 crackers
Prep Time: 15 minutes
Cooking Time: 60 minutes
Ingredients:

- ¾ cup almond flour
- ¼ cup coconut four
- ¼ cup coconut flour
- ½ teaspoon paprika
- ½ teaspoon cumin
- 1 ½ teaspoons chili pepper spice
- 1 teaspoon onion powder
- ½ teaspoon sunflower seeds
- 1 whole egg
- ¼ cup unsalted almond butter

How To:

1. Preheat your oven to 350 degrees F.
2. Line a baking sheet with parchment paper and keep it on the side.
3. Add ingredients to your kitchen appliance and pulse until you've got a pleasant dough.
4. Divide dough into two equal parts.
5. Place one ball on a sheet of parchment paper and canopy with another sheet; roll it out.
6. dig crackers and repeat with the opposite ball.
7. Transfer the prepped dough to a baking tray and bake for 8-10 minutes.
8. Remove from oven and serve.
9. Enjoy!

Nutrition (Per Serving)
Total Carbs: 2.8g

Fiber: 1g
Protein: 1.6g
Fat: 4.1g
Golden Eggplant Fries
Serving: 8
Prep Time: 10 minutes
Cook Time: 15 minutes
Ingredients:

- 2 eggs
- 2 cups almond flour
- 2 tablespoons coconut oil, spray
- 2 eggplant, peeled and cut thinly Sunflower seeds and pepper

How To:

1. Preheat your oven to 400 degrees F.
2. Take a bowl and blend with sunflower seeds and black pepper.
3. Take another bowl and beat eggs until frothy.
4. Dip the eggplant pieces into the eggs.
5. Then coat them with the flour mixture.
6. Add another layer of flour and egg.
7. Then, take a baking sheet and grease with copra oil on top.
8. Bake for about quarter-hour .
9. Serve and enjoy!

Nutrition (Per Serving)
Calories: 212
Fat: 15.8g
Carbohydrates: 12.1g
Protein: 8.6g
Traditional Black Bean Chili
Serving: 4
Prep Time: 10 minutes
Cooking Time: 4 hours
Ingredients:

- 1 ½ cups red bell pepper, chopped
- 1 cup yellow onion, chopped
- 1 ½ cups mushrooms, sliced
- 1 tablespoon olive oil
- 1 tablespoon chili powder
- 2 garlic cloves, minced
- 1 teaspoon chipotle chili pepper, chopped

- ½ teaspoon cumin, ground
- 16 ounces canned black beans, drained and rinsed
- 2 tablespoons cilantro, chopped
- 1 cup tomatoes, chopped

How To:

1. Add red bell peppers, onion, dill, mushrooms, flavor, garlic, chili pepper, cumin, black beans, tomatoes to your Slow Cooker.
2. Stir well.
3. Place lid and cook on HIGH for 4 hours.
4. Sprinkle cilantro on top.
5. Serve and enjoy!

Nutrition (Per Serving)
Calories: 211
Fat: 3g
Carbohydrates: 22g
Protein: 5g
Very Wild Mushroom Pilaf
Serving: 4
Prep Time: 10 minutes
Cooking Time: 3 hours
Ingredients:

- 1 cup wild rice
- 2 garlic cloves, minced
- 6 green onions, chopped
- 2 tablespoons olive oil
- ½ pound baby Bella mushrooms
- 2 cups water

How To:

1. Add rice, garlic, onion, oil, mushrooms and water to your Slow Cooker.
2. Stir well until mixed.
3. Place lid and cook on LOW for 3 hours.
4. Stir pilaf and divide between serving platters.
5. Enjoy!

Nutrition (Per Serving)
Calories: 210
Fat: 7g

Carbohydrates: 16g
Protein: 4g
Green Palak Paneer
Serving: 4
Prep Time: 5 minutes
Cook Time: 10 minutes
Ingredients:

- 1-pound spinach
- 2 cups cubed paneer (vegan)
- 2 tablespoons coconut oil
- 1 teaspoon cumin
- 1 chopped up onion
- 1-2 teaspoons hot green chili minced up
- 1 teaspoon minced garlic
- 15 cashews
- 4 tablespoons almond milk
- 1 teaspoon Garam masala
- Flavored vinegar as needed

How To:

1. Add cashews and milk to a blender and blend well.
2. Set your pot to Sauté mode and add coconut oil; allow the oil to heat up.
3. Add cumin seeds, garlic, green chilies, ginger and sauté for 1 minute.
4. Add onion and sauté for two minutes.
5. Add chopped spinach, flavored vinegar and a cup of water.
6. Lock up the lid and cook on high for 10 minutes.
7. Quick-release the pressure.
8. Add ½ cup of water and blend to a paste.
9. Add cashew paste, paneer and Garam Masala and stir thoroughly.
10. Serve over hot rice!

Nutrition (Per Serving)
Calories: 367
Fat: 26g
Carbohydrates: 21g
Protein: 16g
Sporty Baby Carrots
Serving: 4
Prep Time: 5 minutes
Cook Time: 5 minutes
Ingredients:

- 1-pound baby carrots
- 1 cup water
- 1 tablespoon clarified ghee
- 1 tablespoon chopped up fresh mint leaves
- Sea flavored vinegar as needed

How To:

1. Place a steamer rack on top of your pot and add the carrots.
2. Add water .
3. Lock the lid and cook at high for two minutes.
4. Do a fast release.
5. Pass the carrots through a strainer and drain them.
6. Wipe the insert clean.
7. Return the insert to the pot and set the pot to Sauté mode.
8. Add drawn butter and permit it to melt.
9. Add mint and sauté for 30 seconds.
10. Add carrots to the insert and sauté well.
11. Remove them and sprinkle with little bit of flavored vinegar on top.
12. Enjoy!

Nutrition (Per Serving)
Calories: 131
Fat: 10g
Carbohydrates: 11g
Protein: 1g
Saucy Garlic Greens
Serving: 4
Prep Time: 5 minutes
Cook Time: 20 minutes
Ingredients:

- 1 bunch of leafy greens Sauce
- ½ cup cashews soaked in water for 10 minutes
- ¼ cup water
- 1 tablespoon lemon juice
- 1 teaspoon coconut aminos
- 1 clove peeled whole clove
- 1/8 teaspoon of flavored vinegar

How To:

1. Make the sauce by draining and discarding the soaking water from your cashews and add the cashews to a blender.

2. Add water , juice , flavored vinegar, coconut aminos, garlic.
3. Blitz until you've got a smooth cream and transfer to bowl.
4. Add ½ cup of water to the pot.
5. Place the steamer basket to the pot and add the greens within the basket.
6. Lock the lid and steam for 1 minute.
7. Quick-release the pressure.
8. Transfer the steamed greens to strainer and extract excess water.
9. Place the greens into a bowl .
10. Add lemon aioli and toss.
11. Enjoy!

Nutrition (Per Serving)
Calories: 77
Fat: 5g
Carbohydrates: 0g
Protein: 2g
Garden Salad
Serving: 6
Prep Time: 5 minutes
Cook Time: 20 minutes
Ingredients:

- 1 pound raw peanuts in shell
- 1 bay leaf
- 2 medium-sized chopped up tomatoes
- ½ cup diced up green pepper
- ½ cup diced up sweet onion
- ¼ cup finely diced hot pepper
- ¼ cup diced up celery
- 2 tablespoons olive oil
- ¾ teaspoon flavored vinegar
- ¼ teaspoon freshly ground black pepper

How To:

1. Boil your peanuts for 1 minute and rinse them.
2. The skin are going to be soft, so discard the skin.
3. Add 2 cups of water to the moment Pot.
4. Add herb and peanuts.
5. Lock the lid and cook on high for 20 minutes.
6. Drain the water.
7. Take an outsized bowl and add the peanuts, diced up vegetables.
8. Whisk in vegetable oil , juice , pepper in another bowl.

9. Pour the mixture over the salad and blend .
10. Enjoy!

Nutrition (Per Serving)
Calories: 140
Fat: 4g
Carbohydrates: 24g
Protein: 5g
Spicy Cabbage Dish
Serving: 4
Prep Time: 10 minutes
Cooking Time: 4 hours
Ingredients:

- 2 yellow onions, chopped
- 10 cups red cabbage, shredded
- 1 cup plums, pitted and chopped
- 1 teaspoon cinnamon powder
- 1 garlic clove, minced
- 1 teaspoon cumin seeds
- ¼ teaspoon cloves, ground
- 2 tablespoons red wine vinegar
- 1 teaspoon coriander seeds
- ½ cup water

How To:

1. Add cabbage, onion, plums, garlic, cumin, cinnamon, cloves, vinegar, coriander and water to your Slow Cooker.
2. Stir well.
3. Place lid and cook on LOW for 4 hours.
4. Divide between serving platters.
5. Enjoy!

Nutrition (Per Serving)
Calories: 197
Fat: 1g
Carbohydrates: 14g
Protein: 3g
Extreme Balsamic Chicken
Serving: 4
Prep Time: 10 minutes
Cook Time: 35 minutes
Ingredients:

- 3 boneless chicken breasts, skinless
- Sunflower seeds to taste
- ¼ cup almond flour
- 2/3 cups low-fat chicken broth
- 1 ½ teaspoons arrowroot
- ½ cup low sugar raspberry preserve
- 1 ½ tablespoons balsamic vinegar

How To:

1. Cut pigeon breast into bite-sized pieces and season them with seeds.
2. Dredge the chicken pieces in flour and shake off any excess.
3. Take a non-stick skillet and place it over medium heat.
4. Add chicken to the skillet and cook for quarter-hour , ensuring to show them half-way through.
5. Remove chicken and transfer to platter.
6. Add arrowroot, broth, raspberry preserve to the skillet and stir.
7. Stir in balsamic vinegar and reduce heat to low, stir-cook for a couple of minutes.
8. Transfer the chicken back to the sauce and cook for quarter-hour more.
9. Serve and enjoy!

Nutrition (Per Serving)
Calories: 546
Fat: 35g
Carbohydrates: 11g
Protein: 44g
Enjoyable Spinach and Bean Medley
Serving: 4
Prep Time: 10 minutes
Cooking Time: 4 hours
Ingredients:

- 5 carrots, sliced
- 1 ½ cups great northern beans, dried
- 2 garlic cloves, minced
- 1 yellow onion, chopped
- Pepper to taste
- ½ teaspoon oregano, dried
- 5 ounces baby spinach
- 4 ½ cups low sodium veggie stock
- 2 teaspoons lemon peel, grated

- 3 tablespoon lemon juice

How To:

1. Add beans, onion, carrots, garlic, oregano and stock to your Slow Cooker.
2. Stir well.
3. Place lid and cook on HIGH for 4 hours.
4. Add spinach, juice and lemon rind .
5. Stir and let it sit for five minutes.
6. Divide between serving platters and enjoy!

Nutrition (Per Serving)
Calories: 219
Fat: 8g
Carbohydrates: 14g
Protein: 8g
Tantalizing Cauliflower and Dill Mash
Serving: 6
Prep Time: 10 minutes
Cooking Time: 6 hours
Ingredients:

- 1 cauliflower head, florets separated
- 1/3 cup dill, chopped
- 6 garlic cloves
- 2 tablespoons olive oil
- Pinch of black pepper

How To:

1. Add cauliflower to Slow Cooker.
2. Add dill, garlic and water to hide them. 3. Place lid and cook on HIGH for five hours.
3. Drain the flowers.
4. Season with pepper and add oil, mash using potato masher.
5. Whisk and serve.
6. Enjoy!

Nutrition (Per Serving)
Calories: 207
Fat: 4g
Carbohydrates: 14g
Protein: 3g

Secret Asian Green Beans
Serving: 10
Prep Time: 10 minutes
Cooking Time: 2 hours
Ingredients:

- 16 cups green beans, halved
- 3 tablespoons olive oil
- ¼ cup tomato sauce, salt-free
- ½ cup coconut sugar
- ¾ teaspoon low sodium soy sauce
- Pinch of pepper

How To:

1. Add green beans, coconut sugar, pepper spaghetti sauce , soy sauce, oil to your Slow Cooker.
2. Stir well.
3. Place lid and cook on LOW for 3 hours.
4. Divide between serving platters and serve.
5. Enjoy!

Nutrition (Per Serving)
Calories: 200
Fat: 4g
Carbohydrates: 12g
Protein: 3g

Excellent Acorn Mix
Serving: 10
Prep Time: 10 minutes
Cooking Time: 7 hours
Ingredients:

- 2 acorn squash, peeled and cut into wedges
- 16 ounces cranberry sauce, unsweetened
- ¼ teaspoon cinnamon powder Pepper to taste

How To:

1. Add acorn wedges to your Slow Cooker.
2. Add condiment , cinnamon, raisins and pepper.
3. Stir.
4. Place lid and cook on LOW for 7 hours.
5. Serve and enjoy!

Nutrition (Per Serving)
Calories: 200
Fat: 3g
Carbohydrates: 15g
Protein: 2g

Crunchy Almond Chocolate Bars
Serving: 12
Prep Time: 10 minutes
Cooking Time: 2 hours 30 minutes

Ingredients:

- 1 egg white
- ¼ cup coconut oil, melted
- 1 cup coconut sugar
- ½ teaspoon vanilla extract
- 1 teaspoon baking powder
- 1 ½ cups almond meal
- ½ cup dark chocolate chips

How To:

1. Take a bowl and add sugar, oil, vanilla , egg white, almond flour, leaven and blend it well.
2. Fold in chocolate chips and stir.
3. Line Slow Cooker with parchment paper.
4. Grease.
5. Add the cookie mix and continue bottom.
6. Place lid and cook on LOW for two hours half-hour .
7. Take cooking utensil out and let it cool.
8. Cut in bars and enjoy!

Nutrition (Per Serving)
Calories: 200
Fat: 2g
Carbohydrates: 13g
Protein: 6g

Lettuce and Chicken Platter
Serving: 6
Prep Time: 10 minutes
Cook Time: nil

Ingredients:

- 2 cups chicken, cooked and coarsely chopped
- ½ head ice berg lettuce, sliced and chopped

- 1 celery rib, chopped
- 1 medium apple, cut
- ½ red bell pepper, deseeded and chopped
- 6-7 green olives, pitted and halved
- 1 red onion, chopped

For dressing

- 1 tablespoon raw honey
- 2 tablespoons lemon juice
- Salt and pepper to taste

How To:

1. Cut the vegetables and transfer them to your Salad Bowl.
2. Add olives.
3. Chop the cooked chicken and transfer to your Salad bowl.
4. Prepare dressing by mixing the ingredients listed under Dressing.
5. Pour the dressing into the Salad bowl.
6. Toss and enjoy!

Nutrition (Per Serving)
Calories: 296
Fat: 21g
Carbohydrates: 9g
Protein: 18g
Greek Lemon Chicken Bowl
Serving: 6
Prep Time: 10 minutes
Cook Time: 15 minutes
Ingredients:

- 2 cups chicken, cooked and chopped
- 2 cans chicken broth, fat free
- 2 medium carrots, chopped
- ¼ teaspoon pepper
- 2 tablespoons parsley, snipped
- ¼ cup lemon juice
- 1 can cream chicken soup, fat free, low sodium
- ½ cup onion, chopped
- 1 garlic clove, minced

How To:

1. Take a pot and add all the ingredients except parsley into it.
2. Season with salt and pepper.
3. Bring the combination to a overboil medium-high heat.
4. Reduce the warmth and simmer for quarter-hour .
5. Garnish with parsley.
6. Serve hot and enjoy!

Nutrition (Per Serving)
Calories: 520
Fat: 33g
Carbohydrates: 31g
Protein: 30g

Chilled Chicken, Artichoke and Zucchini Platter
Serving: 4
Prep Time: 10 minutes
Cook Time: 5 minutes
Ingredients:

- 2 medium chicken breasts, cooked and cut into 1-inch cubes
- ¼ cup extra virgin olive oil
- 2 cups artichoke hearts, drained and roughly chopped
- 3 large zucchini, diced/cut into small rounds
- 1 can (15 ounce) chickpeas
- 1 cup Kalamata olives
- ½ teaspoon Fresh ground black pepper
- ½ teaspoon Italian seasoning
- ¼ cup parmesan, grated

How To:

1. Take an outsized skillet and place it over medium heat, heat up vegetable oil .
2. Add zucchini and sauté for five minutes, season with salt and pepper.
3. Remove from heat and add all the listed ingredients to the skillet.
4. Stir until combined.
5. Transfer to glass container and store.
6. Serve and enjoy!

Nutrition (Per Serving)
Calories: 457
Fat: 22g
Carbohydrates: 30g
Protein: 24g

Chicken and Carrot Stew

Serving: 6
Prep Time: 15 minutes
Cook Time: 6 hours

Ingredients:

- 4 chicken breasts, boneless and cubed
- 2 cups chicken broth
- 1 cup tomatoes, chopped
- 3 cups carrots, peeled and cubed
- 1 teaspoon thyme dried
- 1 cup onion, chopped
- 2 garlic clove, minced
- Pepper to taste

How To:

1. Add all the ingredients to the Slow Cooker.
2. Stir and shut the lid.
3. Cook for six hours.
4. Serve hot and enjoy!

Nutrition (Per Serving)

Calories: 182
Fat: 4g
Carbohydrates: 10g
Protein: 39g

Tasty Spinach Pie

Serving: 2
Prep Time: 10 minutes
Cooking Time: 4 hours

Ingredients:

- 10 ounces spinach
- 2 cups baby Bella mushrooms, chopped
- 1 red bell pepper, chopped
- 1 ½ cups low-fat cheese, shredded
- 8 whole eggs
- 1 cup coconut cream
- 2 tablespoons chives, chopped
- Pinch of pepper
- ½ cup almond flour
- ¼ teaspoon baking soda

How To:

1. Take a bowl and add eggs, coconut milk , chives, pepper and whisk well.
2. Add almond flour, bicarbonate of soda , cheese, mushrooms bell pepper, spinach and toss well.
3. Grease your cooker and transfer mix to the Slow Cooker.
4. Place lid and cook on LOW for 4 hours.
5. Slice and enjoy!

Nutrition (Per Serving)
Calories: 201
Fat: 6g
Carbohydrates: 8g
Protein: 5g
Mesmerizing Carrot and Pineapple Mix
Serving: 10
Prep Time: 10 minutes
Cooking Time: 6 hours
Ingredients:

- 1 cup raisins 6 cups water
- 23 ounces natural applesauce
- 2 tablespoons stevia
- 2 tablespoons cinnamon powder
- 14 ounces carrots, shredded
- 8 ounces canned pineapple, crushed
- 1 tablespoon pumpkin pie spice

How To:

1. Add carrots, applesauce, raisins, stevia, cinnamon, pineapple, pie spice to your Slow Cooker and gently stir.
2. Place lid and cook on LOW for six hours .
3. Serve and enjoy!

Nutrition (Per Serving)
Calories: 179
Fat: 5g
Carbohydrates: 15g
Protein: 4g
Blackberry Chicken Wings
Serving: 4
Prep Time: 35 minutes

Cook Time: 50minutes
Ingredients:

- 3 pounds chicken wings, about 20 pieces
- ½ cup blackberry chipotle jam
- Sunflower seeds and pepper to taste
- ½ cup water

How To:

1. Add water and jam to a bowl and blend well.
2. Place chicken wings during a zip bag and add two-thirds of the marinade.
3. Season with sunflower seeds and pepper.
4. Let it marinate for half-hour .
5. Pre-heat your oven to 400 degrees F.
6. Prepare a baking sheet and wire rack, place chicken wings in wire rack and bake for quarter-hour .
7. Brush remaining marinade and bake for half-hour more.
8. Enjoy!

Nutrition (Per Serving)
Calories: 502
Fat: 39g
Carbohydrates: 01.8g
Protein: 34g
Generous Lemon Dredged Broccoli
Serving: 4
Prep Time: 10 minutes
Cook Time: 15 minutes
Ingredients:

- 2 heads broccoli, separated into florets
- 2 teaspoons extra virgin olive oil
- 1 teaspoon sunflower seeds
- ½ teaspoon pepper
- 1 garlic clove, minced
- ½ teaspoon lemon juice

How To:

1. Pre-heat your oven to a temperature of 400 degrees F.
2. Take an outsized sized bowl and add broccoli florets with some extra virgin vegetable oil , pepper, sea sunflower seeds and garlic.

3. Spread the broccoli call at one even layer on a fine baking sheet.
4. Bake in your pre-heated oven for about 15-20 minutes until the florets are soft enough to be pierced with a fork.
5. Squeeze juice over them generously before serving.
6. Enjoy!

Nutrition (Per Serving)
Calories: 49
Fat: 2g
Carbohydrates: 4g
Protein: 3g
Tantalizing Almond butter Beans
Serving: 4
Prep Time: 5 minutes
Cook Time: 12 minutes
Ingredients:

- 2 garlic cloves, minced
- Red pepper flakes to taste
- Sunflower seeds to taste
- 2 tablespoons clarified butter
- 4 cups green beans, trimmed

How To:

1. Bring a pot of water to boil, with added seeds for taste.
2. Once the water starts to boil, add beans and cook for 3 minutes.
3. Take a bowl of drinking water and drain beans, plunge them into the drinking water .
4. Once cooled, keep them on the side.
5. Take a medium skillet and place it over medium heat, add ghee and melt.
6. Add red pepper, sunflower seeds, garlic.
7. Cook for 1 minute.
8. Add beans and toss until coated well, cook for 3 minutes.
9. Serve and enjoy!

Nutrition (Per Serving)
Calories: 93
Fat: 8g
Carbohydrates: 4g
Protein: 2g
Healthy Chicken Cream Salad
Serving: 3

Prep Time: 5 minutes
Cook Time: 50 minutes

Ingredients:

- 2 chicken breasts
- 1 ½ cups low fat cream
- 3 ounces celery
- 2 ounce green pepper, chopped
- ½ ounce green onion, chopped
- ½ cup low fat mayo
- 3 hard-boiled eggs, chopped

How To:

1. Pre-heat your oven to 350 degrees F.
2. Take a baking sheet and place chicken, cover with cream.
3. Bake for 30-40 minutes.
4. Take a bowl and blend within the chopped celery, peppers, onions.
5. Chop the baked chicken into bite-sized portions.
6. Peel and chop the hard boiled eggs.
7. Take an outsized salad bowl and blend in eggs, veggies and chicken.
8. Toss well and serve.
9. Enjoy!

Nutrition (Per Serving)
Calories: 415
Fat: 24g
Carbohydrates: 4g
Protein: 40g

Generously Smothered Pork Chops
Serving: 4
Prep Time: 10 minutes
Cook Time: 30 minutes

Ingredients:

- 4 pork chops, bone-in
- 2 tablespoons of olive oil
- ¼ cup vegetable broth
- ½ pound Yukon gold potatoes, peeled and chopped
- 1 large onion, sliced
- 2 garlic cloves, minced
- 2 teaspoon rubbed sage
- 1 teaspoon thyme, ground
- Pepper as needed

How To:

1. Pre-heat your oven to 350 degrees F.
2. Take an outsized sized skillet and place it over medium heat.
3. Add a tablespoon of oil and permit the oil to heat up.
4. Add pork chops and cook them for 4-5 minutes per side until browned.
5. Transfer chops to a baking dish.
6. Pour broth over the chops.
7. Add remaining oil to the pan and sauté potatoes, onion, garlic for 3-4 minutes.
8. Take an outsized bowl and add potatoes, garlic, onion, thyme, sage, pepper.
9. Transfer this mixture to the baking dish (wish pork).
10. Bake for 20-30 minutes.
11. Serve and enjoy!

Nutrition (Per Serving)
Calorie: 261
Fat: 10g
Carbohydrates: 1.3g
Protein: 2g

Crazy Lamb Salad
Serving: 4
Prep Time: 10 minutes
Cook Time: 35 minutes

Ingredients:

- 1 tablespoon olive oil
- 3 pound leg of lamb, bone removed, leg butterflied
- Salt and pepper to taste
- 1 teaspoon cumin
- Pinch of dried thyme
- 2 garlic cloves, peeled and minced

For Salad

- 4 ounces feta cheese, crumbled
- ½ cup pecans
- 2 cups spinach
- 1 ½ tablespoons lemon juice
- ¼ cup olive oil
- 1 cup fresh mint, chopped

How To:

1. Rub lamb with salt and pepper, 1 tablespoon oil, thyme, cumin, minced garlic.
2. Pre-heat your grill to medium-high and transfer lamb.
3. Cook for 40 minutes, ensuring to flip it once.
4. Take a lined baking sheet and spread the pecans.
5. Toast in oven for 10 minutes at 350 degree F.
6. Transfer grilled lamb to chopping board and let it cool.
7. Slice.
8. Take a salad bowl and add spinach, 1 cup mint, feta cheese, ¼ cup vegetable oil , juice , toasted pecans, salt, pepper and toss well.
9. Add lamb slices on top.
10. Serve and enjoy!

Nutrition (Per Serving)
Calories: 334
Fat: 33g
Carbohydrates: 5g
Protein: 7g
Hearty Roasted Cauliflower
Serving: 8
Prep Time: 5 minutes
Cook Time: 30 minutes
Ingredients:

- 1 large cauliflower head
- 2 tablespoons melted coconut oil
- 2 tablespoons fresh thyme
- 1 teaspoon Celtic sea sunflower seeds
- 1 teaspoon fresh ground pepper
- 1 head roasted garlic
- 2 tablespoons fresh thyme for garnish

How To:

1. Pre-heat your oven to 425 degrees F.
2. Rinse cauliflower and trim, core and sliced.
3. Lay cauliflower evenly on rimmed baking tray.
4. Drizzle copra oil evenly over cauliflower, sprinkle thyme leaves .
5. Season with pinch of sunflower seeds and pepper.
6. Squeeze roasted garlic.
7. Roast cauliflower until slightly caramelized for about half-hour , ensuring to show once.

8. Garnish with fresh thyme leaves.
9. Enjoy!

Nutrition (Per Serving)
Calories: 129
Fat: 11g
Carbohydrates: 6g
Protein: 7g

Cool Cabbage Fried Beef
Serving: 4
Prep Time: 5 minutes
Cook Time: 15 minutes

Ingredients:

- 1-pound beef, ground and lean
- ½ pound bacon
- 1 onion
- 1 garlic clove, minced
- ½ head cabbage
- pepper to taste

How To:

1. Take skillet and place it over medium heat.
2. Add chopped bacon, beef and onion until slightly browned.
3. Transfer to a bowl and keep it covered.
4. Add minced garlic and cabbage to the skillet and cook until slightly browned.
5. Return the bottom beef mix to the skillet and simmer for 3-5 minutes over low heat.
6. Serve and enjoy!

Nutrition (Per Serving)
Calories: 360
Fat: 22g
Net Carbohydrates: 5g
Protein: 34g

Fennel and Figs Lamb
Serving: 2
Prep Time: 10 minutes
Cook Time: 40 minutes

Ingredients:

- 6 ounces lamb racks 1 fennel bulbs, sliced pepper to taste

- 1 tablespoon olive oil
- 2 figs, cut in half
- 1/8 cup apple cider vinegar
- 1/2 tablespoon swerve

How To:

1. Take a bowl and add fennel, figs, vinegar, swerve, oil and toss.
2. Transfer to baking dish.
3. Season with sunflower seeds and pepper.
4. Bake for quarter-hour at 400 degrees F.
5. Season lamb with sunflower seeds and pepper and transfer to a heated pan over medium-high heat.
6. Cook for a couple of minutes.
7. Add lamb to the baking dish with fennel and bake for 20 minutes.
8. Divide between plates and serve.
9. Enjoy!

Nutrition (Per Serving)
Calories: 230
Fat: 3g
Carbohydrates: 5g
Protein: 10g
Black Berry Chicken Wings
Serving: 4
Prep Time: 35 minutes
Cook Time: 50minutes
Ingredients:

- 3 pounds chicken wings, about 20 pieces
- ½ cup blackberry chipotle jam
- Pepper to taste
- ½ cup water

How To:

1. Add water and jam to a bowl and blend well.
2. Place chicken wings during a zip bag and add two-thirds of marinade.
3. Season with pepper.
4. Let it marinate for half-hour .
5. Pre-heat your oven to 400 degrees F.
6. Prepare a baking sheet and wire rack, place chicken wings in wire rack and bake for quarter-hour .

7. Brush remaining marinade and bake for half-hour more.
8. Enjoy!

Nutrition (Per Serving)
Calories: 502
Fat: 39g
Carbohydrates: 01.8g
Protein: 34g
Mushroom and Olive "Mediterranean" Steak
Serving: 2
Prep Time: 10 minutes
Cook Time: 14 minutes
Ingredients:

- 1/2-pound boneless beef sirloin steak, ¾ inch thick, cut into 4 pieces
- 1/2 large red onion, chopped
- 1/2 cup mushrooms
- 2 garlic cloves, thinly sliced
- 2 tablespoons olive oil
- 1/4 cup green olives, coarsely chopped
- 1/2 cup parsley leaves, finely cut

How To:
Take an outsized sized skillet and place it over medium-high heat.

1. Add oil and let it heat up.
2. Add beef and cook until each side are browned, remove beef and drain fat.
3. Add the remainder of the oil to the skillet and warmth .
4. Add onions, garlic and cook for 2-3 minutes.
5. Stir well.
6. Add mushrooms, olives and cook until the mushrooms are thoroughly done.
7. Return the meat to the skillet and reduce heat to medium.
8. Cook for 3-4 minutes (covered).
9. Stir in parsley.
10. Serve and enjoy!

Nutrition (Per Serving)
Calories: 386
Fat: 30g
Carbohydrates: 11g
Protein: 21g
Hearty Chicken Fried Rice

Serving: 4
Prep Time: 10 minutes
Cook Time: 12 minutes

Ingredients:

- 1 teaspoon olive oil
- 4 large egg whites
- 1 onion, chopped
- 2 garlic cloves, minced
- 12 ounces skinless chicken breasts, boneless, cut into ½ inch cubes
- ½ cup carrots, chopped
- ½ cup frozen green peas
- 2 cups long grain brown rice, cooked
- 3 tablespoons soy sauce, low sodium

How To:

1. Coat skillet with oil, place it over medium-high heat.
2. Add egg whites and cook until scrambled .
3. Sauté onion, garlic and chicken breasts for six minutes.
4. Add carrots, peas and keep cooking for 3 minutes.
5. Stir in rice, season with soy .
6. Add cooked egg whites, stir for 3 minutes.
7. Enjoy!

Nutrition (Per Serving)
Calories: 353
Fat: 11g
Carbohydrates: 30g
Protein: 23g

Veggie Quesadillas with Cilantro Yogurt Dip
Ingredients

- 1 cup beans, black or pinto
- 2 Tablespoons cilantro, chopped
- ½ bell pepper, finely chopped
- ½ cup corn kernels
- 1 cup low-fat shredded cheese
- Six soft corn tortillas
- One medium carrot, shredded
- ½ jalapeno pepper, finely minced (optional)
- CILANTRO YOGURT DIP
- 1 cup plain nonfat yogurt
- 2 Tablespoons cilantro, finely chopped

- Juice from ½ of a lime

Instructions

1. Preheat large skillet over low heat.
2. Line up three tortillas. Spread cheese, corn, beans, cilantro, shredded carrots, and peppers over the tortillas.
3. Cover all sides with a 2nd tortilla.
4. Place a tortilla on a dry plate and warmth until cheese is melted and tortilla is slightly golden after 3 minutes.
5. Flip and cook another side until golden, about 1 minute.
6. Inside a small bowl, mix the nonfat yogurt, cilantro, and juice.
7. Cut each quesadilla into four wedges (12 wedges total) and serve three wedges per person with about ¼ cup of the dip.
8. Refrigerate leftovers within 2 hours.

Yogurt with Almonds & Honey
Ingredients

- Non-fat greek yoghurt-Nonfat, plain-16 oz-453 grams
- Almonds-Nuts, raw-1/4 cup, whole-35.8 grams
- Honey-2 tsp-14.1 grams

Directions
Rough-chop almonds and blend into yogurt and honey. Enjoy!
Nutrition
Calories 517 Carbs 36g Fat 20g Protein 54g Fiber 5g Net carbs 31g Sodium 164mg Cholesterol 23mg
Quick Buffalo Chicken Salad
Ingredients

- Pepper or hot sauce-Ready-to-serve-4 tbsp-57.6 grams
- Canned chicken-No broth-1 cup-205 grams
- Spinach-Raw-2 cup-60 grams
- Tomatoes-Green, raw-Two medium-246 grams

Directions
Mix hot sauce with chicken. Spread spinach and tomatoes on the top. Toss together and enjoy it!
Nutrition
Calorie 456 Carbs 18g Fat 18g Protein 57g Fiber 4g Net carbs 13g Sodium 2590mg Cholesterol 103mg
All American Tuna
Ingredients

- Tuna-Fish, light, canned in water, drained solids-Two can-330 grams
- Light mayonnaise-Salad dressing, light-2 tbsp-30 grams
- Celery-Cooked, boiled, drained, without a salt-1/4 cup, diced-37.5 grams
- Pickles-Cucumber, dill or kosher dill-One large (4" long)-135 grams
- Wheat bread-Two slice-50 grams

Directions

1. Mix all ingredients in a bowl.
2. Serve with bread.

Nutrition
Calories 512 Carbs 32g Fat 12g Protein 71g Fiber 4g Net carbs 28g Sodium 2443mg Cholesterol 124mg

Pimento Cheese Sandwich
Ingredients

- Pimento cheese-Pasteurized process-2 oz-56.7 grams
- Multi-grain bread-Four slices regular-104 grams

Directions

1. Spread the pimento cheese over the bread.
2. Then, a slice of bread to form a sandwich. Enjoy!

Nutrition
Calories 488 Carbs 46g Fat 22g Protein 26g Fiber 8g Net carbs 38g Sodium 915mg Cholesterol 53mg

Coconut Oil Fat Bombs
Ingredients

- Coconut oil-1 1/2 tbsp-20.8 grams
- Cocoa-Dry powder, unsweetened-3/4 tbsp-4.1 grams
- Honey-5/16 tsp-2 grams
- Salt-Table-1/8 tsp-0.57 grams

Directions

1. Mix all the ingredients during a processor until the mixture is smooth and creamy.
2. Pour into small-sized cube trays or silicone moulds and freeze.
3. Once frozen, pop the copra oil fat bombs out of the pictures and store them during a freezer zip-top bag or jar. Enjoy!

Nutrition
Calories 194 Carbs 4g Fat 21g Protein 1g Fiber 2g Net carbs 3g Sodium 222mg Cholesterol 0mg

Apricot Jam and Almond Butter Sandwich
Ingredients

- Multi-grain bread-Two slices regular-52 grams
- Jams and preserves-1 tbsp-20 grams
- Almond butter-Nuts, every day, without salt, added-1 tbsp-16 grams

Directions

1. Toast the bread optionally.
2. Spread almond butter on one side and jam on the other side.

Nutrition
Calories 292 Carbs 39g Fat 11g Protein 10g Fiber 6g Net carbs 34g Sodium 206mg Cholesterol 0mg

Peanut Butter and Honey Toast
Ingredients

- Multi-grain bread-Two slices regular-52 grams
- Peanut butter-Smooth style, without salt-3 tbsp-48 grams
- Honey-2 tbsp-42 grams

Directions

1. Toast the bread, and it is optionally.
2. Spread peanut butter on the bread and sprinkle with honey. Enjoy!

Nutrition
Calories 553 Carbs 68g Fat 27g Protein 18g Fiber 6g Net carbs 62g Sodium 208mg
Cholesterol 0mg

Cucumber & Hummus
Ingredients

- Hummus-Commercial-1/4 cup-61.5 grams
- Cucumber-With peel, raw-1 cup slices-104 grams

Directions
Cut the cucumber into round slices and eat with hummus.
Nutrition
Calories 118

Carbs13g
Fat6g
Protein6g
Fiber4g
Net carbs8g

Carrot and Hummus Snack

Ingredients

- Hummus-Commercial-2 tbsp-30 grams
- Baby carrots-Baby, raw-1 cup-246 grams

Directions

Dip carrots into hummus and enjoy!

Nutrition

Calories136Carbs25gFat3gProtein4gFiber9gNet   carbs16gSodium306mgC-holesterol0mg

Yogurt with Walnuts & Honey

Ingredients

- Walnuts-Nuts, black, dried-1/4 cup, chopped-31.3 grams
- Non-fat greek yoghurt-Nonfat, plain-480cup-480 grams
- Honey-2 tsp-14.1 gram

Directions

1. Rough-chop walnuts and mix into yogurt.
2. Top with honey and enjoy!

Nutrition

Calories520Carbs32gFat20gProtein56gFiber2gNet   carbs30gSodium174mg-Cholesterol24mg

Simple Caprese Sandwich

Ingredients

- Sourdough bread, French or Vienna, Two slices, 192 grams
- Mozzarella cheese
- Whole milk 2 oz 56.7 grams
- Tomatoes - Red, ripe, raw, year-round average
- Four slices, medium (1/4" thick)

Instructions

Cut a large slice of sourdough in half (or use two small slices). Top one slice with 1oz of sliced mozzarella and then two slices of tomatoes. The flavor is mild, so season with salt pepper if desired.

Nutrition
Calories707Carbs104gFat17gProtein34gFiber5gNet   carbs99gSodi-
um1515mgCholesterol45mg

Cottage Cheese Honey Toast

Ingredients

- Whole-wheat bread-Commercially prepared-Two slice-56 grams
- Cottage cheese- 1% milkfat-1 cup, (not packed)-226 grams
- Honey-2 tbsp-42 grams

Directions
Toast bread to your liking. Spread with cottage cheese and drizzle with
honey. Enjoy!

Nutrition
Calories432Carbs65gFat4gProtein35gFiber3gNet carbs61gSodium1174mgC-
holesterol9mg

Pimento Cheese Sandwich

Ingredients

- Pimento cheese-Pasteurized process-2 oz-56.7 grams
- Multi-grain bread-Four slices regular-104 grams

Directions

1. Spread the pimento cheese on each side of bread. And then on the
   other slice of bread to form a sandwich. Enjoy!

Nutrition
Calories488Carbs46gFat22gProtein26gFiber8gNet   carbs38gSodium915mg-
Cholesterol53mg

Tomato Salad

Ingredients

- Vinegar-Cider-2 2/3 tbsp-39.4 grams
- Cucumber-Peeled, raw-Two medium-402 grams
- Onions-Raw-1/2 large-75 grams
- Tomatoes-Red, ripe, fresh, year-round average
- Three medium whole (2-3/5" dia)-369 grams
- Water-Plain, clean water-1/2 cup-118 grams

Directions
Peel and slice cucumbers into coins. Cut tomatoes into pieces. Dice red
onion. Add vinegar and water and mix well.

Nutrition

Calories153Carbs31gFat1gProtein6gFiber9gNet carbs22gSodium32mgCholesterol0mg

Tomato and Cheese Wrap
Ingredients

- Tortillas-2 tortilla -92 grams
- mayonnaise-like dressing-Regular, with salt-2 tbsp-29.4 grams
- Tomatoes-Two medium whole -246 grams
- Lettuce-2 cup shredded-144 grams
- Cheddar cheese-2 oz-56.7 grams

Directions

1. Lightly spread mayo on tortilla shell.
2. Cut tomatoes however you like them.
3. Layer ingredients, spreading them over the tortilla.
4. Tuck up about an inch the side of the shell you've decided is the bottom and roll up the wrap. Enjoy!

Nutrition
Calories638Carbs66gFat32gProtein25gFiber7gNet carbs59gSodium1236mgCholesterol63mg

Peanut butter yogurt
Ingredients

- Nonfat greek yogurt-1 cup-240 grams
- Peanut butter-2 tbsp-32 grams
- Vanilla extract-1 tsp-2.2 grams

Directions
Combine ingredients and enjoy it!

Nutrition
Calories345Carbs16gFat17gProtein32gFiber2gNet carbs15gSodium223mgCholesterol12mg

Peanut Butter & Carrots
Ingredients

- Peanut butter-4 tbsp-64 grams
- Carrots-2 cup chopped-256 grams

Directions
Spread peanut butter on carrots and enjoy!
Nutrition

Calories482Carbs38gFat33gProtein18gFiber12gNet   carbs26gSodium188mg-Cholesterol0mg

Cucumber Tomato Salad with Tuna
Ingredients

- Tomatoes-Two medium whole -246 grams
- Lettuce-1 cup shredded-36 grams
- Cucumber-With peel, raw-One cucumber-301 grams
- Tuna-One can-165 grams

Directions

1. Chop vegetables and lettuce.
2. Toss together with the tuna and enjoy it!

Nutrition
Calories237Carbs22gFat2gProtein37gFiber5gNet   carbs17gSodium436mgC-holesterol59mg

Peanut butter and Jelly
Ingredients

- Multi-grain bread-Four slices regular-104 grams
- Butter-Unsalted-2 tsp-9.5 grams
- Peanut butter-Smooth style, without salt-3 tbsp-48 grams
- Jams and preserves-2 tbsp-40 grams

Directions

1. Toast the bread, and it's optionally. Drizzle1/2 teaspoon of butter on all sides of the bread.
2. Spread butter on one side and jam on another side.

Nutrition
Calories742Carbs83gFat37gProtein25gFiber11gNet   carbs73gSodium418mg-Cholesterol20mg

Chicken Scampi Pasta
Ingredients

- 1 pound of thinly-sliced chicken cutlets, cut into 1/2-inch-thick strips
- Three tablespoons olive oil
- Eight tablespoons unsalted butter, cubed
- Six cloves garlic, sliced
- 1/2 teaspoon crushed red pepper flakes

- 1/2 cup dry white wine
- 12 ounces angel hair pasta
- One teaspoon lemon zest plus the juice of 1 large lemon
- 1/2 cup freshly grated Parmesan
- 1/2 cup chopped fresh Italian parsley

Directions

1. Take a huge pot of salted water to a boil for the pasta. Sprinkle the chook with a couple of salts. Heat a huge skillet over medium-high warmth until hot, then upload the oil. Working in 2 batches, brown the chook until golden however not cooked through, 2 to a couple of minutes keep with batch. Remove the chicken to a plate.
2. Melt four tablespoons of the butter within the skillet. Add the garlic and crimson pepper flakes and cook dinner until the garlic begins to show golden at the sides , 30 seconds to 1 minute. Add the wine, deliver to a simmer, and cook dinner till reduced by using half, approximately 2 minutes. Remove from the heat .
3. Meanwhile, cook dinner the pasta till very hard , reserving 1 cup of the pasta water. Add the pasta and 3/four cup pasta water to the skillet alongside the hen, lemon peel and juice, and therefore the last four tablespoons butter. Return the skillet to medium-low warmness and gently stir the pasta until the butter is melted, including the last word 1/four pasta water if the pasta appears too dry. Remove the skillet from the heat, sprinkle with the cheese and parsley and toss before serving.

Chapter Twelve

DINNER RECIPES

Zucchini Pasta with Pesto Sauce
Nutritional Facts

servings per container

5

Prep Total

10 min

Serving Size 2/3 cup (20g)

AMOUNT PER SERVING

Calories

100

% DAILY VALUE

Total Fat 8g

12%

Saturated Fat 1g

2%

Trans Fat 0g

20%

Cholesterol

2%

Sodium 10mg

7%
Total Carbohydrate 7g
2%
Dietary Fiber 2g
14%
Total Sugar 1g
01.20%
Protein 3g

Vitamin C 2mcg
10%
Calcium 240mg
1%
Iron 2mg
2%
Potassium 25mg
6%
Ingredients

- 1 to 2 medium zucchini (make noodles with a mandoline or Spiralizer)
- 1/2 teaspoon of salt
- For Pesto
- soaked 1/4 cup cashews
- soaked 1/4 cup pine nuts
- 1/2 cup spinach
- 1/2 cup peas you can make it fresh or frozen one
- 1/4 cup broccoli
- 1/4 cup basil leaves
- 1/2 avocado
- 1 or 2 tablespoons original olive oil
- 2 tablespoons nutritional yeast
- 1/2 teaspoon salt
- Pinch black pepper

Instructions:

1. Place zucchini noodles in a strainer over a clean bowl
2. Include 1/2 teaspoon of salt & let it set while preparing the pesto sauce
3. Mix all the ingredients for the pesto sauce
4. Extract excess water from zucchini noodles & place them in a clean bowl

5. Pour the sauce on top & garnish with some basil leaves & pine nut

Balsamic BBQ Seitan And Tempeh Ribs
Nutritional Facts
servings per container
4
Prep Total
10 min
Serving Size 2/3 cup (56g)

AMOUNT PER SERVING
Calories
100

% DAILY VALUE
Total Fat 7g
1%
Saturated Fat 1g
2%
Trans Fat 0g
20%
Cholesterol
2%
Sodium 160mg
7%
Total Carbohydrate 37g
2%
Dietary Fiber 2g
1%
Total Sugar 2g
01.20%
Protein 14g

Vitamin C 1mcg
10%
Calcium 450mg
1%
Iron 2mg
2%
Potassium 35mg
7%

Ingredients
For the spice rub
Minced ¼ cup fresh parsley
Instructions:

1. In a clean bowl, join the ingredients for the spice rub. Blend well & put aside.
2. In a small saucepan over medium heat, combine the apple juice vinegar, balsamic vinegar, maple syrup, ketchup, red onion, garlic, and chile. Mix & let stew, revealed, for around 60 minutes. Increase the level of the heat to medium-high & cook for 15 additional minutes until the sauce thickens. Mix it frequently. In the event that it appears to be excessively thick, include some water.
3. Preheat the oven to 350 degrees. In a clean bowl, join the dry ingredients for the seitan & blend well. In a clean bowl, add the wet ingredients. Add the wet ingredients to the dry & blend until simply consolidated. Manipulate the dough gently until everything is combined & the dough feels elastic.
4. Grease or shower a preparing dish. Include the dough to the baking dish, smoothing it & stretching it to fit the dish. Cut the dough into 7 to 9 strips & afterward down the middle to make 16 thick ribs.
5. Top the dough with the flavor rub & back rub it in a bit. Heat the seitan for 40 minutes to an hour or until the seitan has a strong surface to it. Remove the dish from the heater. Recut the strips & cautiously remove them from the baking dish.
6. Increase the oven temperature to about 400 degrees. Slather the ribs with BBQ sauce & lay them on a baking sheet. Set the ribs back in the heater for pretty much 12 minutes so the sauce can get a bit roasted. Then again, you can cook the sauce-covered ribs on a grill or in a grill pan.

Green Bean Casserole
Nutritional Facts
servings per container
2
Prep Total
10 min
Serving Size 2/3 cup (5g)

AMOUNT PER SERVING
Calories
100

. . .

% DAILY VALUE

Total Fat 10g
12%
Saturated Fat 2g
2%
Trans Fat 4g
20%
Cholesterol
2%
Sodium 70mg
7%
Total Carbohydrate 18g
2%
Dietary Fiber 9g
10%
Total Sugar 16g
01.20%
Protein 2g

Vitamin C 9mcg
10%
Calcium 720mg
1%
Iron 6mg
2%
Potassium 150mg
6%
Ingredients

- Diced 1 large onion
- 3 tablespoons of original olive oil
- ¼ cup flour
- 2 cups of water
- 1 tablespoon of salt
- ½ tablespoons of garlic powder
- 1 or 2 bags frozen green beans (10 ounces each)
- 1 fried onion

Instructions:

1. Preheat oven to 350 degrees.

2. Heat original olive oil in a shallow pan. Include onion & stir occasionally while the onions soften and turn translucent. This takes about 15 to 20 minutes, don't rush it because it gives so much flavor! Once onion is well cooked, include flour & stir well to cook flour. It will be a dry mixture. Include salt & garlic powder. Add some water. Let simmer for about 1 – 2 minutes & allow mixture to thicken. Immediately remove from heat

3. Pour green beans into a square baking dish & add 2/3 can of onions. Include all of the gravy & stir well to together

4. Place in oven & cook for 25 to 30 minutes, gravy mixture will be bubbly. Top with remaining fried onions & cook for 4 to 12 minutes more. Serve immediately and enjoy your dinner.

Socca Pizza [Vegan]
Nutritional Facts
servings per container
2
Prep Total
10 min
Serving Size 2/3 cup (78g)

AMOUNT PER SERVING
Calories
120

% DAILY VALUE
Total Fat 10g
20%
Saturated Fat 5g
7%
Trans Fat 6g
27%
Cholesterol
5%
Sodium 10mg
10%
Total Carbohydrate 4g
20%
Dietary Fiber 9g
15%
Total Sugar 12g
01.70%

Protein 6g

Vitamin C 7mcg
10%
Calcium 290mg
20%
Iron 4mg
2%
Potassium 240mg
7%

Ingredients
Socca Base

- 1 cup chickpea (garbanzo bean) flour – I used bob's Red Mill Garbanzo Fava Flour
- 1 or 2 cups of cold, filtered water
- 1 to 2 tablespoons minced garlic
- ½ tablespoon of sea salt
- 2 tablespoons coconut oil (for greasing)

Toppings

- Add Tomato-paste
- Add Dried Italian herbs (oregano, basil, thyme, rosemary, etc.)
- Add Mushrooms
- Add Red onion
- Add Capsicum/bell pepper
- Add Sun-dried tomatoes
- Add Kalamata olives
- Add Vegan Cheese & Chopped Fresh basil leaves

Instructions:

1. Pre-heat oven to 350F
2. In a clean mixing bowl, whisk together garbanzo bean flour & water until there are no lumps remaining. Stir together in garlic 7 sea salt. Allow resting for about 12 minutes to thicken.
3. Grease 2 - 4 small, shallow dishes/tins with original coconut oil
4. Pour mixture into a clean dish & bake for about 20 - 15 minutes or until golden brown.
5. Remove dishes from oven, top with your favorite toppings & vegan cheese (optional) & return to the oven for another 7 - 10 minutes or so.

6. Remove dishes from oven & allow to sit for a about 2 − 5 minutes before removing pizzas from the dishes. Enjoy your dinner!

Rainbow Nourishment Bowl
Nutritional Facts
servings per container
5
Prep Total
10 min
Serving Size 2/3 cup (77g)

AMOUNT PER SERVING
Calories
20

% DAILY VALUE
Total Fat 2g
0%
Saturated Fat 7g
2%
Trans Fat 0g
10%
Cholesterol
5%
Sodium 55mg
20%
Total Carbohydrate 9g
200%
Dietary Fiber 7g
1%
Total Sugar 36g
2%
Protein 1g

Vitamin C 6mcg
21%
Calcium 160mg
2%
Iron 7mg
2%
Potassium 320mg

10%
Ingredients

- 2 cups spinach
- 1/2 cup corn kernels
- 1/2 cup edamame beans
- 1/2 cup cabbage, shredded
- 1/4 cup carrots, sliced
- 1/2 cup quinoa, cooked
- 1 radish, sliced
- Handful pea shoot sprouts (or another type of sprouts)
- 1/2 avocado, sliced
- Sesame seeds
- Juice of 1/2 lemon

Instructions:

1. Start by filling the bottom of the Coconut Bowls with spinach.
2. Place the corn, edamame, cabbage, carrots, cooked quinoa, radish, sprouts, & avocado in small piles on top of the bowls.
3. Sprinkle with sesame seeds.
4. Dress with some lemon juice if desired

Caramelized Banana & Blueberry Tacos
Nutritional Facts
servings per container
7
Prep Total
10 min
Serving Size 2/3 cup (51g)

Amount per serving
Calories
11

% Daily Value
Total Fat 2g
2%
Saturated Fat 7g
10%
Trans Fat 3g
8%

**Cholesterol
9%
Sodium 470mg
2%
Total Carbohydrate 20g
200%**
Dietary Fiber 10g
20%
Total Sugar 9g
1%
Protein 6g

Vitamin C 1mcg
20%
Calcium 700mg
7%
Iron 7mg
2%
Potassium 470mg
9%
Ingredients

- 4 flour tortillas
- 1 Teaspoon coconut oil
- 2 ripe bananas, peeled and sliced lengthways into 0.5cm / 0.2″ slices
- 100g / 3.5oz fresh blueberries
- 1 Teaspoon maple syrup
- 3 Teaspoon vanilla favored coconut or soy yogurt
- 1 heaped teaspoon tahini
- 1.5 Teaspoon shredded coconut or coconut flakes
- 1 Teaspoon cacao nibs

Instructions:

1. You will need to preheat the oven to 160°C / 320°F.
2. Kindly wrap the tortillas in foil & heat in the oven for 6 minutes.
3. Heat a medium-sized, heavy-based, non-stick or cast-iron skillet on medium heat on the stove. Add original coconut oil & once it's melted, add the sliced clean bananas.
4. Fry the bananas until they are golden brown on both sides, making sure to rotate them frequently so they won't stick to the pan.
5. You need to top the warm tortillas with the fried bananas and drizzle with tahini, yogurt, and maple syrup.

6. Kindly top with blueberries and sprinkle with coconut and cacao nibs.
7. Serve and enjoy

Decent Beef and Onion Stew
Serving: 4
Prep Time: 10 minutes
Cook Time 1-2 hours
Ingredients:

- 2 pounds lean beef, cubed
- 3 pounds shallots, peeled
- 5 garlic cloves, peeled, whole
- 3 tablespoons tomato paste
- 1 bay leaves
- ¼ cup olive oil
- 3 tablespoons lemon juice

How To:

1. Take a stew pot and place it over medium heat.
2. Add vegetable oil and let it heat up.
3. Add meat and brown.
4. Add remaining ingredients and canopy with water.
5. Bring the entire mix to a boil.
6. Reduce heat to low and canopy the pot.
7. Simmer for 1-2 hours until beef is cooked thoroughly.
8. Serve hot!

Nutrition (Per Serving)
Calories: 136
Fat: 3g
Carbohydrates: 0.9g
Protein: 24g
Clean Parsley and Chicken Breast
Serving: 2
Prep Time: 10 minutes
Cook Time: 40 minutes
Ingredients:

- 1/2 tablespoon dry parsley
- 1/2 tablespoon dry basil
- 2 chicken breast halves, boneless and skinless
- 1/4 teaspoon sunflower seeds

- 1/4 teaspoon red pepper flakes, crushed
- 1 tomato, sliced

How To:

1. Pre-heat your oven to 350 degrees F.
2. Take a 9x13 inch baking dish and grease it up with cooking spray.
3. Sprinkle 1 tablespoon of parsley, 1 teaspoon of basil and spread the mixture over your baking dish.
4. Arrange the pigeon breast halves over the dish and sprinkle garlic slices on top.
5. Take a little bowl and add 1 teaspoon parsley, 1 teaspoon of basil, sunflower seeds, basil, red pepper and blend well. Pour the mixture over the pigeon breast .
6. Top with tomato slices and canopy , bake for 25 minutes.
7. Remove the duvet and bake for quarter-hour more.
8. Serve and enjoy!

Nutrition (Per Serving)
Calories: 150
Fat: 4g
Carbohydrates: 4g
Protein: 25g
Zucchini Beef Sauté with Coriander Greens
Serving: 4
Prep Time: 10 minutes
Cook Time: 10 minutes
Ingredients:

- 10 ounces beef, sliced into 1-2-inch strips
- 1 zucchini, cut into 2-inch strips
- ¼ cup parsley, chopped
- 3 garlic cloves, minced
- 2 tablespoons tamari sauce
- 4 tablespoons avocado oil

How To:

1. Add 2 tablespoons avocado oil during a frypan over high heat.
2. Place strips of beef and brown for a couple of minutes on high heat.
3. Once the meat is brown, add zucchini strips and sauté until tender.
4. Once tender, add tamari sauce, garlic, parsley and allow them to sit for a couple of minutes more.
5. Serve immediately and enjoy!

Nutrition (Per Serving)

- Calories: 500
- Fat: 40g
- Carbohydrates: 5g
- Protein: 31g

Hearty Lemon and Pepper Chicken
Serving: 4
Prep Time: 5 minutes
Cook Time: 15
Ingredients:

- 2 teaspoons olive oil
- 1 ¼ pounds skinless chicken cutlets
- 2 whole eggs
- ¼ cup panko crumbs
- 1 tablespoon lemon pepper
- Sunflower seeds and pepper to taste
- 3 cups green beans
- ¼ cup parmesan cheese
- ¼ teaspoon garlic powder

How To:

1. Pre-heat your oven to 425 degrees F.
2. Take a bowl and stir in seasoning, parmesan, lemon pepper, garlic powder, panko.
3. Whisk eggs in another bowl.
4. Coat cutlets in eggs and press into panko mix.
5. Transfer coated chicken to a parchment lined baking sheet.
6. Toss the beans in oil, pepper, add sunflower seeds, and lay them on the side of the baking sheet.
7. Bake for quarter-hour .
8. Enjoy!

Nutrition (Per Serving)

- Calorie: 299
- Fat: 10g
- Carbohydrates: 10g
- Protein: 43g

Walnuts and Asparagus Delight

Serving: 4
Prep Time: 5 minutes
Cook Time: 5 minutes
Ingredients:

- 1 ½ tablespoons olive oil
- ¾ pound asparagus, trimmed
- ¼ cup walnuts, chopped
- Sunflower seeds and pepper to taste

How To:

1. Place a skillet over medium heat add vegetable oil and let it heat up.
2. Add asparagus, sauté for five minutes until browned.
3. Season with sunflower seeds and pepper.
4. Remove heat.
5. Add walnuts and toss.
6. Serve warm!

Nutrition (Per Serving)
Calories: 124
Fat: 12g
Carbohydrates: 2g
Protein: 3g
Healthy Carrot Chips
Serving: 4
Prep Time: 10 minutes
Cook Time: 10 minutes
Ingredients:

- 3 cups carrots, sliced paper-thin rounds
- 2 tablespoons olive oil
- 2 teaspoons ground cumin
- ½ teaspoon smoked paprika Pinch of sunflower seeds

How To:

1. Pre-heat your oven to 400 degrees F.
2. Slice carrot into thin shaped coins employing a peeler.
3. Place slices during a bowl and toss with oil and spices.
4. Lay out the slices on a parchment paper, lined baking sheet during a single layer.
5. Sprinkle sunflower seeds.

6. Transfer to oven and bake for 8-10 minutes.
7. Remove and serve.

Enjoy!
Nutrition (Per Serving)
Calories: 434
Fat: 35g
Carbohydrates: 31g
Protein: 2g
Beef Soup
Serving: 4
Prep Time: 10 minutes
Cook Time: 40 minutes
Ingredients:

- 1-pound ground beef, lean
- 1 cup mixed vegetables, frozen
- 1 yellow onion, chopped
- 6 cups vegetable broth
- 1 cup low-fat cream Pepper to taste

How To:

1. Take a stockpot and add all the ingredients the except cream , salt, and black pepper.
2. bring back a boil.
3 Reduce heat to simmer.
4. Cook for 40 minutes.
5. Once cooked, warm the cream .
6. Then add once the soup is cooked.
7. Blend the soup till smooth by using an immersion blender.
8. Season with salt and black pepper.
9. Serve and enjoy!

Nutrition (Per Serving)
Calories: 270
Fat: 14g
Carbohydrates: 6g
Protein: 29g
Amazing Grilled Chicken and Blueberry Salad
Serving: 5
Prep Time: 10 minutes
Cook Time: 25 minutes
Smart Points: 9

Ingredients:

- 5 cups mixed greens
- 1 cup blueberries
- ¼ cup slivered almonds
- 2 cups chicken breasts, cooked and cubed

For dressing

- ¼ cup olive oil
- ¼ cup apple cider vinegar
- ¼ cup blueberries
- 2 tablespoons honey
- Sunflower seeds and pepper to taste

How To:

1. Take a bowl and add greens, berries, almonds, chicken cubes and blend well.
2. Take a bowl and blend the dressing ingredients, pour the combination into a blender and blitz until smooth.
3. Add dressing on top of the chicken cubes and toss well.
4. Season more and enjoy!

Nutrition (Per Serving)
Calories: 266
Fat: 17g
Carbohydrates: 18g
Protein: 10g

Clean Chicken and Mushroom Stew
Serving: 4
Prep Time: 10 minutes
Cook Time: 35 minutes

Ingredients:

- 4 chicken breast halves, cut into bite sized pieces
- 1 pound mushrooms, sliced (5-6 cups)
- 1 bunch spring onion, chopped
- 4 tablespoons olive oil
- 1 teaspoon thyme
- Sunflower seeds and pepper as needed

How To:

1. Take an outsized deep frypan and place it over medium-high heat.
2. Add oil and let it heat up.
3. Add chicken and cook for 4-5 minutes per side until slightly browned.
4. Add spring onions and mushrooms, season with sunflower seeds and pepper consistent with your taste.
5. Stir.
6. Cover with lid and convey the combination to a boil.
7. Reduce heat and simmer for 25 minutes.
8. Serve!

Nutrition (Per Serving)
Calories: 247
Fat: 12g
Carbohydrates: 10g
Protein: 23g
Elegant Pumpkin Chili Dish
Serving: 4
Prep Time: 10 minutes
Cook Time: 15 minutes
Ingredients:

- 3 cups yellow onion, chopped
- 8 garlic cloves, chopped
- 1 pound turkey, ground
- 2 cans (15 ounces each) fire roasted tomatoes
- 2 cups pumpkin puree
- 1 cup chicken broth
- 4 teaspoons chili spice
- 1 teaspoon ground cinnamon
- 1 teaspoon sea sunflower seeds

How To:

1. Take an outsized sized pot and place it over medium-high heat.
2. Add copra oil and let the oil heat up.
3. Add onion and garlic, sauté for five minutes.
4. Add ground turkey and break it while cooking, cook for five minutes.
5. Add remaining ingredients and convey the combination to simmer.
6. Simmer for quarter-hour over low heat (lid off).
7. Pour chicken stock .
8. Serve with desired salad.
9. Enjoy!

Nutrition (Per Serving)
Calories: 312
Fat: 16g
Carbohydrates: 14g
Protein: 27g
Zucchini Zoodles with Chicken and Basil
Serving: 2
Prep Time: 10 minutes
Cook Time: 10 minutes
Ingredients:

- 2 chicken fillets, cubed
- 2 tablespoons ghee
- 1-pound tomatoes, diced
- ½ cup basil, chopped
- ¼ cup coconut almond milk
- 1 garlic clove, peeled, minced
- 1 zucchini, shredded

How To:

1. Sauté cubed chicken in ghee until not pink.
2. Add tomatoes and season with sunflower seeds.
3. Simmer and reduce the liquid.
4. Prepare your zucchini Zoodles by shredding zucchini during a kitchen appliance .
5. Add basil, garlic, coconut almond milk to chicken and cook for a couple of minutes.
6. Add half the zucchini Zoodles to a bowl and top with creamy tomato basil chicken.
7. Enjoy!

Nutrition (Per Serving)
Calories: 540
Fat: 27g
Carbohydrates: 13g
Protein: 59g
Tasty Roasted Broccoli
Serving: 4
Prep Time: 5 minutes
Cook Time: 20 minutes
Ingredients:

- 4 cups broccoli florets

- 1 tablespoon olive oil
- Sunflower seeds and pepper to taste

How To:

1. Pre-heat your oven to 400 degrees F.
2. Add broccoli during a zip bag alongside oil and shake until coated.
3. Add seasoning and shake again.
4. Spread broccoli out on baking sheet, bake for 20 minutes.
5. Let it cool and serve.
6. Enjoy!

Nutrition (Per Serving)

- Calories: 62
- Fat: 4g
- Carbohydrates: 4g
- Protein: 4g

The Almond Breaded Chicken Goodness
Serving: 3
Prep Time: 15 minutes
Cook Time: 15 minutes
Ingredients:

- 2 large chicken breasts, boneless and skinless
- 1/3 cup lemon juice
- 1 ½ cups seasoned almond meal
- 2 tablespoons coconut oil
- Lemon pepper, to taste
- Parsley for decoration

How To:

1. Slice pigeon breast in half.
2. Pound out each half until ¼ inch thick.
3. Take a pan and place it over medium heat, add oil and warmth it up.
4. Dip each pigeon breast slice through juice and let it sit for two minutes.
5. Turnover and therefore the let the opposite side sit for two minutes also .
6. Transfer to almond meal and coat each side .
7. Add coated chicken to the oil and fry for 4 minutes per side, ensuring to sprinkle lemon pepper liberally.

8. Transfer to a paper lined sheet and repeat until all chicken are fried.
9. Garnish with parsley and enjoy!

Nutrition (Per Serving)

- Calories: 325
- Fat: 24g
- Carbohydrates: 3g
- Protein: 16g

South-Western Pork Chops

Serving: 4
Prep Time: 10 minutes
Cook Time: 15 minutes
Smart Points: 3
Ingredients:

- Cooking spray as needed
- 4-ounce pork loin chop, boneless and fat rimmed
- 1/3 cup salsa
- 2 tablespoons fresh lime juice
- ¼ cup fresh cilantro, chopped

How To:

1. Take an outsized sized non-stick skillet and spray it with cooking spray.
2. Heat until hot over high heat.
3. Press the chops together with your palm to flatten them slightly.
4. Add them to the skillet and cook on 1 minute for every side until they're nicely browned.
5. Lower the warmth to medium-low.
6. Combine the salsa and juice .
7. Pour the combination over the chops.
8. Simmer uncovered for about 8 minutes until the chops are perfectly done.
9. If needed, sprinkle some cilantro on top.
10. Serve!

Nutrition (Per Serving)

- Calorie: 184
- Fat: 4g
- Carbohydrates: 4g

- Protein: 0.5g

Almond butter Pork Chops

Serving: 2
Prep Time: 5 minutes
Cook Time: 25 minutes
Ingredients:

- 1 tablespoon almond butter, divided
- 2 boneless pork chops
- Pepper to taste
- 1 tablespoon dried Italian seasoning, low fat and low sodium
- 1 tablespoon olive oil

How To:

1. Pre-heat your oven to 350 degrees F.
2. Pat pork chops dry with a towel and place them during a baking dish.
3. Season with pepper, and Italian seasoning.
4. Drizzle vegetable oil over pork chops.
5. Top each chop with ½ tablespoon almond butter.
6. Bake for 25 minutes.
7. Transfer pork chops on two plates and top with almond butter juice.
8. Serve and enjoy!

Nutrition (Per Serving)

Calories: 333
Fat: 23g
Carbohydrates: 1g
Protein: 31g

Chicken Salsa

Serving: 1
Prep Time: 4 minutes
Cook Time: 14 minutes
Ingredients:

- 2 chicken breasts
- 1 cup salsa
- 1 taco seasoning mix
- 1 cup plain Greek Yogurt
- ½ cup of kite ricottta/cashew cheese, cubed

How To:

1. Take a skillet and place over medium heat.
2. Add pigeon breast , ½ cup of salsa and taco seasoning.
3. Mix well and cook for 12-15 minutes until the chicken is completed
.
4. Take the back off and cube them.
5. Place the cubes on toothpick and top with cheddar.
6. Place yogurt and remaining salsa in cups and use as dips.
7. Enjoy!

Nutrition (Per Serving)
Calories: 359
Fat: 14g
Net Carbohydrates: 14g
Protein: 43g
Healthy Mediterranean Lamb Chops
Serving: 4
Prep Time: 10 minutes
Cook Time: 10 minutes
Ingredients:

- 4 lamb shoulder chops, 8 ounces each
- 2 tablespoons Dijon mustard
- 2 tablespoons Balsamic vinegar
- ½ cup olive oil
- 2 tablespoons shredded fresh basil

How To:

1. Pat your lamb chop dry employing a kitchen towel and arrange them on a shallow glass baking dish.
2. Take a bowl and a whisk in Dijon mustard, balsamic vinegar, pepper and blend them well.
3. Whisk within the oil very slowly into the marinade until the mixture is smooth
4. Stir in basil.
5. Pour the marinade over the lamb chops and stir to coat each side well.
6. Cover the chops and permit them to marinate for 1-4 hours (chilled).
7. Take the chops out and leave them for half-hour to permit the temperature to succeed in a traditional level.
8. Pre-heat your grill to medium heat and add oil to the grate.

9. Grill the lamb chops for 5-10 minutes per side until each side are browned.

10. Once the middle reads 145 degrees F, the chops are ready, serve and enjoy!

Nutrition (Per Serving)
Calories: 521
Fat: 45g
Carbohydrates: 3.5g
Protein: 22g

Amazing Sesame Breadsticks
Serving: 5 breadsticks
Prep Time: 10 minutes
Cooking Time: 20 minutes

Ingredients:

- 1 egg white
- 2 tablespoons almond flour
- 1 teaspoon Himalayan pink sunflower seeds
- 1 tablespoon extra-virgin olive oil
- ½ teaspoon sesame seeds

How To:

1. Pre-heat your oven to 320 degrees F.
2. Line a baking sheet with parchment paper and keep it on the side.
3. Take a bowl and whisk in egg whites, add flour and half sunflower seeds and vegetable oil .
4. Knead until you've got a smooth dough.
5. Divide into 4 pieces and roll into breadsticks.
6. Place on prepared sheet and brush with vegetable oil , sprinkle sesame seeds and remaining sunflower seeds.
7. Bake for 20 minutes.
8. Serve and enjoy!

Nutrition (Per Serving)
Total Carbs: 1.1g
Fiber: 1g
Protein: 1.6g
Fat: 5g

Brown Butter Duck Breast
Serving: 3
Prep Time: 5 minutes
Cook Time: 25 minutes

Ingredients:

- 1 whole 6 ounce duck breast, skin on
- Pepper to taste
- 1 head radicchio, 4 ounces, core removed
- ¼ cup unsalted butter
- 6 fresh sage leaves, sliced

How To:

1. Pre-heat your oven to 400 degree F.
2. Pat duck breast dry with towel .
3. Season with pepper.
4. Place duck breast in skillet and place it over medium heat, sear for 3-4 minutes all sides
5. Turn breast over and transfer skillet to oven.
6. Roast for 10 minutes (uncovered).
7. Cut radicchio in half.
8. Remove and discard the woody white core and thinly slice the leaves.
9. Keep them on the side.
10. Remove skillet from oven.
11. Transfer duck breast, fat side up to chopping board and let it rest.
12. Re-heat your skillet over medium heat.
13. Add unsalted butter, sage and cook for 3-4 minutes.
14. Cut duck into 6 equal slices.
15. Divide radicchio between 2 plates, top with slices of duck breast and drizzle browned butter and sage.
16. Enjoy!

Nutrition (Per Serving)
Calories: 393
Fat: 33g
Carbohydrates: 2g
Protein: 22g
Generous Garlic Bread Stick
Serving: 8 breadsticks
Prep Time: 15 minutes
Cooking Time: 15 minutes
Ingredients:

- ¼ cup almond butter, softened
- 1 teaspoon garlic powder
- 2 cups almond flour

- ½ tablespoon baking powder
- 1 tablespoon Psyllium husk powder
- ¼ teaspoon sunflower seeds
- 3 tablespoons almond butter, melted
- 1 egg
- ¼ cup boiling water

How To:

1. Pre-heat your oven to 400 degrees F.
2. Line baking sheet with parchment paper and keep it on the side.
3. Beat almond butter with garlic powder and keep it on the side.
4. Add almond flour, leaven , husk, sunflower seeds during a bowl and blend in almond butter and egg, mix well.
5. Pour boiling water within the mix and stir until you've got a pleasant dough.
6. Divide the dough into 8 balls and roll into breadsticks.
7. Place on baking sheet and bake for quarter-hour .
8. Brush each persist with garlic almond butter and bake for five minutes more.
9. Serve and enjoy!

Nutrition (Per Serving)
Total Carbs: 7g
Fiber: 2g
Protein: 7g
Fat: 24g
Cauliflower Bread Stick
Serving: 5 breadsticks
Prep Time: 10 minutes
Cooking Time: 48 minutes
Ingredients:

- 1 cup cashew cheese/ kite ricotta cheese
- 1 tablespoon organic almond butter
- 1 whole egg
- ½ teaspoon Italian seasoning
- ¼ teaspoon red pepper flakes
- 1/8 teaspoon kosher sunflower seeds
- 2 ups cauliflower rice, cooked for 3 minutes in microwave
- 3 teaspoons garlic, minced
- Parmesan cheese, grated

How To:

1. Pre-heat your oven to 350 degrees F.
2. Add almond butter during a small pan and melt over low heat
3. Add red pepper flakes, garlic to the almond butter and cook for 2-3 minutes.
4. Add garlic and almond butter mix to the bowl with cooked cauliflower and add the Italian seasoning.
5. Season with sunflower seeds and blend , refrigerate for 10 minutes.
6. Add cheese and eggs to the bowl and blend .
7. Place a layer of parchment paper at rock bottom of a 9 x 9 baking dish and grease with cooking spray, add egg and mozzarella cheese mix to the cauliflower mix.
8. Add mix to the pan and smooth to a skinny layer with the palms of your hand.
9. Bake for half-hour , remove from oven and top with few shakes of parmesan and mozzarella.
10. Cook for 8 minutes more.
11. Enjoy!

Nutrition (Per Serving)
Total Carbs: 11.5g
Fiber: 2g
Protein: 10.7g
Fat: 20g
Bacon and Chicken Garlic Wrap
Serving: 4
Prep Time: 15 minutes
Cook Time: 10 minutes
Ingredients:

- 1 chicken fillet, cut into small cubes
- 8-9 thin slices bacon, cut to fit cubes
- 6 garlic cloves, minced

How To:

1. Pre-heat your oven to 400 degrees F.
2. Line a baking tray with aluminum foil .
3. Add minced garlic to a bowl and rub each chicken piece with it.
4. Wrap a bacon piece around each garlic chicken bite.
5. Secure with toothpick.
6. Transfer bites to baking sheet, keeping a touch little bit of space between them.
7. Bake for about 15-20 minutes until crispy.
8. Serve and enjoy!

Nutrition (Per Serving)
Calories: 260
Fat: 19g
Carbohydrates: 5g
Protein: 22g
Chipotle Lettuce Chicken
Serving: 6
Prep Time: 10 minutes
Cook Time: 25 minutes
Ingredients:

- 1-pound chicken breast, cut into strips
- Splash of olive oil
- 1 red onion, finely sliced
- 14 ounces tomatoes
- 1 teaspoon chipotle, chopped
- ½ teaspoon cumin
- Lettuce as needed
- Fresh coriander leaves
- Jalapeno chilies, sliced
- Fresh tomato slices for garnish
- Lime wedges

How To:

1. Take a non-stick frypan and place it over medium heat.
2. Add oil and warmth it up.
3. Add chicken and cook until brown.
4. Keep the chicken on the side.
5. Add tomatoes, sugar, chipotle, cumin to an equivalent pan and simmer for 25 minutes until you've got a pleasant sauce.
6. Add chicken into the sauce and cook for five minutes.
7. Transfer the combination to a different place.
8. Use lettuce wraps to require some of the mixture and serve with a squeeze of lemon.
9. Enjoy!

Nutrition (Per Serving)
Calories: 332
Fat: 15g
Carbohydrates: 13g
Protein: 34g
Balsamic Chicken and Vegetables
Serving: 2

Prep Time: 15 minutes
Cook Time: 25 minutes
Ingredients:

- 4 chicken thigh, boneless and skinless
- 5 stalks of asparagus, halved
- 1 pepper, cut in chunks
- 1/2 red onion, diced
- ½ cup carrots, sliced
- 1 garlic cloves, minced
- 2-ounces mushrooms, diced
- ¼ cup balsamic vinegar
- 1 tablespoon olive oil
- ½ teaspoon stevia
- ½ tablespoon oregano
- Sunflower seeds and pepper as needed

How To:

1. Pre-heat your oven to 425 degrees F.
2. Take a bowl and add all of the vegetables and blend .
3. Add spices and oil and blend .
4. Dip the chicken pieces into spice mix and coat them well.
5. Place the veggies and chicken onto a pan during a single layer.
6. Cook for 25 minutes.
7. Serve and enjoy!

Nutrition (Per Serving)
Calories: 401
Fat: 17g
Net Carbohydrates: 11g
Protein: 48g
Cream Dredged Corn Platter
Serving: 3
Prep Time: 10 minutes
Cook Time: 4 hours
Ingredients:

- 3 cups corn
- 2 ounces cream cheese, cubed
- 2 tablespoons milk
- 2 tablespoons whipping cream
- 2 tablespoons butter, melted
- Salt and pepper as needed

- 1 tablespoon green onion, chopped

How To:

1. Add corn, cheese , milk, light whipping cream , butter, salt and pepper to your Slow Cooker.
2. provides it a pleasant toss to combine everything well.
3. Place lid and cook on LOW for 4 hours.
4. Divide the combination amongst serving platters.
5. Serve and enjoy!

Nutrition (Per Serving)
Calories: 261
Fat: 11g
Carbohydrates: 17g
Protein: 6g
Exuberant Sweet Potatoes
Serving: 4
Prep Time: 5 minutes
Cook Time: 7-8 hours
Ingredients:

- 6 sweet potatoes, washed and dried

How To:

1. Loosely botch 7-8 pieces of aluminium foil within the bottom of your Slow Cooker, covering about half the area .
2. Prick each potato 6-8 times employing a fork.
3. Wrap each potato with foil and seal them.
4. Place wrapped potatoes within the cooker on top of the foil bed.
5. Place lid and cook on LOW for 7-8 hours.
6. Use tongs to get rid of the potatoes and unwrap them.
7. Serve and enjoy!

Nutrition (Per Serving)
Calories: 129
Fat: 0g
Carbohydrates: 30g
Protein: 2g
Ethiopian Cabbage Delight
Serving: 6
Prep Time: 15 minutes
Cook Time: 6- 8 hours

Ingredients:

- ½ cup water
- 1 head green cabbage, cored and chopped
- 1-pound sweet potatoes, peeled and chopped
- 3 carrots, peeled and chopped
- 1 onion, sliced
- 1 teaspoon extra virgin olive oil
- ½ teaspoon ground turmeric
- ½ teaspoon ground cumin
- ¼ teaspoon ground ginger

How To:

1. Add water to your Slow Cooker.
2. Take a medium bowl and add cabbage, carrots, sweet potatoes, onion and blend .
3. Add vegetable oil , turmeric, ginger, cumin and toss until the veggies are fully coated.
4. Transfer veggie mix to your Slow Cooker.
5. Cover and cook on LOW for 6-8 hours.
6. Serve and enjoy!

Nutrition (Per Serving)
Calories: 155
Fat: 2g
Carbohydrates: 35g
Protein: 4g
The Vegan Lovers Refried Beans
Serving: 12
Prep Time: 5 minutes
Cook Time: 10 hours
Ingredients:

- 4 cups vegetable broth
- 4 cups water
- 3 cups dried pinto beans
- 1 onion, chopped
- 2 jalapeno peppers, minced
- 4 garlic cloves, minced
- 1 tablespoon chili powder
- 2 teaspoon ground cumin
- 1 teaspoon sweet paprika
- 1 teaspoon salt

- ½ teaspoon fresh ground black pepper

How To:

1. Add the listed ingredients to your Slow Cooker.
2. Cover and cook on HIGH for 10 hours .
3. If there's any extra liquid, ladle the liquid up and reserve it during a bowl .
4. Use an immersion blender to blend the mixture (in the Slow Cooker) until smooth.
5. Add the reserved liquid.
6. Serve hot and enjoy!

Nutrition (Per Serving)
Calories: 91
Fat: 0g
Carbohydrates: 16g
Protein: 5g
Cool Apple and Carrot Harmony
Serving: 6
Prep Time: 10 minutes
Cook Time: 10 minutes
Ingredients:

- 1 cup apple juice
- 1 pound baby carrots
- 1 tablespoon cornstarch
- 1 tablespoon mint, chopped

How To:

1. Add fruit juice , carrots, cornstarch and mint to your Instant Pot.
2. Stir and lock the lid.
3. Cook on high for 10 minutes.
4. Perform a fast release.
5. Divide the combination amongst plates and serve.
6. Enjoy!

Nutrition (Per Serving)
Calories: 161
Fat: 2g
Carbohydrates: 9g
Protein: 8g
Mac and Chokes

Serving: 6
Prep Time: 5 minutes
Cook Time: 20 minutes
Ingredients:

- 1 tablespoon of olive oil
- 1 large sized diced onion
- 10 minced garlic cloves
- 1 can artichoke hearts
- 1-pound uncooked macaroni shells
- 12-ounce baby spinach
- 4 cups vegetable broth
- 1 teaspoon red pepper flakes
- 4 ounces vegan cheese
- ¼ cup cashew cream

How To:

1. Set the pot to Sauté mode and add oil, allow the oil to heat up and add onions.
2. Cook for two minutes.
3. Add garlic and stir well.
4. Add artichoke hearts and sauté for 1 minute more.
5. Add uncooked pasta and three cups of broth alongside 2 cups of water.
6. Mix well.
7. Lock the lid and cook on high for 4 minutes.
8. Quick release the pressure.
9. Open the pot and stir.
10. Add extra water, fold in spinach and cook on Sauté mode for a couple of minutes.
11. Add cashew cream and grated vegan cheese.
12. Add pepper flakes and blend well.
13. Enjoy!

Nutrition (Per Serving)
Calories: 649
Fat: 29g
Carbohydrates: 64g
Protein: 34g
Black Eyed Peas and Spinach Platter
Serving: 4
Prep Time: 10 minutes
Cook Time: 8 hours

Ingredients:

- 1 cup black eyed peas, soaked overnight and drained
- 2 cups low-sodium vegetable broth
- 1 can (15 ounces) tomatoes, diced with juice
- 8 ounces ham, chopped
- 1 onion, chopped
- 2 garlic cloves, minced
- 1 teaspoon dried oregano
- 1 teaspoon salt
- ½ teaspoon freshly ground black pepper
- ½ teaspoon ground mustard
- 1 bay leaf

How To:

1. Add the listed ingredients to your Slow Cooker and stir.
2. Place lid and cook on LOW for 8 hours.
3. Discard the herb .
4. Serve and enjoy!

Nutrition (Per Serving)
Calories: 209
Fat: 6g
Carbohydrates: 22g
Protein: 17g
Humble Mushroom Rice
Serving: 3
Prep Time: 10 minutes
Cook Time: 3 hours
Ingredients:

- ½ cup rice
- 2 green onions chopped
- 1 garlic clove, minced
- ¼ pound baby Portobello mushrooms, sliced
- 1 cup vegetable stock

How To:

1. Add rice, onions, garlic, mushrooms, stock to your Slow Cooker.
2. Stir well and place lid.
3. Cook on LOW for 3 hours..
4. Stir and divide amongst serving platters.

5. Enjoy!

Nutrition (Per Serving)
Calories: 200
Fat: 6g
Carbohydrates: 28g
Protein: 5g
Sweet and Sour Cabbage and Apples
Serving: 4
Prep Time: 15 minutes
Cook Time: 8 hours
Ingredients:

- ¼ cup honey
- ¼ cup apple cider vinegar
- 2 tablespoons Orange Chili-Garlic Sauce
- 1 teaspoon sea salt
- 3 sweet tart apples, peeled, cored and sliced
- 2 heads green cabbage, cored and shredded
- 1 sweet red onion, thinly sliced

How To:

1. Take alittle bowl and whisk in honey, orange-chili aioli , vinegar.
2. Stir well.
3. Add honey mix, apples, onion and cabbage to your Slow Cooker and stir.
4. Close lid and cook on LOW for 8 hours.
5. Serve and enjoy!

Nutrition (Per Serving)
Calories: 164
Fat: 1g
Carbohydrates: 41g
Protein: 4g
Delicious Aloo Palak
Serving: 6
Prep Time: 10 minutes
Cook Time: 6-8 hours
Ingredients:

- 2 pounds red potatoes, chopped
- 1 small onion, diced
- 1 red bell pepper, seeded and diced

- ¼ cup fresh cilantro, chopped
- 1/3 cup low-sodium veggie broth
- 1 teaspoon salt
- ½ teaspoon Garam masala
- ½ teaspoon ground cumin
- ¼ teaspoon ground turmeric
- ¼ teaspoon ground coriander
- ¼ teaspoon freshly ground black pepper
- 2 pounds fresh spinach, chopped

How To:

1. Add potatoes, bell pepper, onion, cilantro, broth and seasoning to your Slow Cooker.
2. Mix well.
3. Add spinach on top.
4. Place lid and cook on LOW for 6-8 hours.
5. Stir and serve.
6. Enjoy!

Nutrition (Per Serving)
Calories: 205
Fat: 1g
Carbohydrates: 44g
Protein: 9g

Orange and Chili Garlic Sauce
Serving. 5 cups
Prep Time: 15 minutes
Cook Time: 8 hours
Ingredients:

- ½ cup apple cider vinegar
- 4 pounds red jalapeno peppers, stems, seeds and ribs removed, chopped
- 10 garlic cloves, chopped
- ½ cup tomato paste
- Juice of 1 orange zest
- ½ cup honey
- 2 tablespoons soy sauce
- 2 teaspoons salt

How To:

1. Add vinegar, garlic, peppers, ingredient , fruit juice , honey, zest, soy

and salt to your Slow Cooker.
2. Stir and shut lid.
3. Cook on LOW for 8 hours.
4. Use as required !

Nutrition (Per Serving)
Calories: 33
Fat: 1g
Carbohydrates: 8g
Protein: 1g
Tantalizing Mushroom Gravy
Serving: 2 cups
Prep Time: 5 minutes
Cook Time: 5-8 hours
Ingredients:

- 1 cup button mushrooms, sliced
- ¾ cup low-fat buttermilk
- 1/3 cup water
- 1 medium onion, finely diced
- 2 garlic cloves, minced
- 2 tablespoons extra virgin olive oil
- 2 tablespoons all-purpose flour
- 1 tablespoon fresh rosemary, minced Freshly ground black pepper

How To:

1. Add the listed ingredients to your Slow Cooker.
2. Place lid and cook on LOW for 5-8 hours.
3. Serve warm and use as needed!

Nutrition (Per Serving)
Calories: 54
Fat: 4g
Carbohydrates: 4g
Protein: 2g
Everyday Vegetable Stock
Serving: 10 cups
Prep Time: 5 minutes
Cook Time: 8-12 hours
Ingredients:

- 2 celery stalks (with leaves), quartered
- 4 ounces mushrooms, with stems

- 2 carrots, unpeeled and quartered
- 1 onion, unpeeled, quartered from pole to pole
- 1 garlic head, unpeeled, halved across middle
- 2 fresh thyme sprigs
- 10 peppercorns
- ½ teaspoon salt
- Enough water to fill 3 quarters of Slow Cooker

How To:

1. Add celery, mushrooms, onion, carrots, garlic, thyme, salt, peppercorn and water to your Slow Cooker.
2. Stir and canopy .
3. Cook on LOW for 8-12 hours.
4. Strain the stock through a fine mesh cloth/metal mesh and discard solids.
5. Use as needed.

Nutrition (Per Serving)
Calories: 38
Fat: 5g
Carbohydrates: 1g
Protein: 0g
Grilled Chicken with Lemon and Fennel
Serving: 4
Prep Time: 5 minutes
Cook Time: 25 minutes
Ingredients:

- 2 cups chicken fillets , cut and skewed
- 1 large fennel bulb
- 2 garlic cloves
- 1 jar green olives
- 1 lemon

How To:

1. Pre-heat your grill to medium-high.
2. Crush garlic cloves.
3. Take a bowl and add vegetable oil and season with sunflower seeds and pepper.
4. Coat chicken skewers with the marinade.
5. Transfer them under the grill and grill for 20 minutes, ensuring to show them halfway through until golden.

6. Zest half the lemon and cut the opposite half into quarters.
7. Cut the fennel bulb into similarly sized segments.
8. Brush vegetable oil everywhere the clove segments and cook for 3-5 minutes.
9. Chop them and add them to the bowl with the marinade.
10. Add lemon peel and olives.
11. Once the meat is prepared , serve with the vegetable mix.
12. Enjoy!

Nutrition (Per Serving)
Calories: 649
Fat: 16g
Carbohydrates: 33g
Protein: 18g
Caramelized Pork Chops and Onion
Serving: 4
Prep Time: 5 minutes
Cook Time: 40 minutes
Ingredients:

- 4-pound chuck roast
- 4 ounces green Chili, chopped
- 2 tablespoons of chili powder
- ½ teaspoon of dried oregano
- ½ teaspoon of cumin, ground
- 2 garlic cloves, minced

How To:

1. Rub the chops with a seasoning of 1 teaspoon of pepper and a couple of teaspoons of sunflower seeds.
2. Take a skillet and place it over medium heat, add oil and permit the oil to heat up
3. Brown the seasoned chop each side .
4. Add water and onion to the skillet and canopy , lower the warmth to low and simmer for 20 minutes.
5. Turn the chops over and season with more sunflower seeds and pepper.
6. Cover and cook until the water fully evaporates and therefore the beer [MOU1]shows a rather brown texture.
7. Remove the chops and serve with a topping of the caramelized onion.
8. Serve and enjoy!

Nutrition (Per Serving)
Calorie: 47
Fat: 4g
Carbohydrates: 4g
Protein: 0.5g
Hearty Pork Belly Casserole
Serving: 4
Prep Time: 5 minutes
Cook Time: 25 minutes
Ingredients:

- 8 pork belly slices, cut into small pieces
- 3 large onions, chopped
- 4 tablespoons lemon
- Juice of 1 lemon
- Seasoning as you needed

How To:

1. Take an outsized autoclave and place it over medium heat.
2. Add onions and sweat them for five minutes.
3. Add side of pork slices and cook until the meat browns and onions become golden.
4. Cover with water and add honey, lemon peel , sunflower seeds, pepper, and shut the pressure seal.
5. Pressure cook for 40 minutes.
6. Serve and luxuriate in with a garnish of fresh chopped parsley if you favor .

Nutrition (Per Serving)
Calories: 753
Fat: 41g
Carbohydrates: 68g
Protein: 30g
Apple Pie Crackers
Serving: 100 crackers
Prep Time: 10 minutes
Cooking Time: 120 minutes
Ingredients:

- 2 tablespoons + 2 teaspoons avocado oil
- 1 medium Granny Smith apple, roughly chopped
- ¼ cup Erythritol
- 1/4 cup sunflower seeds, ground

- 1 ¾ cups roughly ground flax seeds
- 1/8 teaspoon Ground cloves
- 1/8 teaspoon ground cardamom
- 3 tablespoons nutmeg
- ¼ teaspoon ground ginger

How To:

1. Pre-heat your oven to 225 degrees F.
2. Line two baking sheets with parchment paper and keep them on the side.
3. Add oil, apple, Erythritol to a bowl and blend .
4. Transfer to kitchen appliance and add remaining ingredients, process until combined.
5. Transfer batter to baking sheets, spread evenly and dig crackers.
6. Bake for 1 hour, flip and bake for an additional hour.
7. allow them to cool and serve.
8. Enjoy!

Nutrition (Per Serving)
Total Carbs: 0.9g (%)
Fiber: 0.5g
Protein: 0.4g (%)
Fat: 2.1g (%)
Paprika Lamb Chops
Serving: 4
Prep Time: 10 minutes
Cook Time: 15 minutes
Ingredients:

- 1 lamb rack, cut into chops pepper to taste 1 tablespoon paprika
- 1/2 cup cumin powder
- 1/2 teaspoon chili powder

How To:

1. Take a bowl and add paprika, cumin, chili, pepper, and stir.
2. Add lamb chops and rub the mixture.
3. Heat grill over medium-temperature and add lamb chops, cook for five minutes.
4. Flip and cook for five minutes more, flip again.
5. Cook for two minutes, flip and cook for two minutes more.
6. Serve and enjoy!

Nutrition (Per Serving)
Calories: 200
Fat: 5g
Carbohydrates: 4g
Protein: 8g
Chicken & Goat Cheese Skillet
Ingredients

- 1/2 pound of boneless skinless chicken breasts, cut into 1-inch pieces
- 1/4 teaspoon salt
- 1/8 teaspoon pepper
- Two teaspoons olive oil
- 1 cup sliced fresh asparagus (1-inch pieces)
- One garlic clove, minced
- Three plum tomatoes, chopped
- Three tablespoons 2% milk
- Two tablespoons herbed fresh goat cheese, crumbled
- Hot cooked rice or pasta
- Additional goat cheese, optional

Directions

1. Toss chicken with salt and pepper. Heat oil at medium heat; saute chicken until not pink, 4-6 minutes. Remove from pan; keep warm.
2. Add asparagus to skillet; cook and blend at medium-high heat 1 minute. Add garlic; cook and stir 30 seconds. Stir in tomatoes, milk, and two tablespoons cheese; cook, covered, over medium heat until cheese begins to melt, 2-3 minutes. Stir in chicken. Serve with rice. If desired, top with additional cheese.

Nutrition

251 calories, 11g fat, 74mg cholesterol, 447mg sodium, 8g carbohydrate (5g sugars, 3g fiber), 29g protein. Diabetic Exchanges: 4 lean meat, two fat, one vegetable.
Green Curry Salmon with Green Beans
Ingredients

- Four salmon fillets (4 ounces each)
- 1 cup light coconut milk
- Two tablespoons green curry paste
- 1 cup uncooked instant brown rice
- 1 cup reduced-sodium chicken broth
- 1/8 teaspoon pepper

- 3/4 pound fresh green beans, trimmed
- One teaspoon sesame oil
- One teaspoon sesame seeds, toasted
- Lime wedges

Directions

1. Preheat oven to 400°. Place salmon in an 8-in. Square baking dish.
   Mix together coconut milk and curry paste; pour over salmon.
   Bake, uncovered, till fish simply starts offevolved to flake
   effortlessly with a fork, 15-20 minutes.
2. Meanwhile, during a small saucepan, integrate rice, broth and
   pepper; convey to a boil. Reduce warmth; simmer, covered, 5
   minutes. Remove from heat; let stand five minutes.
3. In a big saucepan, area steamer basket over 1 in. Of water. Place
   inexperienced beans inside the basket; convey water to a boil.
   Reduce heat to take care of a simmer; steam, covered, till beans are
   crisp-tender, 7-10 minutes. Toss with vegetable oil and sesame
   seeds.
4. Serve salmon with rice, beans and lime wedges. Spoon coconut
   sauce over the salmon.

Nutrition Facts
366 calories, 17g fat (5g saturated fat), 57mg cholesterol, 340mg sodium, 29g carbohydrate (5g sugars, 4g fibre), 24g protein.

Chicken Veggie Packets
Ingredients

- Four boneless and skinless chicken breast halves (4 ounces each)
- 1/2 pound sliced fresh mushrooms
- 1-1/2 cups fresh baby carrots
- 1 cup pearl onions
- 1/2 cup julienned sweet red pepper
- 1/4 teaspoon pepper
- Three teaspoons minced fresh thyme
- 1/2 teaspoon salt, optional
- Lemon wedges, optional

Directions

1. Flatten bird breasts to 1/2-in. Thickness; vicinity every on a touch
   of industrial quality foil (about 12 in. Square). Layer the mushrooms,
   carrots, onions and pink pepper over bird; sprinkle with pepper,
   thyme and salt if desired.

2. Fold foil around hen and greens and seal tightly. Place on a baking sheet. Bake at 375° for a half-hour or until chook juices run clear. If desired, serve with lemon wedges.

Nutrition Facts

175 calories, 3g fat (1g saturated fat), 63mg cholesterol, 100mg sodium, 11g carbohydrate (6g sugars, 2g fibre), 25g protein.

Sweet Onion & Sausage Spaghetti
Ingredients

- 6 ounces uncooked whole-wheat spaghetti
- 3/4 pound Italian turkey sausage links, casings removed
- Two teaspoons olive oil
- One sweet onion, thinly sliced
- 1-pint cherry tomatoes halved
- One and a half cup of fresh basil leaves (sliced)
- 1/2 cup half-and-half cream
- Shaved Parmesan cheese, optional

Directions

1. Cook spaghetti consistent with directions given. At an equivalent time, during a large nonstick skillet over medium heat, cook sausage in oil for five minutes. Add onion; bake 8-10 minutes longer or until meat is not any longer pink and onion is tender.
2. Stir in tomatoes and basil; heat through. Add cream; bring back a boil. Drain spaghetti; toss with sausage mixture. Garnish with cheese if desired.

Nutrition Facts

334 calories, 12g fat (4g saturated fat), 46mg cholesterol, 378mg sodium, 41g carbohydrate (8g sugars, 6g fibre), 17g protein.

Beef and Blue Cheese Penne with Pesto
Ingredients

- 2 cups uncooked whole wheat penne pasta
- Two beef tenderloin steaks (6 ounces each)
- 1/4 teaspoon salt
- 1/4 teaspoon pepper
- 5 ounces of fresh baby spinach (about 6 cups), coarsely chopped
- 2 cups grape tomatoes, halved
- 1/3 cup prepared pesto
- 1/4 cup chopped walnuts
- 1/4 cup crumbled Gorgonzola cheese

Directions

1. Cook pasta consistent with package directions.
2. Meanwhile, sprinkle steaks with salt and pepper. Grill steaks, covered, over medium heat. Heat for 5-7 mins on all sides or until meat reaches desired doneness.
3. Drain pasta; transfer to an outsized bowl. Add spinach, tomatoes, pesto and walnuts; toss to coat. Cut steak into thin slices. Serve pasta mixture with beef; sprinkle with cheese.

Nutrition Facts

532 calories, 22g fat (6g saturated fat), 50mg cholesterol, 434mg sodium, 49g carbohydrate (3g sugars, 9g fibre), 35g protein.

Asparagus Turkey Stir-Fry
Ingredients

- Two teaspoons cornstarch
- 1/4 cup chicken broth
- One tablespoon lemon juice
- One teaspoon soy sauce
- 1 pound of turkey breast tenderloins, cut into 1/2-inch strips
- One garlic clove, minced
- Two tablespoons canola oil, divided
- 1 pound of asparagus, cut into 1-1/2-inch pieces
- One jar (2 ounces) sliced pimientos, drained

Instructions

1. In a little bowl, mix the cornstarch, broth, juice and soy until smooth; put aside . during a large skillet orwok, stir-fry turkey and garlic in 1 tablespoon oil until meat is not any longer pink; remove and keep warm.
2. Stir-fry asparagus in remaining oil until crisp-tender. Add pimientos. Stir the mixture and increase the pan; cook andstir for 1 minute or until thickened. Return turkey to the pan; heat through.

Nutrition Facts

205 calories, 9g fat (1g saturated fat), 56mg cholesterol, 204mg sodium, 5g carbohydrate (1g sugars, 1g fibre), 28g protein.

Chicken with Celery Root Puree
Ingredients

- Four boneless skinless chicken breast halves (6 ounces each)
- 1/2 teaspoon pepper

- 1/4 teaspoon salt
- Three teaspoons canola oil, divided
- One large celery root, peeled and chopped (about 3 cups)
- 2 cups diced peeled butternut squash
- One small onion, chopped
- Two garlic cloves, minced
- 2/3 cup unsweetened apple juice

Instructions

1. Sprinkle chicken with pepper and salt. Take an outsized skillet and coat with cooking spray, heat two teaspoons oil over medium heat. Brown chicken on each side . Remove chicken from pan.
2. Heat the remaining oil over medium-high within the same pan. Add celery root, squash and onion; cook and stir until squash is crisp-tender. Add garlic; cook 1 minute longer.
3. Return chicken to pan; add fruit juice . bring back a boil. Reduce heat; simmer, covered, 12-15 minutes or until a thermometer inserted in chicken reads 165°.
4. Remove chicken; keep warm. Cool vegetable mixture slightly. Process during a kitchen appliance until smooth. Return to pan and warmth through. Serve with chicken.

Nutrition Facts
328 calories, 8g fat (1g saturated fat), 94mg cholesterol, 348mg sodium, 28g carbohydrate (10g sugars, 5g fibre), 37g protein.

Apple-Cherry Pork Medallions
Ingredients

- One pork tenderloin (1 pound)
- One teaspoon minced fresh rosemary or 1/4 teaspoon dried rosemary, crushed
- One teaspoon minced fresh thyme or 1/4 teaspoon dried thyme
- 1/2 teaspoon celery salt
- One tablespoon olive oil
- One large apple, sliced
- 2/3 cup unsweetened apple juice
- Three tablespoons dried tart cherries
- One tablespoon honey
- One tablespoon cider vinegar
- One package (8.8 ounces) ready-to-serve brown rice

Instructions

1. Cut tenderloin crosswise into 12 slices; sprinkle with rosemary, thyme and flavorer . during a huge skillet, heat oil over medium-excessive heat. Brown pork on both sides; do away with from pan.
2. In the equal skillet, combine apple, fruit juice , cherries, honey and vinegar. Boil it and stirring to loosen browned bits from pan. Reduce warmness; simmer, uncovered, 3-four minutes or simply till apple is tender.
3. Return meat to the pan, turning to coat with sauce; cook, covered, 3-4 minutes or till meat is tender. Meanwhile, put together rice keep with package deal directions; serve with meat mixture.

Nutrition Facts

349 calories, 9g fat (2g saturated fat), 64mg cholesterol, 179mg sodium, 37g carbohydrate (16g sugars, 4g fibre), and 25g protein.

Butternut Turkey Soup
Ingredients

- Three shallots, thinly sliced
- One tsp of olive oil
- 3 cups of reduced-sodium chicken broth
- 3 cups of cubed peeled butternut squash (3/4-inch cubes)
- Two medium-sized red potatoes, cut into 1/2-inch cubes
- 1-1/2 cups of water
- Two teaspoons of minced fresh thyme
- 1/2 teaspoon pepper
- Two whole cloves
- 3 cups cubed cooked turkey breast

Instructions

1. In a large-size saucepan coated with cooking spray, cook dinner shallots in oil over medium heat till tender. Stir within the broth, squash, potatoes, water, thyme and pepper.
2. Place spices on a double thickness of cheesecloth; carry up corners of the material and tie with string to shape a bag. Stir into soup. bring back a boil. Reduce warmness; cowl and simmer for 10-15 mins or till vegetables are tender. Stir in turkey; warmth through. Discard spice bag.

Nutrition

192 calories, 2g fat (0 saturated fat), 60mg cholesterol, 332mg sodium, 20g carbohydrate (3g sugars, 3g fibre), 25g protein.

Black Bean & Sweet Potato Rice Bowls
Ingredients

- 3/4 cup uncooked long-grain rice
- 1/4 teaspoon garlic salt
- 1-1/2 cups water
- Three tablespoons olive oil, divided
- One large sweet potato, peeled and diced
- One medium red onion, finely chopped
- 4 cups chopped fresh kale (sturdy stems removed)
- One can (15 ounces) black beans, rinsed and drained
- Two tablespoons sweet chilli sauce
- Lime wedges, optional
- Additional sweet chilli sauce, optional

Instructions

1. Place rice, flavorer and water during a large saucepan; bring back a boil. Reduce heat; simmer, covered until liquid is absorbed and rice is tender 15-20 minutes. Remove from heat; let stand 5 minutes.
2. At an equivalent time take an outsized pan and warmth two tablespoons oil over medium-high heat; saute sweet potato 8 minutes. Add onion; cook and stir until potato is tender 4-6 minutes. Add kale; cook and stir until tender, 3-5 minutes. Stir in beans; heat through.
3. Gently stir two tablespoons chilli sauce and remaining oil into rice; increase potato mixture. If you would like , serve with lime wedges and extra chilli sauce.

Nutrition

435 calories, 11g fat (2g saturated fat), 0 cholesterol, 405mg sodium, 74g carbohydrate (15g sugars, 8g fibre), 10g protein.

Pepper Ricotta Primavera
Ingredients

- 1 cup part-skim ricotta cheese
- 1/2 cup fat-free milk
- Four teaspoons olive oil
- One garlic clove, minced
- 1/2 teaspoon crushed red pepper flakes
- One medium green pepper, julienned
- One medium sweet red pepper, julienned
- One medium fresh yellow pepper, julienned
- One medium zucchini, sliced
- 1 cup frozen peas, thawed
- 1/4 teaspoon dried oregano
- 1/4 teaspoon dried basil

- 6 ounces fettuccine, cooked and drained

Instructions

1. Whisk together ricotta cheese and milk; put aside . Take an outsized skillet, heat oil over medium heat. Add garlic and pepper; saute 1 minute. Add subsequent seven ingredients. Cook and blend over medium heat until vegetables are crisptender, about 5 minutes.
2. Add cheese mixture to fettuccine; top with vegetables. Toss to coat. Serve immediately.

Nutrition

229 calories, 7g fat (3g saturated fat), 13mg cholesterol, 88mg sodium, 31g carbohydrate (6g sugars, 4g fibre), 11g protein.

Bow Ties with Sausage & Asparagus
Ingredients

- 3 cups of uncooked whole wheat bow tie pasta (about 8 ounces)
- 1 pound of asparagus, cut into 1-1/2-inch pieces
- One package (19-1/2 ounces) Italian turkey sausage links, casings removed
- One medium onion, chopped
- Three garlic cloves, minced
- 1/4 cup shredded Parmesan cheese
- Additional shredded Parmesan cheese, optional

Instructions

1. In a 6-qt. Stockpot, prepare dinner pasta in line with package directions, including asparagus over the last 2-three minutes of cooking. Drain, reserving half cup pasta water; return pasta and asparagus to the pot.
2. Meanwhile, during a big skillet, cook sausage, onion and garlic over medium heat until no pink, 6-8 minutes, breaking sausage into large crumbles. increase stockpot. Stir in 1/four cup cheese and reserved pasta water as desired. Serve with additional cheese if desired.

Nutrition

247 calories, 7g fat (2g saturated fat), 36mg cholesterol, 441mg sodium, 28g carbohydrate (2g sugars, 4g fibre), 17g protein

Pork and Balsamic Strawberry Salad
Ingredients

- One pork tenderloin (1 pound)

- 1/2 cup Italian salad dressing
- 1-1/2 cups halved fresh strawberries
- Two tablespoons balsamic vinegar
- Two teaspoons sugar
- 1/4 teaspoon salt
- 1/4 teaspoon pepper
- Two tablespoons olive oil
- 1/4 cup chicken broth
- One package about 5 ounces spring mix salad greens
- 1/2 cup crumbled goat cheese

Instructions

1. Place pork during a shallow dish. Add salad dressing; flip for coating. Refrigerate and canopy for a minimum of eight hours. Mix strawberries, vinegar and sugar; cover and refrigerate.
2. Preheat oven to 425°. Drain and wipe off meat , discarding marinade. Sprinkle with salt and pepper. during a large cast-iron or every other ovenproof skillet, warmness oil over medium-high warmness. Add beef; brown on all sides.
3. Bake until a thermometer reads 145°, 15-20 minutes. Remove from skillet; permit or stand 5 min. Then, add broth to skillet; cook over medium warmth, stirring to loosen browned bits from pan. bring back a boil. Reduce warmth; add strawberry. Then heat it.
4. Place green vegetables on a serving platter; sprinkle with cheese. Slice pork; found out over veggies. Top with strawberry mixture.

Nutrition
291 calories, 16g fat (5g saturated fat), 81mg cholesterol, 444mg sodium, 12g carbohydrate (7g sugars, 3g fibre), 26g protein.
Peppered Tuna Kabobs
Ingredients

- 1/2 cup frozen corn, thawed Four green onions, chopped
- One jalapeno pepper, seeded and chopped
- Two tablespoons coarsely chopped fresh parsley
- Two tablespoons lime juice
- 1 pound tuna steaks, cut into 1-inch cubes
- One teaspoon coarsely ground pepper
- Two large sweet red peppers, cut into 2x1-inch pieces

Instructions

1. One medium mango, peeled and cut into 1-inch cubes

2. For salsa, during a small bowl, combine the primary five ingredients; put aside .
3. Rub tuna with pepper. On 4metal or soaked wooden skewers, alternately thread red peppers, tuna and mango.
4. Place skewers on greased grill rack. Cook, covered, over medium heat, occasionally turning, until tuna is slightly pink in centre (medium-rare) and peppers are tender 10-12 minutes. Serve with salsa.

Nutrition
205 calories, 2g fat (0 saturated fat), 51mg cholesterol, 50mg sodium, 20g carbohydrate (12g sugars, 4g fibre), 29g protein.

Weeknight Chicken Chop Suey
Ingredients

- Four teaspoons of olive oil
- 1 pound of boneless chicken breast side, cut into 1-inch cubes
- 1/2 teaspoon dried tarragon
- 1/2 teaspoon dried basil
- 1/2 teaspoon dried marjoram
- 1/2 teaspoon grated lemon zest
- 1-1/2 cups chopped carrots
- 1 cup unsweetened pineapple tidbits, drained (reserve juice)
- One can (8 ounces) sliced water chestnuts, drained
- One medium tart apple, chopped
- 1/2 cup chopped onion
- 1 cup cold water, divided
- Three tablespoons unsweetened pineapple juice
- Three tablespoons reduced-sodium teriyaki sauce
- Two tablespoons cornstarch
- 3 cups hot cooked brown rice

Instructions

1. In a massive cast-iron or another heavy skillet, heat oil at medium temperature. Add chicken, herbs and lemon zest; leave it until lightly browned. Add subsequent five ingredients. Stir in 3/four cup water, fruit juice and teriyaki sauce; bring back a boil. Reduce warmness; simmer covered till chicken is not any longer purple, and therefore the carrots are gentle 10-15 minutes.
2. Combine cornstarch and remaining water. Gradually stir into hen mixture. Leave for boiling; cook and stir till thickened, about 2 minutes. Serve with rice.

Nutrition

330 calories, 6g fat, 42mg cholesterol, 227mg sodium, 50g carbohydrate (14g sugars, 5g fibre), 20g protein

Thai Chicken Pasta Skillet

Ingredients

- 6 ounces uncooked whole-wheat spaghetti
- Two teaspoons canola oil
- One package (10 ounces) fresh sugar snap peas, trimmed and cut diagonally into thin strips
- 2 cups julienned carrots (about 8 ounces)
- 2 cups shredded cooked chicken
- 1 cup Thai peanut sauce
- One medium cucumber, halved lengthwise, seeded and sliced diagonally
- Chopped fresh cilantro, optional

Instructions

1. Cook spaghetti according to package directions; drain.
2. Then, during a large skillet, heat oil a medium-high heat. Add snap peas and carrots; stir-fry 6-8 minutes or until crisptender. Add chicken, peanut sauce and spaghetti; heat through, tossing to mix .
3. Transfer to a serving plate. Top with cucumber and, if desired, cilantro.

Nutrition Facts

403 calories, 15g fat (3g saturated fat), 42mg cholesterol, 432mg sodium, 43g carbohydrate (15g sugars, 6g fibre), 25g protein

Spinach-Orzo Salad with Chickpeas

Ingredients

- One 14-1/2 ounces reduced-sodium chicken broth
- 1-1/2 cups of uncooked whole wheat orzo pasta
- 4 cups of fresh baby spinach
- 2 cups of grape tomatoes, halved
- Two cans (15 ounces each) of chickpeas or garbanzo beans, rinsed and drained
- 3/4 cup chopped fresh parsley
- Two green onions, choppedDRESSING:
- 1/4 cup olive oil
- Three tablespoons lemon juice
- 3/4 teaspoon salt
- 1/4 teaspoon garlic powder

- 1/4 teaspoon hot pepper sauce
- 1/4 teaspoon pepper

Instructions

1. Take an outsized saucepan and convey broth to a boil. Stir in orzo; return to a boil. Reduce heat; simmer, covered, until hard , 8-10 minutes.
2. Take an outsized pan and add spinach and warm orzo, allowing the spinach to wilt slightly. Add tomatoes, chickpeas, parsley and green onions.
3. Whisk together dressing ingredients. Toss with salad.

Nutrition

122 calories, 5g fat, o cholesterol, 259mg sodium, 16g carbohydrate (1g sugars, 4g fibre), 4g protein. Diabetic Exchanges: 1 starch, one fat.

Roasted Chicken Thighs with Peppers & Potatoes
Ingredients

- 2 pounds red potatoes (about six medium)
- Two large sweet red peppers
- Two large green peppers
- Two medium onions
- Two tablespoons olive oil, divided
- Four teaspoons minced fresh thyme or 1-1/2 teaspoons dried thyme, divided
- Three teaspoons minced fresh rosemary or one teaspoon dried rosemary, crushed, divided
- Eight boneless skinless chicken thighs (about 2 pounds)
- 1/2 teaspoon salt
- 1/4 teaspoon pepper

Instructions

1. Preheat oven to 450°. Cut potatoes, peppers and onions into 1-in. Pieces. Place vegetables during a roasting pan.Drizzle with one tablespoon oil; sprinkle with two teaspoons each thyme and rosemary and toss to coat. Place chicken over greens. Brush chicken with remaining oil; sprinkle with remaining thyme and rosemary. Drizzle vegetables and chicken with salt and pepper.
2. Roast until a thermometer inserted in chicken reads 170° and green vegetables are tender 35-40 minutes.

Nutrition Facts

308 calories, 12g fat (3g saturated fat), 76mg cholesterol, 221mg sodium, 25g carbohydrate (5g sugars, 4g fibre), 24g protein. Diabetic Exchanges: 3 lean meat, one starch, one vegetable, 1/2 fat.

Spiced Split Pea Soup
Ingredients

- 1 cup dried green split peas
- Two medium potatoes, chopped
- Two medium carrots, halved and thinly sliced
- One medium onion, chopped
- One celery rib, thinly sliced
- Three garlic cloves, minced
- Three bay leaves
- Four teaspoons curry powder
- One teaspoon ground cumin
- 1/2 teaspoon coarsely ground pepper
- 1/2 teaspoon ground coriander
- One carton (32 ounces) reduced-sodium chicken broth
- One can (28 ounces) diced tomatoes, undrained

Instructions

1. In a 4-qt. Slow cooker combines the primary 12 ingredients. Cook, covered, on low until peas are tender, 8-10 hours.
2. Stir in tomatoes; heat through. Discard bay leaves.

Nutrition Facts
139 calories, 0 fat (0 saturated fat), 0 cholesterol, 347mg sodium, 27g carbohydrate (7g sugars, 8g fibre), 8g protein. Diabetic Exchanges: 1 starch, one lean meat, one vegetable.

Escarole and Bean Soup
Ingredients

- Two tablespoons olive oil
- Two chopped garlic cloves
- 1 pound of escarole, chopped
- Salt
- 4 cups of low-salt broth chicken
- 1 can of cannellini beans
- 1 (1-ounce) piece of Parmesan
- Freshly ground black pepper
- Six teaspoons extra-virgin olive oil

Directions

1. Heat vegetable oil during a big heavy pot at normal heat. Add the garlic and sauté till fragrant, for 15 seconds. Add the escarole and sauté till wilted, for 2 min. Add salt. Add the chicken, beans, then Parmesan cheese. Cover and simmer till the beans are heated through, approximately five minutes — season with salt and pepper, to taste.

2. Ladle the soup into six bowls. Sprinkle one teaspoon extra-virgin vegetable oil over each. Serve with crusty bread.

AFTERWORD

In conclusion, the Dash diet instructs people to finish the entire scramble diet program by beginning with stocking up the kitchen with Dash inviting nourishment, getting ready scramble agreeable plans, and performing Dash-accommodating activities. Supper plans proposed by Dash, for the most part, contain fixings high in fiber, calcium, magnesium, and potassium. Dash abstains from food go low on sodium and sugar and accentuate the need to eat green verdant vegetables and natural products.

Avocado plunge, for example, is one of the most popular Dash slims down there is today, as a result of its exceptionally helpful and moderate planning. Avocado, a rich wellspring of monosaturated fat and lutein, (cancer prevention agents that help ensure vision), is among the numerous organic products that are enthusiastically prescribed for the Dash diet. Right now, must be pounded and hollowed, blended in with sans fat harsh cream, onion, and hot sauce.

This plunge will be eaten with tortilla chips or cut vegetables. From this dish, an individual can get a sum of 65 calories, 2 grams protein, 5 grams absolute fat, 4 grams sugar, 172 milligrams potassium and 31 milligrams calcium. From this, we can deduce that an individual is encouraged a lot of fundamental supplements, basic for keeping up a well-adjusted eating regimen that is useful for the heart.

In only 14 days, a Dash diet devotee will encounter typical circulatory strain, with fewer propensities to eat in the middle of dinners, the significant guilty party of weight gain. The Dash diet program additionally instructs people to decide the perfect measure of nourishment consumption, the essential exercise to perform as per age and activity level.

Dash teaches and spurs - one of the significant reasons why individuals think that it's simple to adhere to the diet. Additionally, the eating regimen doesn't expect us to quit any pretense of anything critical in our standard diet; rather, it encourages us to make a procedure of acclimating to little changes so we can effectively support ourselves.